A Guide to Balance and Dizziness

Neurologic Evaluation and Treatment of Vestibular Conditions

Second Edition

Charles M. Plishka

CRC Press
Taylor & Francis Group
Boca Raton London New York

CRC Press is an imprint of the
Taylor & Francis Group, an **Informa** business

Designed cover image: Shutterstock

Second edition published 2026
by CRC Press
2385 NW Executive Center Drive, Suite 320, Boca Raton, FL 33431

and by CRC Press
4 Park Square, Milton Park, Abingdon, Oxon, OX14 4RN

CRC Press is an imprint of Taylor & Francis Group, LLC

© 2026 Charles M. Plishka

First edition originally published by SLACK Incorporated 2015
First edition published by CRC Press 2024

ISBN: 9781032903590 (hbk)
ISBN: 9781638220817 (pbk)
ISBN: 9781003524441 (ebk)

DOI: 10.1201/9781003524441

Typeset in Minion
by Deanta Global Publishing Services, Chennai, India

Access the Support Materials: www.routledge.com/9781638220817

Contents

Foreword

As Dean and Professor of Optometry at Pacific University College of Optometry from 1975 until 1991, and Distinguished University Professor of Optometry and Public Health, 2003–present, I have reviewed many books and research papers. I have been an editorial reviewer of five professional journals in the field of optometry; and an appointed member of the National Advisory Council, Health Professions Education, US Department of Health and Human Services, 1983–1987.

I met the author of this text, Charles "Chuck" Plishka, PT, DPT, NCS, as we are both active in the National Optometric Rehabilitation Association (NORA). This organization includes a "Fellowship" program. Among the requirements is the development of a paper for submission to a professional journal. My role was to supervise the development of these papers. Plishka was one of those candidates. We first connected in 2018.

This book centers upon a well-established and ever-expanding subspecialty. With vestibular issues in mind, the book provides excellent cross-discipline coverage relative to those visual disorders common in vestibular cases. Particular emphasis can be found in areas like ocular anatomy and physiology, along with visual pathways found in the brain. Specifics relate to ocular motility, visual fields, and relationships to the central nervous system. It serves as a reference resource for the identification and follow-up intervention for vestibular conditions.

In short, this book has created an important bridge as to key vestibular issues, relative to case management in other health science disciplines. The emphasis centers upon physical therapy and optometry; other health science disciplines from audiology to general medicine are also pertinent.

Supporting this are the credentials of the author, prior publications on balance/dizziness, and noted speaker, internationally, for both physical therapy and medical conferences. He is often asked to be a guest speaker at schools offering courses in the assessment of the vestibular system and physical therapy.

This book provides an excellent resource for those professions dealing with vestibular issues related to brain function.

Willard B. Bleything, OD, MS, FAAO, FCOVD, FNAPO
Distinguished University Professor of Optometry and Public Health

Preface

As a neurologic physical therapist (PT), I have been interested in balance and dizziness since my days as a volunteer before even applying to PT school. As a practitioner, I have learned there are many disciplines that test and treat balance and dizziness; however, each usually focuses only on a part of the whole picture, lending their expertise. Because of this, there are gaps in understanding of the causes, as well as the treatments, that are available to help the patient. This second edition of the original text, *A Clinician's Guide to Balance and Dizziness: Evaluation and Treatment,* expands our understanding of the anatomy, examination, and treatment of the patient complaining of dizziness and/or balance deficits. As stated in the original text, a review of the anatomy and physiology required for balance will allow you to better understand the evaluation techniques and intervention options available to treat balance. This text is intended for disciplines that evaluate and treat dizziness and balance to share information with which we should all familiarize ourselves. It introduces students to topics of anatomy, physiology, and pathology, as well as treatment options, and may act as a reference for professionals already involved in patient care.

Acknowledgments

I would like to acknowledge the following people for their expertise and advice while writing this text: Willard B. Bleything, OD, MS, FAAO, FCOVD, FAAP; Ken Ciuffreda, OD, PhD; Anne K. Galgon, PT, MPT, PhD, NCS; Susan Jong, OD; Anthony Kincaid, PT, PhD; Andrew E. Littman, PT, PhD; Nguyen Tran, OD, FAAO, FOVDR; and Susan L. Whitney, DPT, PhD, NCS, ATC, FAPTA. I once again thank Madeline Guire, PT, for introducing me to the world of vestibular therapy. Finally, the amazing artwork by Emily Petersen, owner of Em Petersen Art, has been added to this edition.

About the Author

Charles M. Plishka, PT, DPT, NCS, earned his Doctor of Physical Therapy from Creighton University in Omaha, Nebraska, and is a board-certified Neurologic Clinical Specialist in physical therapy. He is the owner of Posture & Balance Concepts, LLC, which offers consulting services, program development, and continuing education courses. He teaches continuing education courses on the topics of vestibular therapy, evaluation and treatment of balance and dizziness, Parkinson's disease, and multiple sclerosis, acquired brain injury, and is an international speaker on topics of vestibular therapy. He is co-owner and operator of a vestibular and balance clinic in Billings, Montana.

Dr. Plishka is a member of the American Physical Therapy Association where he has served as the secretary of the Vestibular Special Interest Group. He is a founder and served as Chair of the Vestibular Special Interest Group for the International Neurologic Physical Therapy Association (INPA), which is part of World Physiotherapy.

He is excited to present *A Guide to Balance and Dizziness: Neurologic Evaluation and Treatment of Vestibular Conditions*, Second Edition, as an introductory text and reference for students and clinicians of different disciplines who evaluate and treat those patients suffering from dizziness and/or disequilibrium.

How to Use This Book

This book will walk the clinician through the thought processes and actual mechanics of performing a thorough examination and creating a plan of care for patients who complain of balance issues and/or dizziness. The chapters of the book focus on how their topics apply to the patient populations experiencing issues of balance and dizziness and do not necessarily address other applications or research information.

For quick reference, at the beginning of each chapter is a box that contains the learning goals for that chapter. There are many video examples. A QR code is displayed when a video is available for the topic being discussed. The QR code will lead you to the complete list of videos available, which can also be accessed via www.routledge.com /9781638220817.

Disclaimer

Research is rapidly expanding our knowledge of the physiology of balance and conditions that present dizziness/vertigo. Even among the experts, there are many differing ideas about the best way to treat or intervene. The information provided in this book is a good baseline of current knowledge regarding examination and intervention. It is by no means meant to be interpreted as the "only way" to arrive at a good patient outcome. It does offer basic skill instruction as well as presenting research to guide practice. Regardless of guideline recommendations, clinicians should always do what they believe is in the best interest of their patient. The information provided in this book is not intended to supersede your own professional judgment.

The Systems of Balance

Chapter Goals

1. Name the body planes
2. Define *limits of stability*
3. List the body systems that give information used to formulate a balance plan
4. List the goals of the balance system

With increasing frequency, we are called upon to evaluate a patient who has balance problems, gait difficulties, dizziness, trouble performing activities of daily living, or has recently fallen. Even if they have not yet fallen, if they are presenting with decreased functional movements. A thorough multisystem evaluation to identify and address physical and functional deficits and impairments is warranted. Often, we find that if we try to strengthen our patients with therapy, this does not always solve the problem of disequilibrium. This happens because there are many contributing systems to balance, and the musculoskeletal system is just *one* of those systems. If we look at only one system, we are limiting our view and understanding of the balance system as a whole. To get a good understanding of why our patient is off-balance, we need to look at each system involved with balance. Two types of balance will be discussed in this text: *static balance*, which is the ability to control your body position when you are not moving, and *dynamic balance*, which is the ability to control your body position when you are moving outside of your base of support.

First, let's review the anatomical planes and phrases we use to describe the body (Figure 1.1). The *coronal* (frontal) *plane* divides the body into dorsal and ventral halves. The *sagittal plane* is 90 degrees to the coronal plane and divides the body lengthwise into right and left halves. The *transverse plane* divides the body into superior and inferior parts. The word *lateral* means that which is away from the body or body segment's midline, while *medial* refers to something that is toward the midline. *Caudal* (and inferior) refers to that which is toward the tail of the body, while *cephalad* (and superior) refers to that which is toward the head. The *anterior* is that which is toward the front (*ventral*) side, and *posterior* refers to that which is toward the back (*dorsal*) side of the body.

If we can identify the specific deficiencies and issues that are contributing to the patient's disequilibrium and/or complaints of dizziness, we have a better opportunity to introduce interventions that will more effectively address, correct, or reduce these deficits and thereby reduce the risk of falls and injuries. A review of the anatomy and physiology required for balance will allow you to better understand and select the evaluation techniques and intervention options needed to address a patient's complaints of disequilibrium and/or dizziness. Here, we will discuss the big picture of how we balance, while subsequent chapters will go into more detail about each system that we use to balance.

Many things impact balance including cognition, vision, vestibular function, somatosensory input, cerebellar function, disease, infections and

DOI: 10.1201/9781003524441-1

Body Planes

Coronal
(Frontal Plane)

Sagittal Plane

Inferior

Superior

Transverse
Plane

Posterior

Anterior

Lateral

Medial

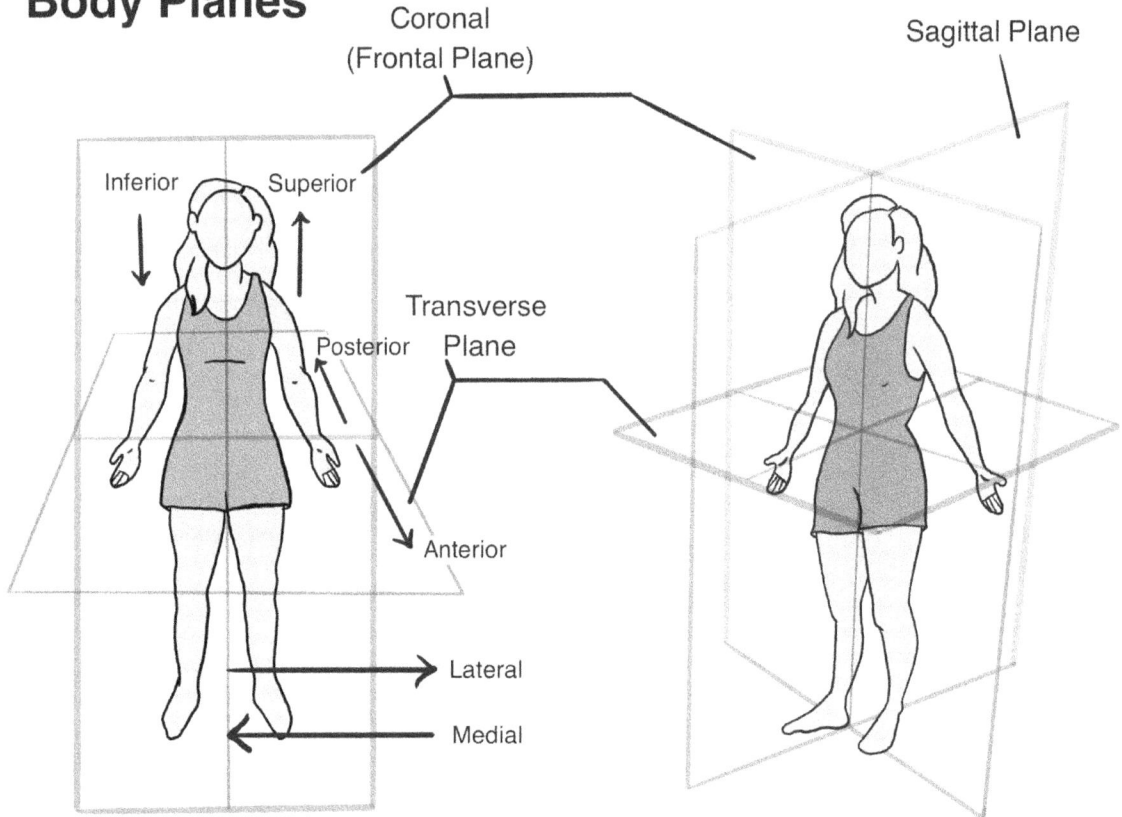

Figure 1.1 Body Planes

inflammations, practice and skill of movement, posture, strength, joint range of motion, neurologic conditions, medications, and use or disuse of body systems. The adage "If you don't use it, you'll lose it" is true in the case of acquired skills. If you do not stand or walk frequently enough, you will lose some level of skill to perform these activities.

There are many steps to complete for performing intended and skilled movements. For planned movement, these include the following:

- Having a goal, desire, or an externally driven need that provides the incentive to move
- Knowing the body's present position and movements
- Being aware of one's environment and any obstacles that would prevent or challenge the body's movements
- The ability to plan muscle activity to move or remain stable/still

- Having the strength and range of motion to carry out the plan
- Knowing how much muscle force will be required and how far the limbs must move to perform the task
- Assessing and adjusting movements based on feedback or environmental changes
- Having some degree of experience performing the chosen movement

Before initiating any intentional plan of movement, one must first start by collecting information, so this is where the review begins. Figure 1.2 is a basic schematic of how the systems of balance interact. As you can see, there is a lot of information sharing. There is information coming into the brain from the vestibular, visual, and somatosensory systems. Often called *input* systems, they give you information about your location, movement, and position as well as that of your surroundings.

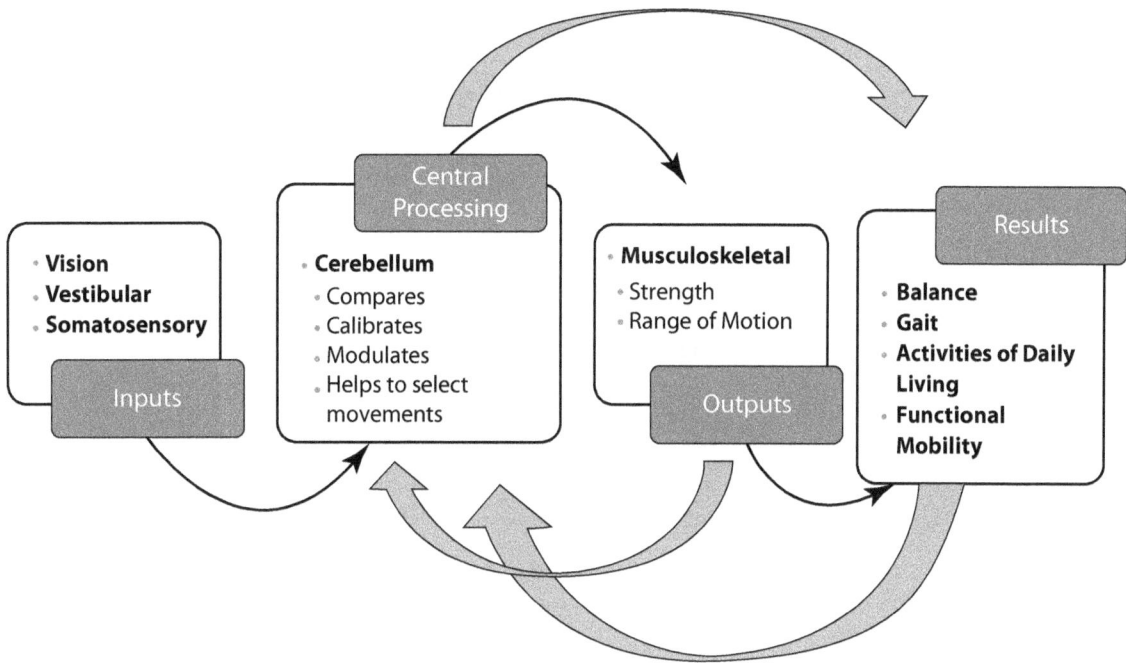

Figure 1.2 Diagram of the Balance System

The cerebellum compares and coordinates information flow; in some cases, it alters signals coming from the input systems. It uses the information it receives from the input systems to help plan and correct movement. Once we have a plan of how we wish to move/balance, the orders are given to the musculoskeletal system from the motor cortex to carry out the plan. How well we perform depends on each system's ability to give accurate information, the brain's ability to assess the information and create a proper plan, the musculoskeletal system being at optimal performance, and the skill we have to perform.

An easier way to imagine how this works is to compare it with baking a pie (Figure 1.3). When making a pie you must start with the ingredients such as apples, eggs, sugar, flour, butter, etc. You must mix these ingredients in just the right amounts to produce what you need—in this case, the apple filling and dough for the crust. Next, you need a pie pan in which to place the ingredients before they are baked to shape the pie. If all goes well, once your pie is done baking it will come out of the oven looking great! To find out how good it is, you will have to perform a taste test. If there is

a problem at *any step* of the process, the pie may either look bad (being burned or misshapen) or taste bad. For example, if you make a pie using rotten apples or spoiled milk, it will taste bad. If the mixer is not working well, you may find lumps of flour or butter in the pie, and again it will taste bad. If the pan is too thin, the pie may burn. If there are only one or two small problems, the pie may still be edible. However, if you have multiple problems or even one large problem (perhaps having forgotten to add sugar), your failure as a baker will be obvious, and the pie will be inedible.

Similar to the list of problems that may arise while baking a pie, if there are deficits in any part of the balance system, one's balance may be compromised. The systems that gather information provide the *ingredients* of balance—visual, vestibular, and somatosensory information. Like the mixer, the brain (especially the cerebellum) combines the information into a useful movement plan and assigns weight to each system's information, depending upon the given activity needs. Your musculoskeletal system shapes balance, just as the pie pan shapes the pie. Finally, to see how well you balance and perform activities that require

Baking a Pie	Balancing
Need fresh ingredients	Need accurate input information: Vision, Vestibular, Somatosensory
Need to blend ingredients in the right amounts	Cerebellum weights the input info and uses them to adjust our balance plan
Ingredients go into a pie pan to shape it	Musculoskeletal systems shape our movements
A taste test lets us know if the pie is good	Standardized tests of balance and fall risk tell us how well we balance

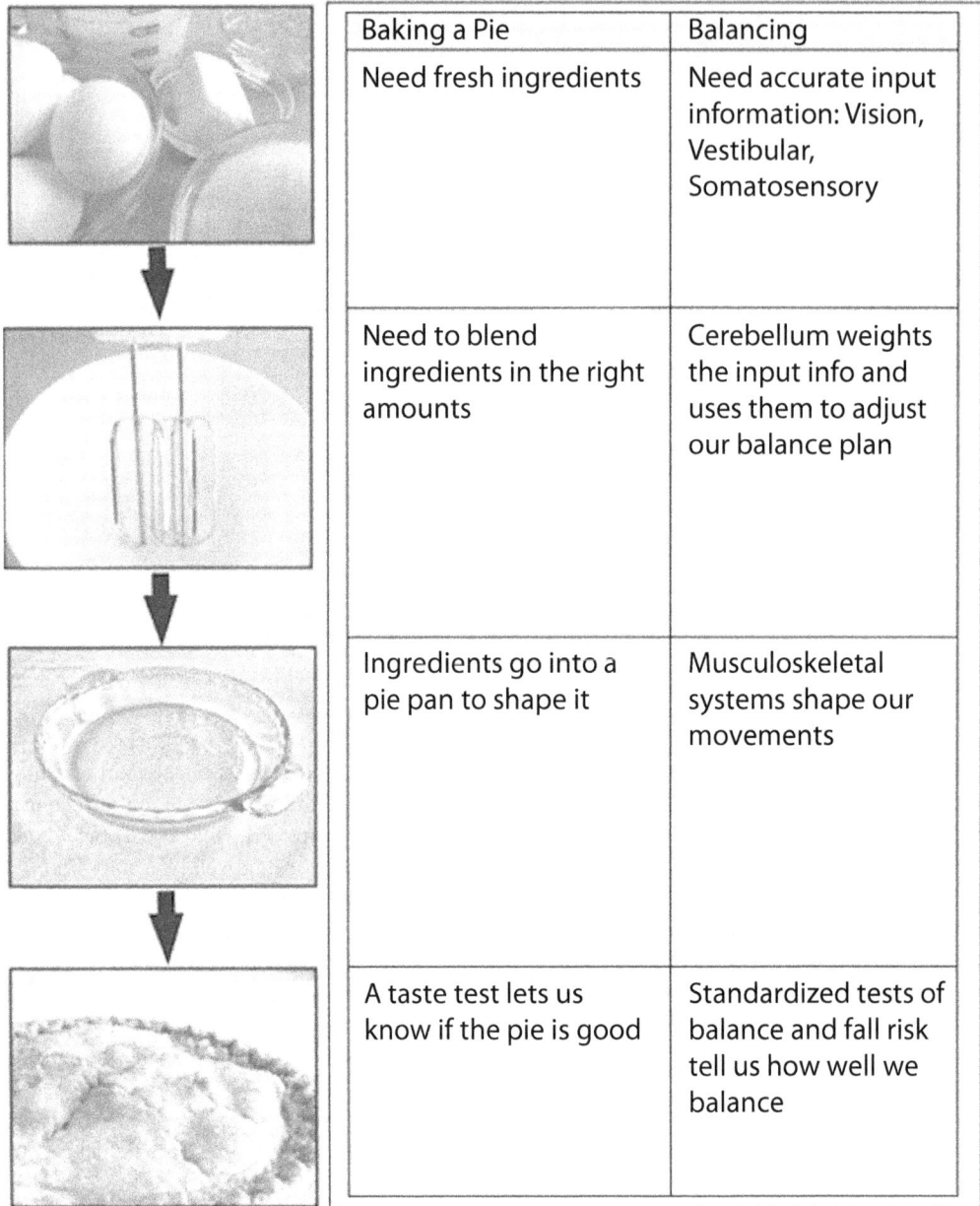

Figure 1.3 Ingredients of Balance

balance, you need a "taste test." You do this by using standardized tests of balance and/or the risk of falling. If there is a problem at *any step* in the balancing process, it may present itself in the form of disequilibrium, difficulty performing the activities of daily living (ADLs), gait deviations, falls, and, in some cases, complaints of dizziness. The more problems that exist, the worse the individual's balance, function, or complaints will be. Just like the pie example, if one small problem exists, the patient may still be able to function. However, the more problems that exist, or if one very large problem such as missing or incorrect information from any given system exists, then the impact on functional movement will be obvious. We can balance with only two working inputs or partially working systems (vision, vestibular, somatosensory). However, we cannot balance using only one of the systems that gives us information used in balancing.

HOW SYSTEM DEFICITS AFFECT PATIENTS

Specific examples of how deficits affect people are as follows:

- *Visual/oculomotor deficits*: These deficits may affect balance, gait, ADLs, and, in the case of the athlete, sports performance. Patients with visual deficits may complain of blurred vision, diplopia, difficulty reading, dizziness, or headaches. They may trip on objects in their path, miss stair steps, or find it difficult to keep their balance. Those with visual field deficits may run into objects while ambulating. For athletes, visual impairments may mean decreased accuracy of depth perception, which causes them to react too soon or too late during sports performance. During throwing or swinging activities, such an athlete may overshoot or undershoot the target.
- *Vestibular deficits*: Acute and chronic vestibular deficits have both similarities and differences regarding signs and symptoms. During acute episodes of vestibular loss, complaints of vertigo, nausea, and balance disturbances are common. These disturbances may cause vomiting and falls. Chronic vestibular issues typically do not present with vertigo (sensations of movement or spinning), but common complaints include dizziness or disequilibrium during quick turns, disequilibrium while in dark environments, or the presence of nausea provoked by visually stimulating environments such as when walking down a grocery store aisle, a moving ceiling fan, moving cars, action movies, video games, or being in a crowd of people. When questioned, many patients who have chronic vestibular loss admit to avoiding these settings. It is also not uncommon for them to avoid head turns while they walk, as they tend to deviate or stumble.

- *Somatosensory deficits*: Those lacking somatosensory information often are balance challenged and stumble/fall more frequently than others. Impaired proprioception, especially of the foot, ankle, knee, and hip, can lead to absent or delayed stepping reactions when off-balance, as well as poor planning for desired movements. Disequilibrium may be more common in the dark or on uneven or compliant (soft) surfaces such as grass, gravel, or thick carpet. Patients lacking ankle proprioception will sway more and often lack a stepping response to perturbations. Those with a lack of visual information combined with an impaired proprioception system will be at a severe disadvantage in knowing their environment.
- *Central processing deficits*: The cerebellum is responsible for the coordination and accuracy of movements. Those with deficits in this part of the brain may present with the inability to coordinate their movements; they may seem clumsy or lacking in accuracy as they move (e.g., trying to touch something with a fingertip and missing the mark). They may be ataxic (uncoordinated) with gait and have severe balance deficits. Memory and cognition deficits may interfere with correct motor-plan choices or may impair the ability to make safe movement choices.
- *Musculoskeletal deficits*: Muscle weaknesses or poor range of motion may impact the patient's ability to perform daily tasks, walk, or even perform simple transfers such as getting out of a chair. Elderly people who stoop (flexed hips and knees) often lean forward, which puts them off-balance. Those with tight leg muscles (especially hip flexors and hamstrings) or weak calves often take short and flat steps, putting them at a higher risk of tripping. When they find themselves off-balance, they may not be able to react quickly enough to step and prevent a fall.

GOALS OF THE BALANCE SYSTEM

The balance system has several jobs. It helps to regulate muscle tone, eye movements, and keep us upright. According to Shepard and Telian,[1] there are three goals of the balance system:

1. To correct any inadvertent displacement of the center of mass from its equilibrium position over the base of support and thus prevent a fall (e.g., if someone nudges you off-center, you can control yourself without falling and bring yourself back to a balanced position)
2. To provide an accurate perception of the body's position in the environment along with perceptions of direction and speed of movement
3. To control eye movements to maintain a clear image of the environment while the individual, the environment, or both are in motion

For most, it may be surprising to find that the balance system assists in the control of eye movements! Most clinicians do not get many hours of education regarding the visual and vestibular systems, but their impact on balance and daily function may be profound. Having even a basic understanding of the systems of balance may guide you to interventions or referrals that otherwise you may not have considered.

There are numerous descriptions and definitions of the word *balance*. The simplest definition is likely "the ability to control oneself against gravity." The definition you will see most in the medical community is "balance is the ability to control the center of gravity over the base of support." To fully appreciate this definition, you need to also understand the concepts of *center of gravity* (COG), *limits of stability* (LOS), and *base of support* (BOS).

The COG is the average location of an object's weight. For example, consider a rectangular or square piece of high-density balance foam, such as used by therapists to test and train balance. These foam pads are rectangular, one solid piece, and comprised of the same material throughout. If you wanted to balance the foam on top of a point (like the top of a pyramid) it would make sense to place the point of the pyramid in the center of the pad. Intuitively, you understand that the pad's center is the spot where you will have the best chance of getting the pad to balance without falling because there are equal amounts of weight on each side of the center.

Now imagine that you have a box that you need to balance on a point. The box is rectangular like the balance pad, but unlike the balance pad, it is not made up of the same material throughout. It may hold a variety of objects, each with a different weight and density. In this example, the left side of the box holds a 50-pound weight, while the right side of the box holds a feather. If you were to try balancing the box on the pyramid point by placing the point in the center of the box's bottom, the box would quickly tilt and fall toward the side of the 50-pound weight. The COG of the box is *not* going to be in the center of the box, since one side of the box is heavier than the other. To balance the box on top of the point, you would need to place the point of the pyramid well toward the side of the box holding the most weight.

The COG of a human body in the anatomical position is located inside the body and in front of the sacrum at about the spinal level of S2.[2] When considering the COG of the human body as compared to the foam pad, you can quickly see how it is different. The human body is not comprised of the same consistent material throughout. The human body has movable parts, each with its own center of gravity. As you move, the COG of your entire body moves as well, with its location depending on your position, activity, and even clothing. It is not static. If your patient has had a limb amputation, their COG will shift toward the side of the body that has the intact limb, since that side of the body weighs more. Depending upon a person's position, the COG may even be outside of the body! Remember, the COG is a calculation that represents the location of the average weight of an object.

When discussing anatomy, clinicians use other concepts to assess and describe the body's alignment. The *line of gravity* (LOG) represents the area of reaction with the ground and allows for analysis of balance to be made.[2-4] The LOG is used to describe the direction of the pull of gravity moving through the COG. The LOG for a human is located frontally and is represented by a vertical line passing through the middle of the sacrum and perpendicular to the ground.[5] For many older adults, the pelvis moves posteriorly compared to the LOG and heels.[3]

Whatever is being used to support the COG to maintain a stable position is known as the base of support. The BOS may change depending on a person's activity, posture, or choice. In standing, the BOS includes the feet and the area between the feet. In sitting, whatever is in contact with the chair is the BOS. This usually is the buttocks and thighs, but may also be the back. Basically, whatever is in contact with a supporting surface and the area between points of contact represents the BOS.

The location of a person's COG (and LOG) can influence a patient's function, as well as the pain the patient may be feeling while attempting to balance. For example, people whose COG is chronically anterior to their pelvis are required to use more muscle torque to counter gravity and prevent falling because of their flexed posture. In a 2019 published study of older adults in Portugal, Carrasco et al. found that gender and lower body strength seemed to be the main factors for falls, with females and weaker subjects being at higher risk.[8]

In Figure 1.6, the flexed person's COG is represented by the dark "X" and LOG is represented by the solid down-arrow. C7 is represented by the gray "X" and the C7 plumb line is represented by the dashed down-arrow. You will notice both are anterior to L3 and the sacrum. This causes a need for more torque at the pelvis to compensate and places the person at a higher risk of falling. This is the reason therapists promote an upright posture during ambulation!

The next concept needed for further discussion of balance is that of limits of stability. The LOS is the area of movement (or trunk excursion) while standing or sitting within which you have balance control without needing to take a step or adding external sources of stability, such as by touching or leaning on something. Under normal circumstances, you are able to move your COG within your BOS without falling or needing to create a new or additional BOS by stepping or propping on an arm. If you move past this invisible boundary of control (the LOS), you begin to fall. The LOS has been described as a "cone of equilibrium" by Kim, Davis, and Menger: "The spine and the body function within a cone of equilibrium with the focus of maintaining sagittal and coronal alignment with minimum energy expenditure. This happens with a harmonious

relationship involving cervical lordosis, thoracic kyphosis, lumbar lordosis, and pelvic anatomy. The purpose is mostly to maintain a mechanical balance in the sagittal plane and coronal plane centered from the center of cranial mass, femoral heads, and lower extremities"[6, 7] (Figure 1.4).

To be stable, the LOG needs to fall inside of the BOS. If it does not, we need to compensate to prevent loss of balance using muscle force, a stepping strategy, or external assistance from a device such as a cane or a walker.

ACTIVITY 1.1 LIMITS OF STABILITY

While guarded, perform the following either without shoes or in shoes that do not have a raised heel. If you wanted to find your LOS in standing, you could do the following: Stand with your feet together and hands at your sides. When moving, do not bend at the waist in any direction. The only joints you should be using are the ankles. Keeping your back straight, shift all your weight as far as you can in the direction indicated as long as you maintain control. First, lean toward your toes without letting your heels lift off the ground. Keeping yourself forward, shift your weight toward your right pinky toe. Again, go as far as you can without bending at the waist or allowing your heels to rise from the floor. Keeping to the right, shift back to your right heel as far as you can. Keeping your weight on your heels, shift to your left heel. Finally, shift to your left pinky toe and then return to the center front. Finally, return to a comfortable stance. You have just found your limits of stability!

When you balance, you do so under variable conditions. Sometimes you are at rest, as you probably are right now sitting in a chair. At other times, however, you are in motion, as when you are walking. The task of walking typically requires you to move your COG outside of your limits of stability. As you walk, you shift your weight from one leg to the other. That is, you transition your COG from one

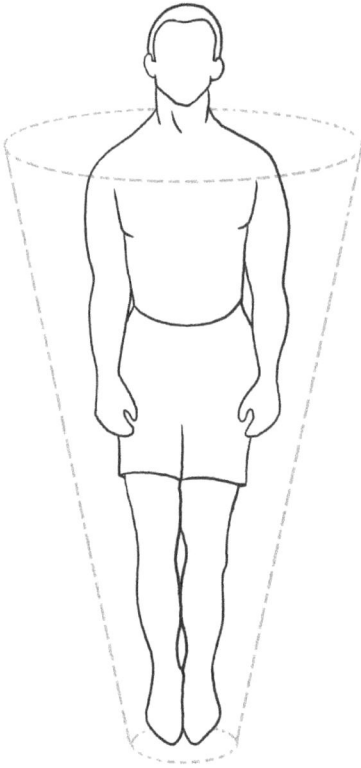

Figure 1.4 Limits of Stability

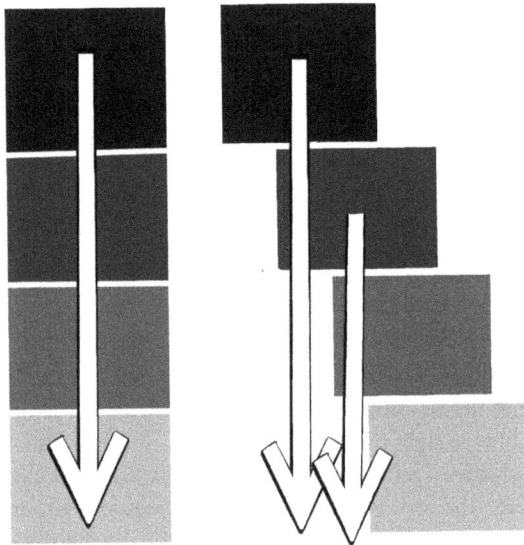

Figure 1.5 Stacked Boxes with Center of Gravity

BOS (say, your left foot) to another BOS (your right foot as it steps forward). Taking a step is an example of creating a new BOS to maintain dynamic standing balance. As you step, your COG moves outside an area of support or control. To avoid falling, you quickly move a leg and take a step in the direction in which you are falling and transition the COG to this foot, which becomes the new BOS. Obviously, this is an oversimplification of gait, but it is basically what occurs when we ambulate. A person who does not move their COG outside of the BOS while ambulating appears to be stiff and to shuffle or take extremely small steps where one foot does not pass the other. People who take short and slow steps are at higher risk of falling.

When the BOS is stable, the person or object(s) (e.g., a stack of boxes) will be stable and will not fall. When the weight of the object (or the COG) is outside of the base, a fall is more likely.

Use the images of the stack of boxes (Figure 1.5) to assist with this concept.

When stacked directly on top of each other, the COG of each box will be directly on top of the one below. The COG of each box is supported. Now imagine that you are stacking boxes, but as you place each new box on the stack, you position it a few inches off-center of the box below. Each box has a COG, and if the COGs are located past the support of the box beneath, the boxes are more likely to fall. Figures 1.4 and 1.5 help to illustrate this concept. Thinking of this example, imagine two people standing next to each other. One is standing straight with their center of gravity within their base of support, and the other has a flexed trunk and is leaning forward with the center of gravity anterior to the base of support (Figure 1.6). Because the second person's COG is shifted in front of the BOS, they are more likely to fall.

Using the concepts discussed up to this point, review the three basic steps of balancing, which are (1) getting the information, (2) processing the information, and (3) carrying out a plan of action.

STEP 1: GETTING THE INFORMATION

As discussed, your body uses three main *input* systems to get the information needed to balance/

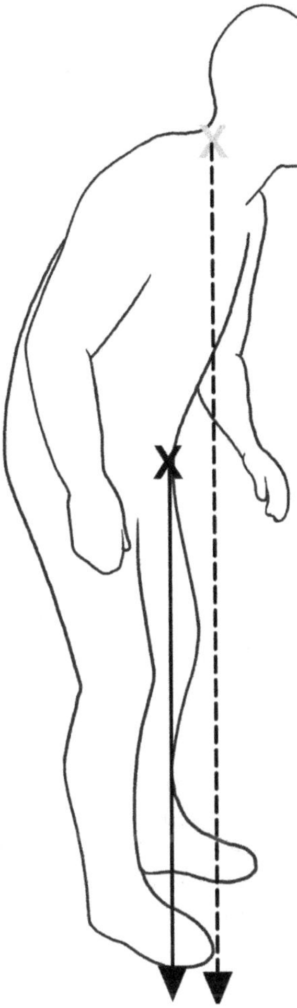

Figure 1.6 Human Posture

of the word. This term may refer to one nystagmus beat or many. There are various types of nystagmus, and unless otherwise stated, in this book *nystagmus* will refer to "jerk nystagmus." Jerk nystagmus moves the eye quickly in one direction and slowly in the reverse direction. Nystagmus occur under different conditions and throughout the day as needed to help keep the eyes on objects of interest or to help a moving person see more clearly. Under normal circumstances, nystagmus are under the control of various reflexes (specifically the optokinetic and vestibulo-ocular reflexes). When there is pathology, nystagmus may sometimes be observed at inappropriate times or directions.

People use visual information to check their head and body positions as well as to see the environment and help plan motor strategies. For example, using visual information you may check if you are standing or sitting straight, tilting, or swaying. While ambulating, as you approach something small in your path, your visual information is used when preprogramming gait and stepping responses. We use peripheral vision to notice things moving in our environment that may be of interest (such as a car driving toward us or a tiger about to pounce) and can then move our eyes or head in the direction of this motion. The discussion of vision can be complex and will be covered more in depth in Chapter 2.

Vestibular System

The vestibular system has two parts: a central vestibular system that includes the vestibular nuclei; and a peripheral vestibular system that includes the vestibular organs (utricle, saccule, and semicircular canals) and the nerves, which are outside of the central nervous system that conducts information to and from these organs. The vestibular organs are found in the inner ear between the eardrum and the cochlea, and their anatomy and physiology are well described in the literature.[1,10–14] The vestibular organs share cranial nerve VIII (the vestibulo-cochlear nerve) with the cochlea and have several jobs, including maintaining posture, regulating muscle tone, maintaining equilibrium, and stabilizing gaze (that is, keeping your eyes steady on a target of interest) when the head is in motion. The vestibular system, along with the somatosensory

move in the desired manner: visual, vestibular, and somatosensory. Our eyes see the environment, our vestibular system tells us if the head is moving or tilted, and the somatosensory system reports on body position and movement. The brain places importance on each of these inputs differently, based on activity.

Vision

Before we begin our discussion on how visual information is used to assist our balance, we must first define the word *nystagmus*, which refers to involuntary rhythmic movements of the eye. Scientific literature uses the singular form of the word *nystagmus* to indicate both singular and plural forms system, is responsible for information regarding head position and motion.

The vestibular system is discussed in depth in Chapter 3.

Somatosensory System

The somatosensory system collects a variety of information such as light touch, pressure, joint position and movement, and temperature (hot/cold) sensations. With regard to balance, it senses body sway using pressure sensation of the feet, light touch sensations of the feet, stretch receptors, and proprioception information from the ankles, knees, and hips. While someone is standing still the somatosensory information is usually given more importance and is used to provide a correct response to small balance challenges. Those with neuropathies, for example, are at a higher risk of fall as they cannot always tell their joint position or if they are swaying/falling until it's too late.

STEP 2: PROCESSING THE INFORMATION

Cerebellum

Once we have gathered information regarding the body's position, motion, and environment, we need to process this information to plan muscle activity to enact a plan to balance and/or move. In our big picture overview of balance, the cerebellum is responsible for comparing information from different systems and correcting movements. The cerebellum is discussed in more detail in Chapter 5. Depending on the activity a person performs, the brain will put more weight on each input system differently. For example, while quietly standing, the cerebellum primarily uses information from the somatosensory system using information received from the proprioceptors (especially the ankle proprioceptors). When a person is moving, however, the importance shifts to the vison and vestibular systems. It is hypothesized that the vestibular system contributes to 65% of dynamic body stability.[9] If two input systems have a conflict (e.g., the vestibular system is telling you that you are spinning in a circle, but your somatosensory system disagrees), the cerebellum decides which

system will have priority. When we have a planned movement, the cerebellum uses the information from each system to compare what was planned with the actual motion and may adjust the movement on the fly.

STEP 3: CARRYING OUT A PLAN OF ACTION

Musculoskeletal System

Finally, once we have a plan of action, we use our musculoskeletal system to carry it out. This is where strength and range of motion are important. The shape of the spine affects balance and the need for compensations to maintain balance. The strength of the muscles to control one's trunk, limbs, head, and eyes is a prerequisite for normal balance. The range of motion of the muscles, regardless of strength, also plays a role in the ability to correctly move or maintain a position of stability while standing still or moving. Looking back at our hypothetical elderly person who sits in a chair all day and has tight hip flexors and tight knee flexors (and likely limited range of motion in the ankles) that when combined prevent them to stand erect, we already know that this person is at a higher risk of falling simply from the anatomical positions of their spine, head, trunk, and limbs due to gravity. If they lack the strength or awareness to perform a sway or stepping strategy to maintain balance, they will likely fall.

SUMMARY

As clinicians, we need to be able to identify deficient systems that may affect our patients' balance. This means we need to learn to assess the systems we use to gather information (vison, vestibular, somatosensory), the cerebellum, and the musculoskeletal system, as well as a person's overall ability to balance, ambulate, and perform functional movement. Up to this point, we have discussed how spinal shape and posture may affect balance. We have also discussed how we use the systems of balance to gather correct information about ourselves and our environments so that we can make appropriate plans of muscle activity to enact a balance strategy, and the importance of strength and range of motion. However, there are other factors that we may use to identify fall risk. As pointed out by Kyrdalen et al., it has been found that gait speed that is slower than 1.0 m/s is a strong predictor of falls in the elderly. Also, there have been many research articles that have identified vision as an independent risk factor.[15] Fear of falling seems to have an impact on balance. In a review of studies involving fear of falling, a positive association was found between fear of falling and the presence of worse physical performance and greater degrees of disability.[16] Another study found that "falling is significantly related to impaired cognition, reduced muscle strength, impaired balance, gait, and activities of daily living abilities, and depression in older adults with dementia."[17]

We will begin our review of each system of balance in the next chapter. Once we understand these systems, we will be ready to assess and treat those complaining of disequilibrium and/or dizziness. There is a learning curve when you are using tests with which you are unfamiliar. It takes time and practice to integrate new tests into your practice, and sometimes the effort required to do so seems overwhelming. If only a portion of these systems are examined or treated (for example, only focusing on the musculoskeletal system), but problems exist in other parts of the balance system, then

patients will most likely not reach their maximum level of function. Refer to Table 1.1 for information gained from an evaluation of the balance system.

Quite often, balance issues or functional motion problems are due to a combination of deficits in multiple systems. It is a fact that aging often brings about changes to our bodies, impacting systems that affect balance and motion. Many elderly patients have poor eyesight, glaucoma, macular degeneration, decreased joint range of motion, neuropathies, arthritis, vestibular weakness, decreased muscle mass and flexibility, postural inadequacies, and memory/dementia deficits. Some of these elderly patients may not choose to move or walk often because of these issues; as a result, they are out of practice with regard to walking or balance. So, with increasing age, people may have more things interfering with the balance process than they did when they were younger. The same holds true for aging athletes, who are less flexible or have decreased visual acuity and muscle mass as compared with their younger selves. The more deficits we can identify affecting balance, the more opportunities we will have to treat patients or refer them to someone who can.

How do we make plans of care for patients with deficient balance or complaints of dizziness? After reviewing the steps involved in the process of balance, you probably agree that it does not make sense for clinicians to give all of their balance patients

Table 1.1 Information Gained from an Evaluation

System	Information Gained
Vison	Are pathologic nystagmus present? Are the eyes aligned and focused on a single target? Do the eyes have a normal range of motion? Do the eyes move conjugately? Is acuity normal? Are there any central signs present?
Vestibular	Is vestibular function grossly normal? Are there any loose otoconia (crystals) causing vertigo?
Somatosensory	Is light touch sensation intact? Is proprioception of joints intact?
Cerebellar screen	Is coordination of joints normal? Are there abnormal reflexes present that may indicate stroke? Are there any eye movements present that may indicate stroke?
Musculoskeletal system	Do weaknesses, limited or excessive motion, or postural issues exist that may be impacting balance and function?

the same exercises. If the patient has a visual or vestibular disorder, obviously long arc quad exercises should not be the first choice as a therapeutic intervention. If the patient is at high risk of falling, will walking them down a hallway yield the desired maximal therapeutic outcomes if the specific reasons the patient has balance issues are not assessed or addressed? When treating athletes, it does not make sense to give the same exercises and drills to players of different sports or even different team positions in the same sport. Customized drills, exercises, and activities will yield a better athlete, and the same is true for the patient with a balance deficit. Someone with an inner ear problem will not need the same exercises as the patient who has weak hip abductors.

A helpful analogy is that of getting your car repaired. Let us say, for example, that you take your car to the shop to have a cracked windshield replaced. After a wait of about 45 minutes, the mechanic tells you that the car is ready; however, you see that the windshield is still cracked. When you ask why this is, the mechanic tells you not to worry because the oil was changed. This was done, the mechanic explains, because "we do that for all our cars." In this situation, would you pay the mechanic? Besides not paying for the wrong service, you would probably have a few choice words to say, and your car would still have the problem—a cracked windshield. If the windshield was broken, should the mechanic not have fixed it?

Now let us apply this analogy to patients. If a patient has a "balance problem," you must first discover *why* that patient has such a problem. You can't simply "change the oil," providing the same interventions you do for every patient with a balance problem. I'm sure you can agree that not everyone will need quad exercises or a dozen or so upper extremity strengthening exercises. With the information you gain in examining each system that contributes to balance and functional movement, you will discover the specific issues that are adding to the imbalance or dizziness. You will have the information you need to create a *specific* and *customized* plan of care that addresses the patient-specific deficits, and you will easily explain why each part of the plan of care is required and how it will help the patient.

You have now learned which systems are involved in the balance process. Further, you also know that practice and skill will affect ability. The remaining chapters will help you to do the following:

- Identify the key points for performing a competent evaluation
- Identify deficiencies contributing to poor balance or complaints of dizziness
- Make a customized plan of care
- Recognize when to refer patients to other specialists

The most effective plans of care, treatments, and therapeutic interventions will be those that address the specific deficits involved in each system and that also address function as a whole. To increase your success in treating balance/dizziness disorders and achieve the best possible outcomes, you must perform a thorough evaluation and refer to other members of the health care team when appropriate to gain further knowledge regarding the patient's complaints, signs, symptoms, and function.

REFERENCES

1. Shepard NT, Telian SA. *Practical Management of the Balance Disorder Patient.* San Diego, CA: Singular Publishing Group, 1996.
2. Heuc JC, Saddiki R, Franke J, Rigal J, Aunoble S. Equilibrium of the human body and gravity line: the basics. *Eur Spine J* 2011;20 (Suppl 5):S558–S563.
3. Schwab F, Lafage V, Boyce R, Skalli W, Farcy JP. Gravity line analysis in adult volunteers: age-related correlation with spinal parameters, pelvic parameters, and foot position. *Spine* 2006;31(25):E959–E967.
4. Roussouly P, Gollogly S, Noseda O, Berthonnaud E, Dimnet J. The vertical projection of the sum of the ground reactive forces of a standing patient is not the same as the C7 plumb line: a radiographic study of the sagittal alignment of 153 asymptomatic volunteers. *Spine* 2006;31(11):E320–E325.

5. Heuc JC, Saddiki R, Franke J, Rigal J, Aunoble S. Equilibrium of the human body and gravity line: the basics. *Eur Spine J* 2011;20 (Suppl 5):S558–S563.

6. Kim D, Davis DD, Menger RP. Spine Sagittal Balance. [Updated 2021 Aug 11]. In: *StatPearls* [Internet]. Treasure Island (FL): StatPearls Publishing;2022 Jan. Available from: https://www.ncbi.nlm.nih.gov/books/NBK534858.

7. Gaillard F, Knipe H. Sagittal balance. Reference article, Radiopaedia.org. (Accessed on 23 Apr 2022) https://doi.org/10.53347/rID-49585).

8. Carrasco C, Tomas-Carus P, Bravo J, Pereira C, Mendes F. Understanding fall risk factors in community-dwelling older adults: a cross-sectional study. *Int J Older People Nurs* 2020 Mar;15(1):e12294. doi: 10.1111/opn.12294. Epub 2019 Dec 5. PMID: 31803994.

9. Allum HJ, Pfaltz CR. Visual and vestibular contributions to pitch sway stabilization in the ankle muscles of normals and patients with bilateral peripheral vestibular deficits. *Exp Brain Res* 1985;58:82–94.

10. Alberstone CD, Benze, EC, Najm IM, Steinmetz MP. *Anatomic Basis of Neurologic Diagnosis*. New York: Thieme; 2009.

11. Herdman S. *Vestibular Rehabilitation*. 3rd ed. Philadelphia: FA Davis; 2007.

12. Baloh R, Honrubia V. *Clinical Neurophysiology of the Vestibular System*. 2nd ed. Philadelphia: FA Davis; 1979.

13. Greenberg D, Aminoff M, Simon R. *Clinical Neurology*. 8th ed. New York: McGraw Hill; 2012.

14. Albert M, McCaig LF, Ashman JJ. Emergency department visits by persons aged 65 and over: United States, 2009-142010. *NCHS Data Brief* 2013;(130):1–8.

15. Kyrdalen IL, Thingstad P, Sandvik L, Ormstad H. Associations between gait speed and well-known fall risk factors among community-dwelling older adults. *Physiother Res Int* 2019 Jan;24(1):e1743. doi: 10.1002/pri.1743. Epub 2018 Sep 10. PMID: 30198603.

16. MacKay S, Ebert P, Harbidge C, Hogan D. Fear of falling in older adults: a scoping review of literature. *Can Geriat J* 2021 Dec;24(4):379–394.

17. Park H, Lee N, Kang T. Fall-related cognition, motor function, functional ability, and depression measure in older adults with dementia. *NeuroRehabilitation* 2020;47:487–494.

2

Vision and the Oculomotor Anatomy

Chapter Goals

1. Describe the anatomy of the orbit
2. Describe the anatomy of the eye
3. List the extraocular eye muscles and actions
4. Explain the visual pathway
5. List and describe eye positions and movements
6. Describe visual reflexes
7. List and explain visual impairments

Vision has been defined as the "act or power of seeing," and "the special sense by which the qualities of an object (such as color, luminosity, shape, and size) constituting its appearance are perceived through a process in which light rays entering the eye are transformed, by the retina, into electrical signals that are transmitted to the brain via the optic nerve."[2] As light enters the eye it passes through the cornea and crystalline lens and comes to a focus on the macular region of the retina. Here, the energy is transformed into electrical signals that travel along ganglion cells to the optic nerve. Following the path of the optic nerve, the electrical signals connect to the lateral geniculate nucleus, then along optic rays to the primary visual cortex found in the occipital lobe of the brain. This process is covered in more detail later in the chapter.

As vision dysfunction directly influences posture, balance, and movement, it is an important link to functional mobility. According to Leigh and Zee, "eye movements provide a powerful research

tool to investigate the workings of the brain." They further state: " abnormalities of ocular motility frequently provide diagnostic clues."[3] When we think of vision, we first think of the eyes. While the eye itself serves as a camera, the brain tells us what we have seen. This is called *perception*. Simply put, each eye captures the scenes around us from a different perspective. To illustrate this, perform Activity 2.1. The eye muscles position each eye so they "look" (point at) the same object. The eyes are positioned so that the image of the object falls onto each retina. The cornea and lens focus the image, which is then relayed to the brain via the optic nerve where it is "perceived."

ACTIVITY 2.1 EYE PERSPECTIVES

Hold up your thumb in front of any object. First, close one eye while keeping the thumb in focus with the other eye. Next, swap the eye that is closed, and now look at the thumb with your other eye. You will notice the background slightly shifts. Our brain puts these two images together, so we only see one scene.

There are several vision specialists and eye care professionals:

- *Ophthalmologist (M.D.):* A medical doctor who specializes in diagnosing, treating, and managing diseases of the eye and provides

DOI: 10.1201/9781003524441-2

medical and surgical treatments for eye conditions. They are listed with the surgical staff in a hospital.

- *Neuro-ophthalmologist (M.D.)*: Has a subspecialty in both neurology and ophthalmology. This medical doctor deals with visual problems caused by nervous system deficits.
- *Optometrist (O.D.)*: The doctor of optometry specializes in the examination, diagnosis, treatment, and management of diseases and disorders of the visual system, the eye, and associated structures, as well as the diagnosis of related systemic conditions. They prescribe corrective lenses and manage the treatment of basic eye disease conditions.
- *Behavioral optometrist*: An optometrist who provides vision therapy to remediate visual problems and/or to enhance visual performance to remediate various binocular vision and related disorders.[4-6] They typically have postdoctoral education. Those optometrists offering vision therapy often complete residencies or are certified by the:
  1. American Academy of Optometry (AAO)
  2. College of Optometrists in Vision Development (COVD)
  3. Neuro-Optometric Rehabilitation Association International (NORA)
  Additionally, the Optometric Extension Program Foundation (OEPF), which is an international organization, offers postgraduate education on vision and the visual process.
- *Optician*: A person qualified to make and supply spectacles and contact lenses for the correction of vision. They do not assess a patient's vision.
- *Vision therapist (VT)*: A person who retrains the learned aspects of vision, develops, and performs rehabilitative therapies under the supervision of an optometrist.
- *Physical therapist (PT) and occupational therapist (OT)*: While not "vision specialists" per se, the PT and OT perform vision screenings in many settings and are often the first to discover a vision/oculomotor deficit. They often work with optometrists to begin vision therapy in acute and rehabilitation settings.

Let us review a few definitions, with additional terminology listed in Tables 2.1, 2.2, and 2.3.

Contrast: The degree of blackness to the whiteness of a particular object.[7]
Contrast sensitivity: The ability to perceive sharp and clear outlines of very small objects and identify minute differences in the shadings and patterns.[7]
Visual accommodation: The adjustment of the eye for various distances whereby it can focus the image of an object on the retina by changing the curvature and thus the lens power of the lens. That is to say, the eyes "focus."
Visual efficiency: How well the visual system supplies clear vision and thus efficiently allows an individual to gather visual information. Visual efficiency skills include eye movements (saccades, pursuit, tracking, fixation), binocular vision, and accommodation.
Visual acuity: Refers to how sharply you can see, or the resolving power of the visual system.

There is an incredible array of neural networks involved in processing vision, with over 300 pathways running between more than 32 visual areas in the cerebral cortex. In addition, there are multiple subcortical areas and six cranial nerves that deal with eye movements.[8] Our perceptions, motor output, body orientation, thinking, and memory all affect where we position our eyes.[8] Neurologic damage often results in abnormal eye position, abnormal eye movements, and/or the perception of vision. If there is neurologic damage, this may result in:

- Reduced accommodation (inability to focus)
- Differences between eyes for accommodation
- Impaired near point of convergence (NPC)
- Impaired pursuit or coordinated pursuit
- Visual field loss
- Photophobia (light sensitivity)
- Increases or decreases in blink rate
- Midline shift syndrome/abnormal egocentric localization
- Diplopia (double vision)
- Impaired hand–eye coordination
- Impaired depth perception
- Impaired visual perception

Table 2.1 Terminology of Eye Movements/Positions

Term	Movement
Duction	Movement of a single eye alone
Abduction	Movement of the cornea away from midline (temporally)
Adduction	Movement of the cornea toward midline (nasally)
Eso-	A posture of the eye where it is pointing nasally and is discovered by a cover and alternating cover test when the eye is seen turning outward
Exo-	A posture of the eye where it is pointing temporally and is discovered by a cover and alternating cover test when the eye is seen turning inward
Elevation	Movement of the eye upward
Depression	Movement of the eye downward
Intorsion	Rotation of the upper pole (portion) of the eye nasally
Extorsion	Rotation of the upper pole (portion) of the eye temporally away from midline
Versions	Conjugate movements of both eyes
Dextroversion	Movement of both eyes to the right (abduction of the patient's right eye, adduction of the left eye)
Levoversion	Movement of both eyes to the left (abduction of the patient's left eye, adduction of the right eye)
Upgaze	Movement of both eyes upward
Downgaze	Movement of both eyes downward
Vergence	Both eyes move, but in equal and opposite directions
Convergence	Both eyes adduct (move nasally)
Divergence	Both eyes abduct (move temporally)
Gaze	Indicates that the eyes are looking in a certain direction
Primary gaze	The eyes are looking straight ahead
Secondary gaze	Up, down, left, or right
Tertiary gaze	Up + in, up + out, down + in, down + out

Table 2.2 Eye Motions Used to See Objects

Eye Motions	Goal
Saccades Smooth pursuit Vergence	Direct the eyes
Fixation Vestibulo-ocular reflex Optokinetics	Hold the images steady

Table 2.3 Visual Fields

Visual Field Area	Typical Degrees of Vision of Each Eye
Nasal	60 degrees medially
Superior	60 degrees upward
Inferior	70 to 75 degrees downward
Temporal	100 degrees laterally

As a result of visual deficits, patients may have difficulty ambulating, balancing, reading, or performing activities of daily living (ADLs), as well as complain of dizziness, nausea, or headaches.

ACTIVITY 2.2 FOVEAL VISION

This activity will help demonstrate the difference between the sharp foveal field dominated by cones and the less sharp areas of vision detected by the rods: straighten your arm and stare at your thumb. The image of your thumb should be sharp. Without taking your eyes off the thumb, pay attention to the peripheral areas of vision. You will notice they are somewhat blurred.

EYE ANATOMY

THE BONY ORBIT

The anatomy of the eye and orbit has been well documented (Figure 2.1).[5,9,10]

The bony orbit is a socket for the eyeball comprised of seven bones: the maxillary, palatine, frontal, sphenoid, zygomatic, ethmoid, and lacrimal bones. The walls of the orbit are comprised of the bones listed in Table 2.4.

The eye socket (or orbit) has a roof, a floor, a medial (nasal) wall, and a lateral (temporal) wall, and is shaped like a pyramid lying on its side with its base positioned anteriorly. The medial walls of the orbit are almost parallel, while the lateral walls are angled about 90 degrees to each other. The lateral wall makes a 45-degree angle with the median plane and faces anteromedially; the apex is toward the back of the head. The eye is positioned in the anterior orbit, nearer to the roof and lateral wall. As you can see in Figure 2.2, the axis of the eye socket is not the same as the axis of the eyes.

The *optic canal* (optic foramen) connects the middle cranial fossa to the apex of the bony orbit and is oriented anterolaterally and slightly downward. The optic nerve, the ophthalmic artery, and branches of the periarterial sympathetic plexus travel through it.

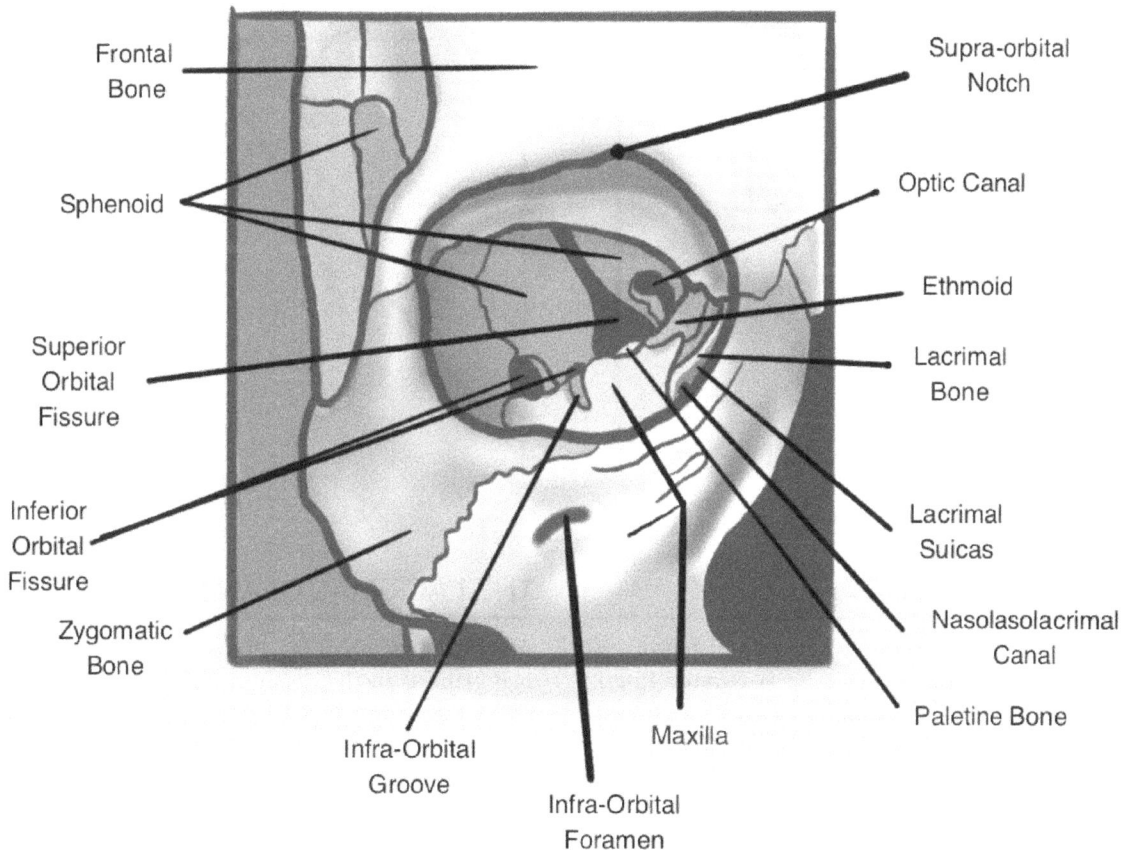

Figure 2.1 The Bony Orbit

Table 2.4 Bony Orbit

Wall	Comprised of the Following Bones	Shape
Roof (vault)	The triangular orbital plate of the **frontal bone** (largest) The lesser wing of the **sphenoid bone**	Triangular
Medial	The frontal process of the **maxilla bone** The **lacrimal bone** The orbital plate of the **ethmoid bone** (largest) A small part of the body of the **sphenoid bone**	Oblong
Floor	The orbital plate of the **maxilla bone** (largest) The orbital surface of the **zygomatic bone** The orbital process of the **palatine bone**	Triangular
Lateral	The orbital surface of the greater wing of the **sphenoid bone** The orbital surface of the **zygomatic bone**	Triangular

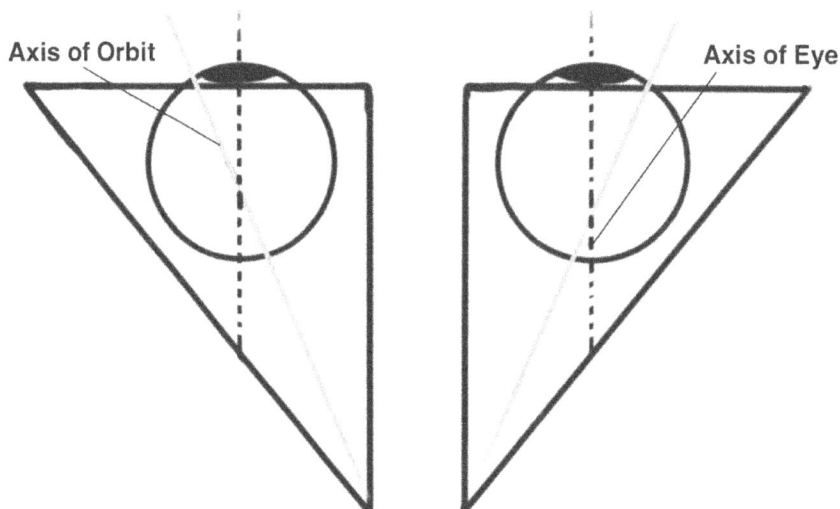

Axis of Orbit   Axis of Eye

Figure 2.2 Axis of the Eye and Orbit

THE EYELID

The *eyelid* protects the eye, keeps it moist, proving a lubrication function. This lid is covered internally by the palpebral conjunctiva and continues onto the eye as the bulbar conjunctiva. The eyelid is opened using the levator palpebrae muscles and is innervated by CN III. You can imagine the Roman numeral III as a brace holding the eyelid open.[5] The facial nerve, CN VII, closes the eye by innervating the orbicularis oculi m. You can imagine the number 7 as a finger pulling the eyelid closed.[5]

THE LACRIMAL GLAND

Innervated by CN VII (facial nerve), the lacrimal gland is in the upper eyelid and conjunctiva above the temporal part of the eye and produces tears that flow down the eye and medially. These drain through small pores called lacrimal puncta on the medial commissure. The puncta lead to lacrimal tubing called the lacrimal canaliculi and into the lacrimal sac through the nasal lacrimal duct, which empties into the nasal cavity at the level of the inferior meatus. This explains why your nose runs when you cry.

THE EYEBALL

The eyeball is suspended in the eye socket of the skull. Bron et al.[9] describe the eye as two modified spheres that are fused together: the larger globe and the smaller cornea. The *limbus* is the border where the spheres meet. The dimensions of the eye are:

* Cornea horizontal diameter: 11.75 mm
* Cornea vertical diameter: 10.6 mm
* Cornea anterior radius of curvature: 7.8 mm
* Globe anterior–posterior diameter (including cornea): 24 mm
* Globe vertical diameter: 23 mm

Six extraocular muscles attach to the eye so that it may move in any direction. The eye is divided into an *anterior chamber* lying between the cornea and iris; the *posterior* chamber, which is between the iris and the lens; and a *vitreous* chamber in the back that is filled with vitreous gel.[5]

The eye has three main layers (Figure 2.3):

* *Outer layer*: Cornea and sclera (covered by the conjunctiva mucus membrane)
* *Middle layer*: Known as the uvea, this heavily pigmented region contains the iris, ciliary body, and choroid
* *Inner layer*: Retina

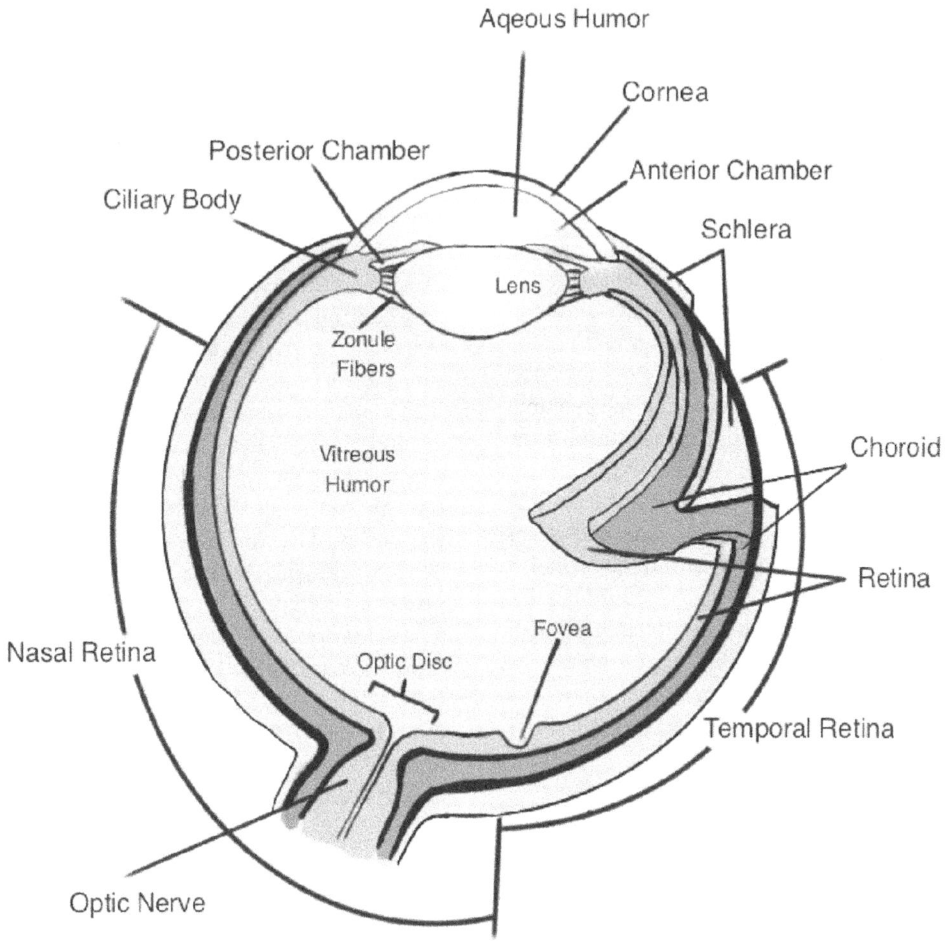

Figure 2.3 Eye Diagram

THE OUTER LAYER

The Cornea

As described by Bron et al.,[9] the anterior one-sixth of the eye is covered by the clear and transparent cornea, which is the clear front surface of the eye. The cornea provides most of the refracting power (~40–45 diopters) of the eye, about 70% of the unaccommodated eye. Therefore, the main function of the cornea is optical. It is 11.7 mm wide and measures 10.6 mm vertically for the front and about 11.7 mm in diameter for the circular posterior surface. There are three layers of the cornea: the *epithelium* (surface), the connective tissue *stroma* (90% of corneal thickness), and the *endothelium* single-cell layer that is in contact with *aqueous humor*, the jelly-like substance that fills most of the eye and provides nutrients to the avascular cornea and lens. The central third of the cornea is called the optical zone and has a radius of curvature of its anterior surface of 7.8 mm, and 6.5 mm for the posterior surface.

Sclera

The sclera is the tough, nonelastic, white portion of the eyeball and covers the posterior five-sixths of the eye structures. Collagen makes up most of the sclera with a small amount of ground substance, along with fibrocytes. It is covered by the conjunctiva, which is a mucus membrane that starts at the edge of the cornea and flows back behind the eye, loops forward, and forms the inside surface of the eyelids. This membrane is continuous and keeps objects from becoming lodged behind the eyeball.[5,9] Posteriorly, near the optic canal, the fibrils of the sclera are continuous with the dural sheath. There is an outer layer of connective tissue that supports the vasculature aspect called the episclera. The sclera is always under slight tension from the intraocular pressure (fluid pressure within the eye).

THE MIDDLE LAYER (UVEA)

Iris

The colored—visible—portion of the eye is called the *iris*. It is about 12 mm in diameter, 0.6 mm thick at its thickest, and 0.5 mm at the periphery. It has a circumference of 38 mm[9] and is located between the cornea and the lens (between the anterior and posterior chambers). The iris is equipped with a diaphragm within a central open area; this is called the *pupil*. The muscles associated with the iris are innervated by CN III. It is covered anteriorly and posteriorly by aqueous humor, but aqueous flow is blocked through the pupil by the contact of the lens with the posterior aspect of the iris. The pupil is located slightly nasal to the center of the iris. The iris forms the posterior boundary of the anterior chamber and helps regulate the amount of light allowed into the eyes. The iris constricts (contracts) with activation of the *sphincter pupillae muscle*, which is flat and encircles the pupil margin. The iris dilates when the *dilator pupillae muscle*, which extends from the iris root toward the pupil, is activated.

The Lens

The lens sits behind the iris and helps focus light upon the retina. It is transparent and flexible, and it has three layers: the outer layer is called the capsule, the middle layer is the cortex (or lens epithelium), and the center is a nucleus (lens fibers). The lens continues to grow throughout life becoming less pliable and more compact, while the lens capsule increases in thickness with age.[10] The lens is held in place by zonular fibers (zonules) that insert around the periphery of the capsule and connect to the ciliary body. It allows the focus of images onto the retina at different distances. To do this, the lens must be transparent and elastic. It is biconvex with the anterior surface less convex than the posterior surface. The center of the anterior surface is known as its *anterior pole*. The lens adds 15 diopters of refractive power at birth and, due to its decreasing ability to deform with accommodation, it decreases to ~7–8 diopters at about 25 years of age; and then to 2 diopters or less at age 50, leading to presbyopia.[9]

Choroid

The *choroid* is a dark brown membrane that covers the entire posterior portion of the eye and attaches to the retina. It then extends to the *ora serrata*, which is the junction between the choroid and ciliary body. The choroid is a key structure as it contains the venous plexuses (a collection of veins clustered together) and layers of capillaries responsible for the nutrition of the retina.

The Ciliary Body

The black-colored *ciliary body* lies between the iris and the choroid, and secretes aqueous humor. It also contains the triangle-shaped ciliary muscle that contracts to permit accommodation (for eye focusing). The ciliary muscles contract to change the shape of the lens to accommodate (focus) the image on the retina, as described earlier.

Aqueous Humor

The aqueous humor is a watery, clear solution that is high in nutrients and supports the cornea and lens. It is produced in the posterior chamber by the ciliary body and flows anteriorly to eventually be drained off via the canal of Schlemm into the venous circulation.[5] An intraocular pressure of 10–21 mmHg is maintained by the constant production and drainage of aqueous humor.[9]

THE INNER LAYER

Vitreous Humor

The *vitreous humor* is a transparent gel that makes up about two-thirds of the eye, contains a mesh of collagen fibrils, and occupies the vitreous cavity. It transmits light, supports the lens, holds the retina in place, acts as a shock absorber, and maintains the shape of the eye. Unlike the aqueous humor that provides nutrients to the lens, the vitreous humor is not replaced and consists of water (~98%), a small percentage of collagen, glycosaminoglycan sugars, electrolytes, and proteins. As we age, the vitreous humor becomes less viscous and shrinks, called vitreous degeneration, causing vitreous floaters (clumps of proteins) that cause floating shadows of lines or circles. When mild, this is a normal part of the aging process for middle-aged or older people. However, when there is a rapid increase in floaters or a person starts to see light flashes, this may indicate a health emergency of a possible vitreous detachment, retinal tear, or retinal detachment.

The Retina

The *retina* is in the posterior portion of the eye and contains the photosensitive layer. Bron et al. describe it as "an outgrowth of the brain."[9] There is a circular depressed area called the *optic disc* where the optic nerve (CN II) enters the eye. The nerve fibers of CN II spread out in the neural layer of the retina. The optic disc has no photoreceptors and only contains nerve fibers.

There are ten layers to the retina (Figure 2.4):

1. *Internal limiting membrane*: Made of Müller cells whose foot plates create a boundary between the vitreous fluid and the retina.
2. *Nerve fiber layer*: Nerve fibers from ganglion cells.
3. *Ganglion cell layer*: Contains the ganglion nuclei and some displaced amacrine cell nuclei.
4. *Inner plexiform layers*: Amacrine cells are interneurons that connect bipolar and ganglion cells to allow cross communication with information from the outer to internal layer.
5. *Inner nuclear layer*: Contains amacrine nuclei, bipolar cell nuclei, horizontal cell nuclei, and Müller cell nuclei. It connects the two plexiform layers with interplexiform cells and uses dopamine as a neurotransmitter.
6. *Outer plexiform layer*: Where horizontal cells make horizontal connections to connect photoreceptor cells with bipolar cells and horizontal cells.
7. *Outer nuclear layer*: The nuclei of rods and cones.
8. *External limiting membrane*: Contains Müller cells creating a lamina-like structure to hold photocells in place and prevents interphotoreceptor extracellular matrix fluid from moving into the inner retina.
9. *Photoreceptors*: Rods and cones convert electromagnetic waves of light into electrochemical changes and produce neural activity, thus converting the optical image into neuronal activity. They are arranged in RBG fashion, meaning (photo) receptor cells, synapsing to

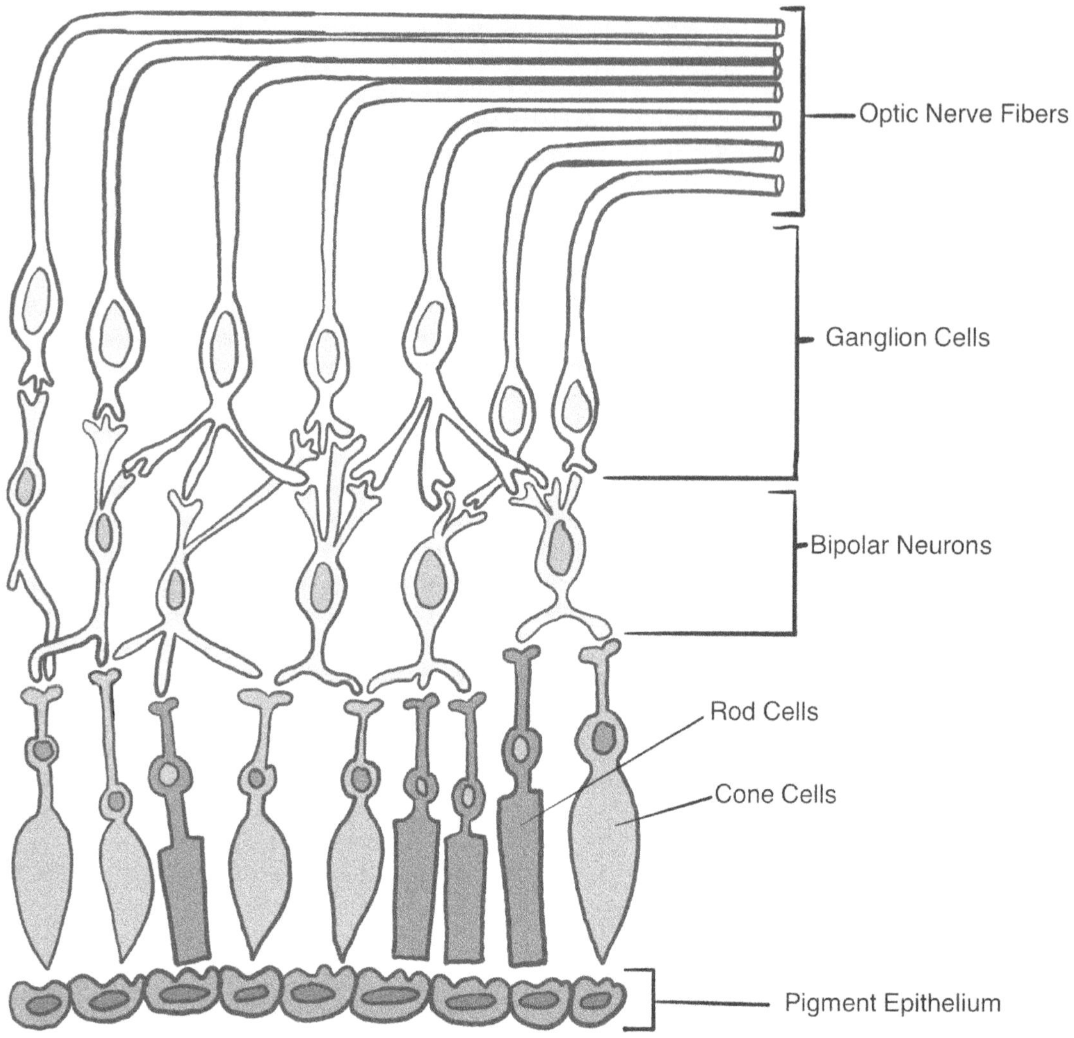

Figure 2.4 Retinal Layers

bipolar cells, then to ganglion cells. Many rods may synapse with one bipolar cell, whereas cones have a 1:1 relationship with bipolar cells. The nerve current moves radially from outer to inner layers using glutamate as a neurotransmitter.

10. *Retinal pigmented epithelial layer*: Cells with tight junctions that have melanin to absorb extra light to prevent internal reflections inside the eye and degradation of the image. These cells use glutamate as a neurotransmitter.

The outer five layers obtain nutrients from diffusion as they do not have capillaries.

Three to 4 mm lateral (temporal) to the optic disc is the high-resolution *fovea*, and it represents about 5% of the visual field.[9] The macula can be separated into three regions: the perifovea, parafovea, and fovea. The macula is about 5.5 mm in diameter and is comprised of three progressively smaller concentric circles: the perifovea, the parafovea, and the foveola. The fovea is approximately 1.5 mm in diameter (Figure 2.5).[11]

At the center of the fovea is a concave indention called the foveola. This part of the retina has the highest visual acuity (sharpest vision) and represents 1% of the visual field and is a deep red color.[9]

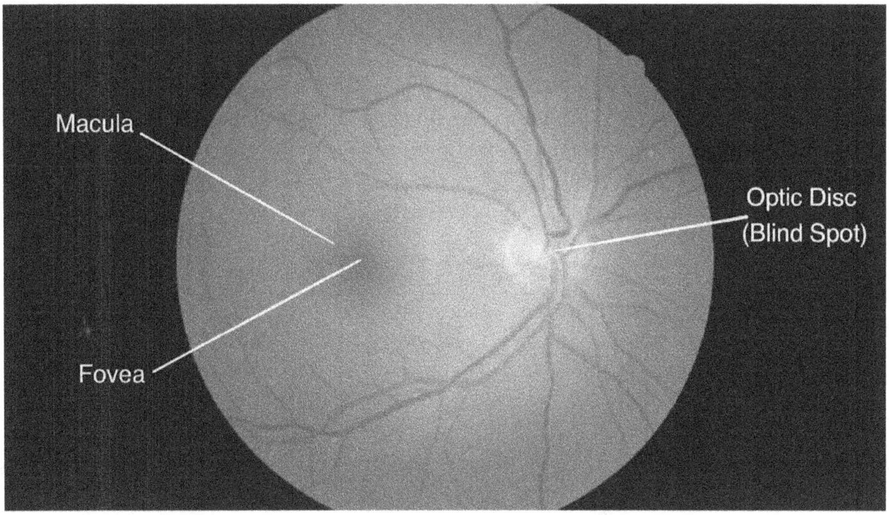

Figure 2.5 Retinal Diagram

Table 2.5 Rods and Cones

Rods	Cones
• Do not detect color • Are 500 to 1,000 times more sensitive to light than cones • Provide low resolution but assist in seeing in decreased illumination • There are about 110 million–125 million rods • There are no rods in the fovea, and rise in number rapidly toward the periphery, then diminish at the extreme periphery	• Are sensitive to color and bright light • Concentrated in the macula; the center of the macula only contains cones • Provide high resolution (sharp vision) • Damage to cones results in color detection deficits and reduced central vision • There are about 6.3 million–9.8 million in each eye • Most dense at the fovea and decrease in the periphery You may remember the cone's function because they come to a sharp point (helping us see sharply) and are shaped like the tip of a pencil.

The fovea contains ganglion cells that are excited by light, bipolar cells that detect movement in the visual field and simultaneously suppress nearby neurons to avoid information overload, and the photoreceptors. There are two types of photoreceptors: *rods* and *cones*. They are named for their shapes and have different functions. Large numbers of rods and cones activate a single axon in the optic nerve (Table 2.5).[1,10]

RODS

Rods are photoreceptors containing a chemical called rhodopsin. Rods are important for retinal sensitivity for *scotopic vision* (or vision in darker environments).

CONES

Cones are photoreceptors containing a chemical called photopsin. There are different types of photopsin that respond to different wavelengths of light, specifically red, blue, and green. Cones are important for photopic vision, or vision in bright light, visual acuity, and color vision (Table 2.6).

Dark to light adaptation sequence:

1. Pupils constrict letting less light into the eye.
2. Bleaching of photopigments (rhodopsin is broken into all-trans retinal and opsin is released).
3. Enzymes regenerate 11-cis-retinal, but this takes time (up to 5–10 minutes to completely adjust).

Table 2.6 Interesting Vision Facts

Here are interesting facts according to the Discovery Eye Foundation:[1]
Men have a higher chance of being color blind.
- The most common type of color blindness is the inability to differentiate between red and green.
- The eye can distinguish between 500 shades of gray.
- A healthy human eye can detect over 10 million different colors.
- Two percent of women have a rare genetic mutation that gives them an extra retinal cone allowing them to see more than 100 million colors.
- During major depressions, people see less contrast, making colors appear dull.

4. Rods are turned off.
5. Less sensitive cones are turned on, and visual acuity increases.

Light to dark adaptation sequence:

1. Pupils dilate allowing more light to enter the eye.
2. Light rays hit all parts of the retina (including the rods in the peripheral retina).
3. Rhodopsin accumulates and is now sensitive to light, and retinal sensitivity increases.
4. Rods turn on.
5. Cones turn off due to a decrease in light intensity and wavelength of light.
6. Visual acuity and color sensitivity decrease.
7. It can take 20–30 minutes to completely adapt.

Nyctalopia (Night Blindness)

The inability to respond to light can be due to a severe decrease in vitamin A intake, which is used to make 11-cis-retinal.

Retinitis Pigmentosa

Rod tips are not regenerated. As rods degenerate, you lose vision.

As mentioned, there are several types of nerve cells that pass visual information. The first in the chain are the *bipolar cells*, of which there are several types:

- *Rod bipolar cells*: Connect several rod cells to one to four ganglion cells.
- *Flat (diffuse) bipolar cells*: Connect many cone cells with many ganglion cells.
- *Midget bipolar cells*: Connect one cone cell with a single midget ganglion cell that provides a direct pathway to a single optic nerve fiber.

Next in the visual pathway are ganglion cells, most of which are midget bipolar neurons. They converge at the exit of the optic nerve at the optic disc.

Horizontal cells are multipolar and run parallel to the retinal surface. When the rods and cones are excited by light, they are believed to release the neurotransmitter GABA to inhibit other bipolar cells, thereby sharpening contrast and increasing spatial resolution.[10] Amacrine cells synapse with one another, with ganglion cells, and with bipolar cells. They are stimulated by bipolar cells, excite ganglion cells, and modulate photoreceptor signals.

EXTRAOCULAR EYE MUSCLES

There are six extraocular eye muscles that are used to move our eyes. They are the superior rectus, inferior rectus, medial rectus, lateral rectus, superior oblique, and inferior oblique. The innervations, actions, and attachments are listed in Table 2.7 (also see Table 2.8).

EXTRAOCULAR MUSCLE INNERVATION

There are a couple of ways to remember the innervation of the extraocular muscles. One way is to think of the innervation as a chemical equation LR_6SO_4, where LR is the lateral rectus muscle and is innervated by CN VI (abducens nerve), and SO is the superior oblique that passes around the "trochlea" like a pulley and is innervated by CN IV (trochlear nerve). All other extraocular muscles are innervated by CN III. Another way to remember the innervations is to recall that the lateral

Table 2.7 Extraocular Muscle Attachments and Innervations

Four Rectus Muscles	Abbreviation	CN	Action(s)	Origin	Insertion
Superior rectus[12]	SR	III	• Primary: Rolls eyes up (superiorly), called elevation • Secondary: Adduction • Tertiary: Intorsion	The annulus of Zinn (common tendinous ring) in the posterior eye socket	The anterior, superior eye
Inferior rectus[13]	IR	III	• Primary: Rolls eyes down, called depression • Secondary: Adduction • Tertiary: Extorsion		The anterior, inferior eye
Medial rectus[14]	MR	III	Rolls eyes in (adducts the eye)		The anterior, medial eye
Lateral rectus[15]	LR	VI	Rolls eyes out (abducts the eye)		The anterior, lateral eye
Two Oblique Muscles					
Superior oblique[16]	SO	IV	Inferolateral eye motion (down and out) • Primary: Intorts • Secondary: Depresses • Tertiary: Abducts	The periosteal covering of the sphenoid above the annulus of Zinn. Passes along the medial border of the roof of the orbit; the tendon passes through the trochlea "pulley"	The posterior, inferolateral eye posterior and deep to the superior rectus muscle
Inferior oblique[17]	IO	III	• Primary: Extorts • Secondary: Elevates • Tertiary: Abducts	The orbital floor, lateral to the nasolacrimal groove in the anterior eye socket	The posterior inferolateral surface of the eye posterior and deep to the lateral rectus

Table 2.8 Extraocular Muscle Blood Supply

Extraocular Muscle	Blood Supply
Superior rectus	Superior muscular branch of the ophthalmic artery
Inferior rectus	Inferior muscular branch of the ophthalmic artery
Medial rectus	Inferior muscular branch of the ophthalmic artery
Lateral rectus	Superior muscular branch of the ophthalmic artery
Superior oblique	Superior muscular branch of the ophthalmic artery
Inferior oblique	Inferior muscular branch of the ophthalmic artery
Levator palpebrae superioris	Superior muscular branch of the ophthalmic artery

rectus muscle "abducts" the eye and is innervated by the abducens nerve (CN VI), and that the superior oblique muscle uses the trochlea as a pulley and is innervated by the trochlear nerve (CN IV). Again, *all other* extraocular eye muscles are innervated by the oculomotor nerve (CN III).

EXTRAOCULAR MUSCLE ATTACHMENTS

The four recti muscles originate posteriorly in the orbit at the annulus of Zinn; this is a tendinous ring that circles the optic nerve. The rectus muscles in Figure 2.6 are depicted in the illustration of the left eye and the oblique muscles on the right. The dashed lines indicate the muscle is below the eye.

The superior oblique originates on the periosteal covering of the sphenoid above the annulus of Zinn posteriorly in the orbit and passes along the medial border of the roof of the orbit. The tendon passes through the trochlea "pulley" and then inserts into the posterior, inferolateral eye, posterior to the superior rectus muscle.

The inferior oblique originates on the maxillary bone on the orbital floor, lateral to the nasolacrimal groove in the anterior eye socket, and inserts onto the inferolateral surface of the eye posterior to the lateral rectus. It is the only extraocular muscle to originate in the anterior orbit.

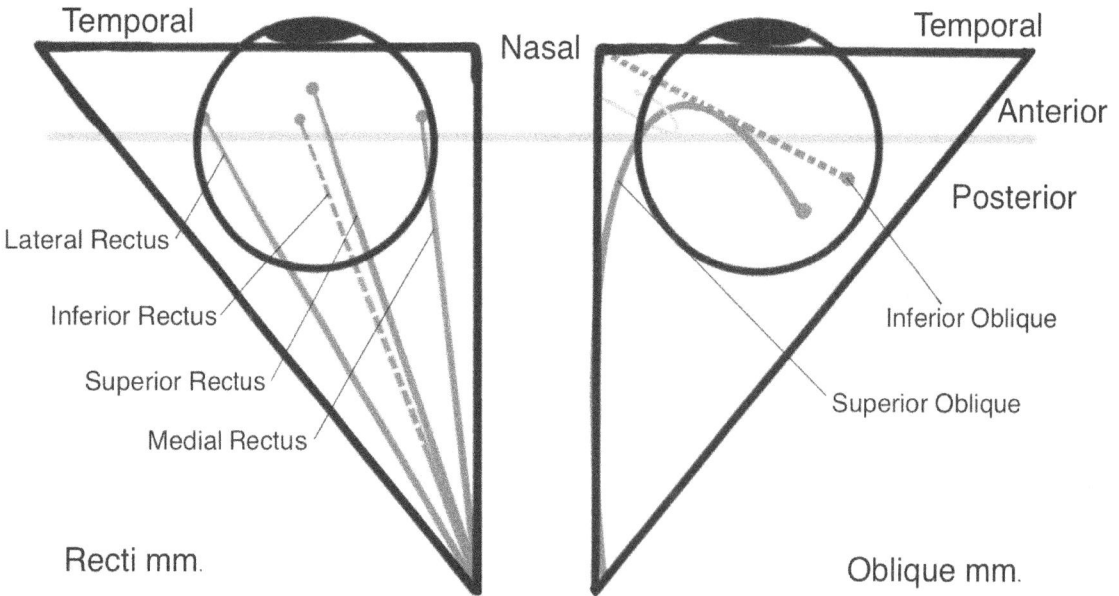

Figure 2.6 Extraocular Muscle Attachments

EXTRAOCULAR MUSCLE ACTIONS

The actions of the recti muscles are straightforward when you consider the eye like a ball rotating in space. The lateral rectus rotates the eye laterally. The medial rectus rotates the eye medially. The superior rectus rotates the eye up and in as well as intorts, while the inferior rectus rotates the eye down and in as well as extorts (Figure 2.7).

The oblique muscles are slightly less straightforward, as the superior oblique rotates the eye down and out, as well as intorts, but does not move the eye superiorly as the name would suggest. The inferior oblique rotates the eye up and out, as well as extorts, but does not move the eye inferiorly as the name would imply (Figure 2.8).

The left and right eye orbits and musculature are mirror images of each other.

When we consider how we move the eyes conjugately (together), we realize that as we look to the right, the right eye is abducted (temporally) by the right LR muscle (CN VI); the left eye is moved medially (nasally) by the MR muscle (CN III). These muscles are called "yoked" muscles as their actions both rotate the eyes to the person's right. Looking to the left, the left LR muscle and the right MR muscle contract. Keep in mind that the extraocular eye muscles do not work independently, but with the other extraocular muscles to control eye movement.

To look up, we use the SR and IO muscles. Considering the origin of the SR and the axis of the eye itself, there is a 23-degree angle of muscle pull. Therefore, the SR not only elevates the eye but also adducts it and causes intorsion (also called internal rotation). When we discuss the intorsion (internal rotation) and extorsion (external rotation) of the eye, think of the iris as being a car's steering wheel that spins one way or another. Intorsion is when the superior pole of the iris is moving nasally, and extorsion is when it moves temporally. Where the SR not only elevates but *add*ucts, the IO elevates and *abd*ucts. By using both the SR and IO muscles,

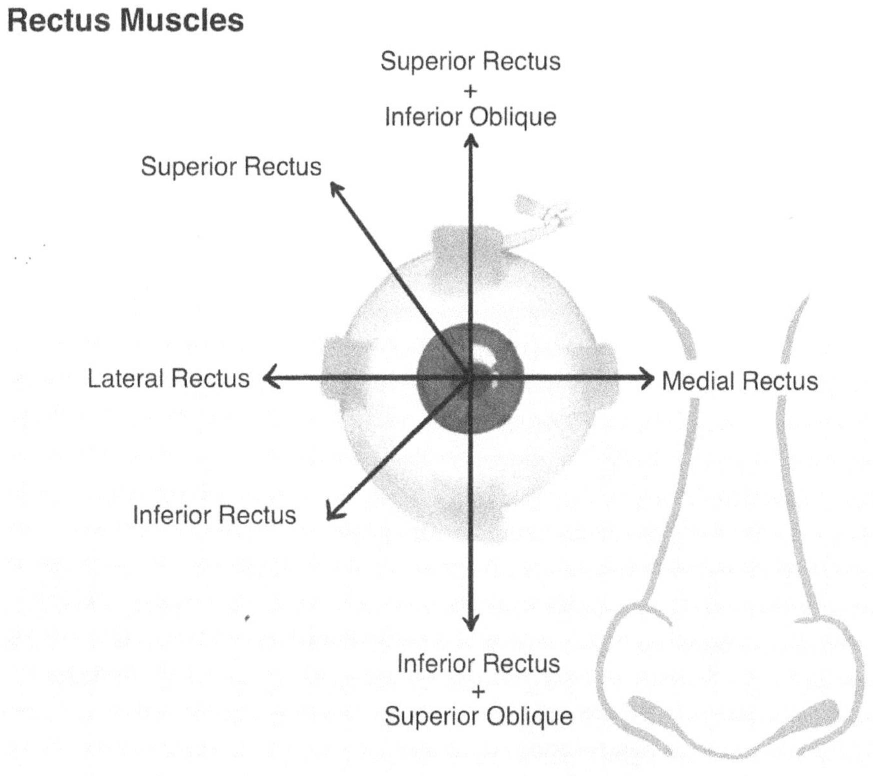

Rectus Muscles

Figure 2.7 Rectus Eye Muscle Actions

Oblique Muscles

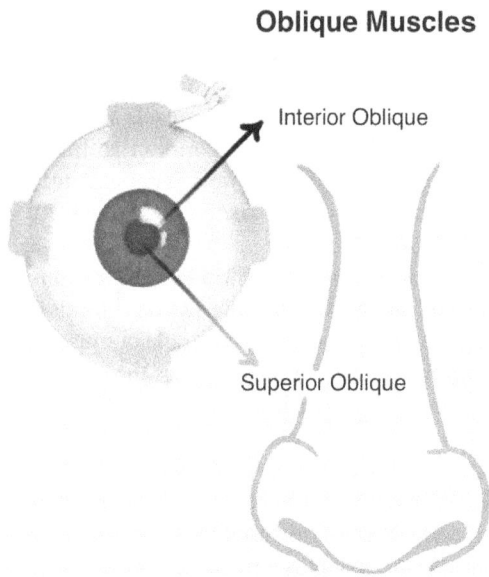

Figure 2.8 Oblique Eye Muscle Actions

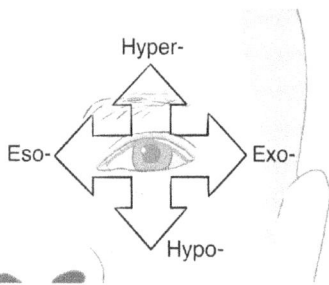

Figure 2.9 Prefixes to Describe Eye Motion/ Position

we are assured the eye will elevate and not deviate laterally or medially.

When the eye is *abducted* at 23 degrees, the SR only acts to elevate the eye, and the IR only acts to depress the eye since the line of muscle pull is now in line with the axis of the eye. The SO acts to intort the eye, while the IO acts to extort it. When the eye is *adducted*, the axis of the eye is more in line with the pull of the SO and IO. Therefore, when the eye is adducted, the superior oblique depresses the eye while the inferior oblique elevates it. The superior rectus now acts to intort the eye while the inferior rectus extorts it.

In the primary position of the eye, to abduct the eye, the lateral rectus muscle is the primary mover; however, it is also assisted by the superior and inferior oblique muscles.

An easy way to remember which muscles create ocular torsion is that both superior muscles (superior rectus and oblique) intort (or medially rotate) the eyes. Both inferior muscles (inferior recutus and oblique) extort (or externally rotate) the eyes.

We use a variety of terms to discuss the movement and position of the eye(s). We use the prefixes in Figure 2.9 and Table 2.9 to describe eye positions.

A *tropia* has been defined as "a deviation of an eye from the normal position with respect to the line of vision when both eyes are open."[18] Tropia signs include the eyes appearing walleyed (one or both eyes pointing temporally) or cross-eyes (one or both eyes pointing nasally). If left untreated it will lead to loss of vision in the strabismic eye (if unilateral) or alternating strabismus if each eye is turned. According to the Mayo Clinic, tropias are the leading cause of decreased vision among children, but treatment can help prevent long-term problems.[19]

Amblyopia, commonly known as lazy eye, is a condition where visual acuity is less than 20/20, but not because of refractive errors or observable eye disease. About 98% of amblyopia is unilateral, and 1–2% bilateral.[20] According to the National Institutes of Health, this usually happens in just

Table 2.9 Tropias and Phorias

Eye Position	Prefix	Chronic Binocular Misalignment Tropias	Misaligned When Binocular Vision Is Prevented. Phorias
Elevated	Hyper-	Hypertropia	Hyperphoria
Depressed	Hypo-	Hypotropia	Hypophoria
Nasally	Eso-	Esotropia	Esophoria
Temporally	Exo-	Exotropia	Exophoria

one eye; less commonly in both eyes. Some premature babies seem to have amblyopia, but in reality, their visual processing and neural circuitry are not fully developed.[20] Children may develop amblyopia. As one eye typically has better visual acuity, over time, the brain tends to ignore signals from the weaker eye. Symptoms of amblyopia in children include squinting, shutting one eye, or tilting the head.[21]

A *phoria* has been defined as "any of various tendencies of the lines of vision to deviate from the normal when binocular fusion of the retinal images is prevented."[22] The average person has a slight exophoria. We become concerned with phorias that are moderate to large.

Convergence insufficiency and *convergence excess* are types of phorias. Convergence insufficiency is the inability to maintain binocular function while working at a near distance (~6 cm distance from the bridge of the nose). Typically, one eye will turn outward when attempting to focus on a nearby object. Convergence excess is an "overconvergence" of the eyes while attempting to focus on an object at a near distance for extended periods, such as while reading or looking at a computer or phone screen. Sometimes this overconvergence causes diplopia. It is present in about 5% of the population. It is commonly seen following a traumatic brain injury or cerebrovascular accident.[23]

Fusional vergence is the movement of both eyes that enables the unification of each monocular image to produce a binocular vision percept. When we converge the eyes to see a near target, it is called *fusional convergence*. When we move each eye outward to see a target (such as when focusing on a distant target or following something moving away from us), it is called *fusional divergence*. Fusional vergence is what improves with vision therapy.[24]

Hypertropia is when one eye is deviated upward in comparison to the other eye. By convention, hypertropia of one eye is the same as a hypotropia (downward deviation) of the other eye. If it behaves the same in all fields of gaze, it is classified as "comitant."

We use the term *comitancy* to describe whether the magnitude of the eye turn is the same in all positions of gaze (tested at 40 cm or 6 m). If we say the eyes are *comitant*, it means the size of the phoria remains constant in all positions of gaze when measured at the same distance. If it behaves differently in different fields of gaze it is termed *incomitant* (or noncomitant). For incomitant phorias (or strabismus), the amount of deviation of the squinting eye varies according to the direction in which the eyes are turned.

BASIC VISUAL PATHWAY

The visual pathway is comprised of the retina, optic nerve, optic chiasm, optic tracts, lateral geniculate bodies, optic radiations, and the visual cortical areas. Snell and Lemp describe the visual pathway as having four parts.[10]

Light enters the eyes and stimulates the rods and cones of the retinas, which send their impulses along the retinal ganglion cells that form the optic nerve. The temporal visual field is projected on the nasal portion of the retina, while the nasal visual field is projected onto the temporal retina. The superior visual field is projected onto the inferior retina, while the inferior visual field is projected onto the superior retina. The optic nerve is covered with the pia, arachnoid, and dura mater sheaths. It is identical to white matter and cannot regenerate. The nerve exits the bony orbit through a foramen in the sphenoid bone called the *optic canal*, and then travels along the surface of the middle cranial fossa near the pituitary gland. The optic nerves from each eye join to form the *optic chiasm*, which is located at the junction of the anterior wall and floor of the third ventricle. Once reaching the optic chiasm, there is a partial decussation of axons with information from the lateral retinas and maculae remaining ipsilaterally, while medial (nasal) retinal and macular information decussate to continue contralaterally. After the optic chiasm, the axons are called the *optic tracts* and emerge from the posterolateral angles of the chiasm. The *left optic tract* carries visual information from the left temporal and right nasal retina, while the *right optic tract* carries visual information from the right temporal and left nasal retina. As the optic tracts move posteriorly, they undergo a 90-degree turn so that the tracts carrying information from the upper retinal quadrants pass to their medial side, and those carrying information from the lower retinal quadrants pass to their lateral side.[10] These optic tracts travel around the midbrain toward the *lateral geniculate nucleus* (LGN) in the thalamus where all but 10% synapse. The remaining 10% pass medially below the pulvinar of the thalamus to enter the *superior colliculus* (which is responsible for reflexive head and eye movements in response to visual stimulus) and *pretectal nucleus* (midbrain before information reaches the Edinger Westphal nucleus), which receive information from the retina as well as the visual cortex. These fibers are concerned with visual body reflexes and light reflexes, respectively.[10] The LGN is located on the undersurface of the pulvinar of the thalamus. Axons spread out from the LGN through the deep white matter and are called *optic Radiations*. Meyer's loop refers to the optic radiations that run through the temporal lobe carrying information from the inferior retina (superior visual field). Baum's loop, which travels around the inferior horn of the lateral ventricle, then on to the visual cortex, is the part of the optic radiation that carries information from the superior retina (inferior visual field).[25] Optic radiation fibers from the lateral portions of the lateral geniculate body receive impulses from the inferior retinal quadrants (superior visual fields). Fibers from the middle portions of the lateral geniculate body receive information from the superior retinal quadrants (inferior visual fields). The optic radiations (also known as geniculocalcarine tracts) travel to the *primary visual cortex (V1)* in the occipital lobe.

Unilateral damage to the visual pathway can cause blindness in one eye, hemianopia (loss of half of the visual field), quadrantanopia (loss of a quarter of the visual field), or scattered scotomas (small blind spots) (Figure 2.10).

Each occipital lobe contains a visual cortex and is divided into five layers that are functionally distinct and specialized. Once the visual cortex processes the information, it is sent to other parts of the brain for further analysis. The five regions of the visual cortex[26] are listed in Table 2.10.

THE VISUAL CORTEX

The visual cortex, which resides in the occipital lobe of the brain, receives, processes, and integrates visual information from the retinas. It is divided into five regions (V1–V5) based on their structure (cell type) and function. These layers[9,26] are described in Table 2.11.

Damage to the visual cortex is referred to as *cortical blindness*, which is typically caused by a stroke in the posterior cerebral artery.[27] Other causes of cortical blindness include infection, eclampsia, traumatic brain injury, encephalitis, meningitis, medications, and hyperammonemia.[26] Damage to bilateral visual cortices can cause complete cortical blindness, which is sometimes accompanied by Anton–Babinski syndrome, when a patient is blind but denies having any visual impairment.[26]

MAGNOCELLULAR AND PARVOCELLULAR PATHWAYS

How do we make sense of the images that we see? The magnocellular and parvocellular pathways are referred to as the "visual attention" pathways because they are the two pathways that process visual information. The parvocellular pathway is involved with seeing in high resolution and in color. One way to remember this is to think of "**p**arvo-" and "**p**igment" (color). The magnocellular pathway has lower acuity resolution but processes faster, so it is used to see motion. One way to remember this is to think of "**m**agno-" and "**m**otion." After leaving the retina, both pathways travel to the LGN of the thalamus, and then on to the primary visual cortex. Each pathway goes to different places in each. It is believed there is early processing for the parvocellular and magnocellular pathways from the retina to the LGN that leads to conscious visual perception. Parvocellular information is sent via midget cells, while magnocellular information is sent via parasol cells. When arriving at the LGN, information is processed in different layers. Magnocellular information is processed through layers 1 and 2, while parvocellular information is processed through layers 3 through 6. From the LGN the pathways travel along the optic radiations to the primary visual cortex (V1).

From the primary visual cortex, the magnocellular pathway fibers travel in a dorsal stream from the occipital cortex to the parietal and then to the

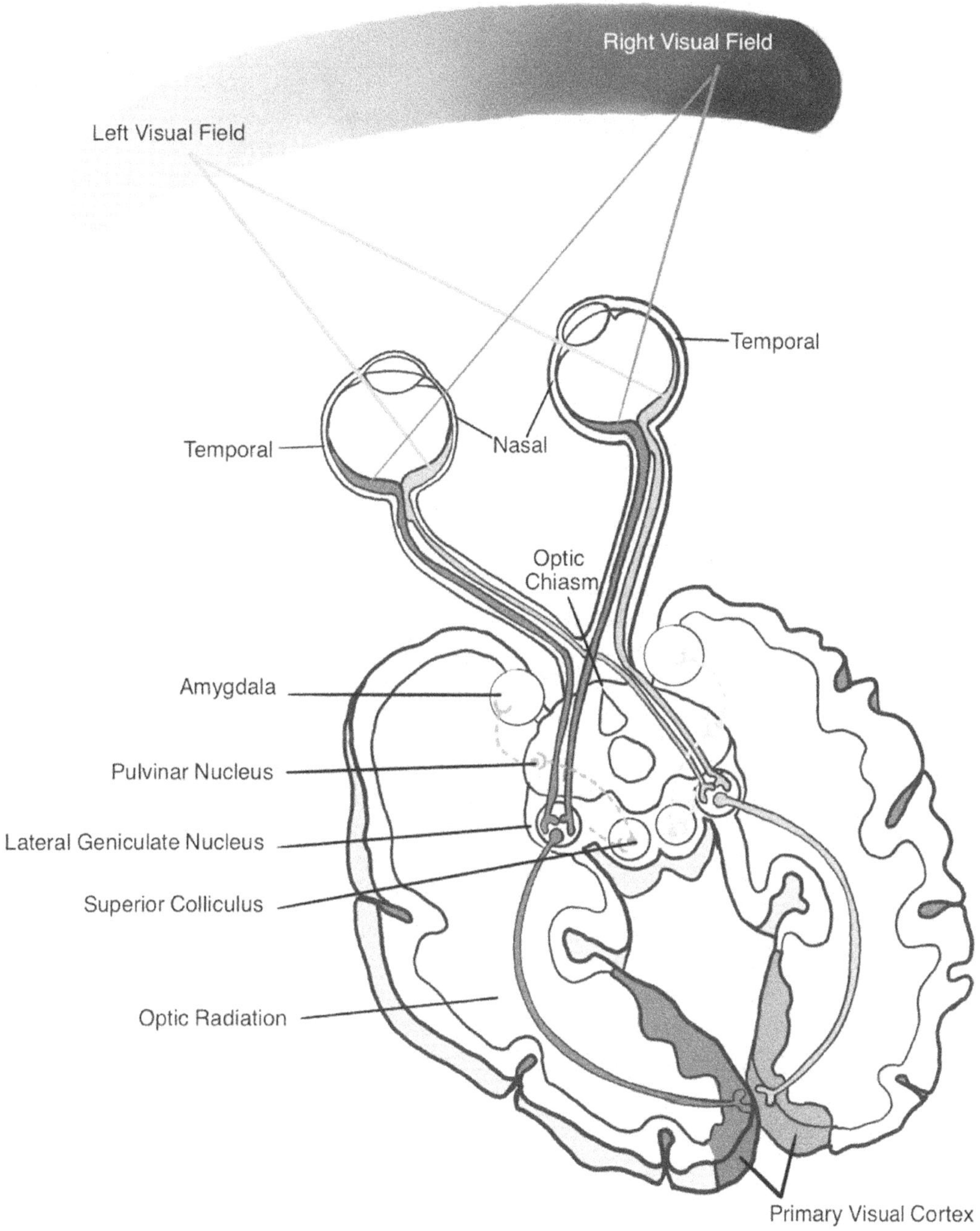

Figure 2.10 Visual Pathway

frontal association areas. Remember, this is the "where is it" pathway. The parvocellular pathway fibers travel in a ventral stream from the occipital cortex to the temporal association areas. The parvocellular pathway is also known as the "what is it" pathway (Figure 2.11).

Twenty percent of the information leaving V2 to these pathways goes to the magnocellular pathway, also called the dorsal stream pathway and deals primarily with peripheral visual information. The name "magnocellular" comes from *magno*, meaning "large," as these retinal cell bodies (rods) are

Table 2.10 Parts of the Visual Pathway

Part	Description
Intraocular	Includes the optic disc and the portion of the optic nerve that lies within the sclera.
Intraorbital	About 25 mm long, it is in this portion that the optic nerve becomes myelinated. This part begins where the optic nerve is formed at the lamina cribrosa (a net-like structure that covers the hold in the posterior sclera through which the optic nerve passes) and ends at the optic canal.
Intracanalicular	The optic nerve passes through the optic canal in the lesser wing of the sphenoid bone. This part is about 5 mm long.
Intracranial	The optic nerve leaves the optic canal and passes within the subarachnoid space to reach the optic chiasm (in the floor of the third ventricle) and travels along the rest of the pathway to the visual cortical areas of the occipital lobes.

Table 2.11 Regions of the Visual Cortex

Visual Cortex Region	Function
V1	V1 is the largest and most important layer of the visual cortex. V1 is divided into six layers, each having a different function. It receives projections from the LGN (thalamus) and responds to specific types of visual cues such as the orientation of edges and lines. It allows you to see, but not recognize what you see. V1 receives input from both magnocellular as well as parvocellular pathways. The output of V1 projects to V2, V3, V4, V5.
V2	V2 is called the secondary visual cortex. It receives information from V1 and responds to differences in color, spatial frequency, moderately complex patterns, object orientation, and recognition. Information leaving V2 splits into magnocellular and parvocellular pathways. It has feedback connections to V1 and feedforward connections to V3–V5.
V3	Along with V4 and V5, this layer is concerned with the recall of visual memory relating to objects (object recognition).
V4	Object orientation, spatial frequency, and color. Along with V3 and V5, V4 is concerned with the recall of visual memory relating to objects (object recognition). The output of V4 is mainly to the inferior temporal cortex.
V5	V5 is called the middle temporal visual area and determines the speed and direction of moving objects. Along with V3 and V4, V5 is also concerned with the recall of visual memory relating to objects (object recognition).

large. The rods give us information about movement and depth and can detect slight differences in brightness. The magnocellular pathway travels dorsally to the parietal cortex. The posterior parietal complex includes parts of the superior parietal lobe, intraparietal sulcus, and part of the frontal cortex that is involved with eye movements and visual perception known as the frontal eye field. Because part of the magnocellular pathway travels through the superior colliculi to the secondary visual cortex, when there is damage to the primary visual cortex or optic radiations, a person may be blind, but still react to lights, motion, or large objects.

The parvocellular pathway, the "what is it" pathway, is also known as the ventral pathway. It travels from V2 of the secondary visual cortex to the inferotemporal cortex. The name comes from *parvo*, meaning "small." The retinal cell bodies the information comes from are small (cones) and give us information about fine detail and color.

The parvocellular pathway is primarily in the right cerebral hemisphere and includes the temporoparietal junction, the intraparietal sulcus, and parts of the frontal cortex.

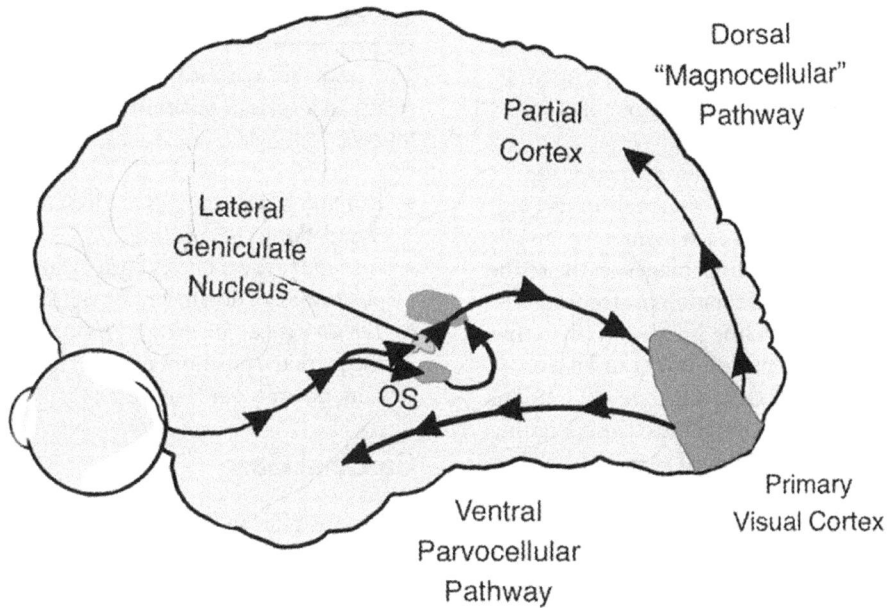

Figure 2.11 Magnocellular and Parvocellular Pathways

SUPERIOR COLLICULUS

The roof of the midbrain is formed by two paired and rounded swellings called the superior and inferior colliculi. The superior colliculi primarily receive information from visual stimuli, while the inferior colliculi primarily receive information from auditory stimuli (see Figure 2.12).

The superior colliculi optimize eye movements in several ways.[28]

They provide vector coordinates for saccades and contribute to saccade velocity. They have premotor preparation, and work on target selection, visual attention, and working memory. They combine saccade and vergence movements and assist in lens accommodation. They also assist in visual fixation and smooth pursuit. These neurons discharge a high-frequency premotor burst before head-restrained saccades as well as just before head-unrestrained gaze shifts. Gandhi and Katnani point out that sometimes gaze shifts are not enough to produce sufficiently large enough changes in gaze (e.g., when trying to look behind you), and you need to coordinate movements across multiple body segments such as the head, trunk, and feet. The superior colliculi assist in the control of these body movements. For reaching

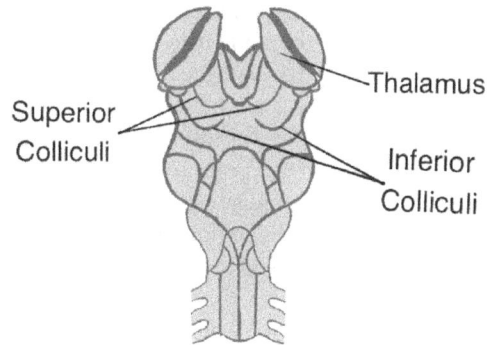

Figure 2.12 Superior and Inferior Colliculi

and catching motions, the superior colliculi and reticular formation (pons and midbrain) are active before the actual movement.[28]

EYE POSITIONS AND MOVEMENT

According to Leigh and Zee, there are seven functional classes of human eye movements:[3]

- *Visual fixation* is holding images of a stationary target on the fovea by minimizing ocular drifts.

- *Saccades* that move the eye to bring images of interest onto the fovea.
- *Smooth pursuit* is holding images of a moving target on the fovea, or on the retina during linear translations.
- *Vergence*, which moves the eyes in opposite directions so that images of a single object are held simultaneously on each fovea.
- *Optokinetic* means holding images on the retina during sustained head rotations or translations.
- *Vestibular* means holding images on the retina during head rotations or linear translations.
- *Nystagmus (quick phase)*, which are eye motions that reset the eye position toward the oncoming visual scene during sustained rotation.

Eye motions may be voluntary using the frontal eye fields (FEF) located in the frontal lobe (that has a role in generating saccades, and controlling pursuits and vergence eye movements), or reflexive using the occipital and parietal lobes. When both eyes are moving in the same direction and velocity, this is described as *conjugate* motion. If they eyes are not moving at the same direction or velocity, this is described as *dysconjugate* (or nonconjugate) motion.

Control centers for the horizontal conjugate gaze pathway are in the pons, while control centers for the vertical conjugate gaze pathway are in the thalamomesencephalic junction (the junction between the midbrain and thalamus):

1. *Supranuclear pathway*: Above the nuclei of midbrain and brainstem, and found in the cerebrum: frontal eye fields, parietal eye fields, visual cortex.
2. *Internuclear*: All the nuclei send information to and from each other in the brainstem (mostly midbrain).
   a. Rostral median longitudinal fasciculus
   b. Interstitial nucleus of Cajal
   c. CN III (oculomotor nerve) nucleus
   d. CN IV (trochlear nerve) nucleus
3. *Infranuclear*
   a. CN III
   b. CN IV
   c. Extraocular eye muscles: Superior rectus, inferior oblique, inferior rectus, superior oblique

GAZE

The term *gaze* indicates that the eyes are held steady in a certain position. Gaze directions are as follows:

- *Primary gaze*: The eyes are looking straight ahead along the midline
- *Secondary gaze:* Gazes away from the primary position: Up, down, left, or right (Figure 2.13)
- *Tertiary gaze (for each eye):* Gazes away from the primary position: up + in, up + out, down + in, down + out (Figure 2.14)

Cardinal Gaze

Clinicians refer to the following six gaze positions as the *cardinal gaze positions*:

1. Right + up
2. Right gaze
3. Right + down
4. Left + up
5. Left gaze
6. Left + down

The activity of different eye muscles, or combinations of eye muscles, produces these motions.[7] In general:

- Horizontal eye movements are generated in the pons.[29]
- Vertical eye movements are generated in the midbrain reticular formation and the pretectal area.[29]

Different types of motion or muscle activity are used to either move or steady the eyes to see clearly and direct the eye to objects of interest. For example, motions that "direct" the eyes include saccades, pursuit, and vergence. Motions that are used to hold the eye "steady" on an object include fixation, optokinetic nystagmus, and the vestibular ocular reflex.

FIXATION

The eye is never truly still, even when it appears to be, as in looking at a still object. To create fixation, we use three miniature eye movements that

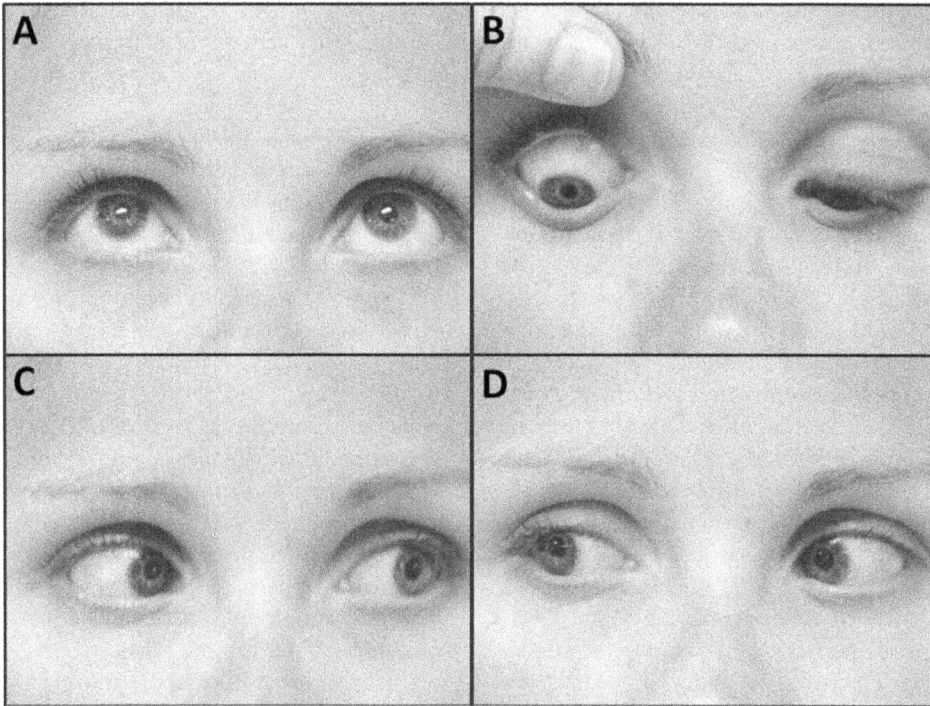

Figure 2.13 Secondary Gazes

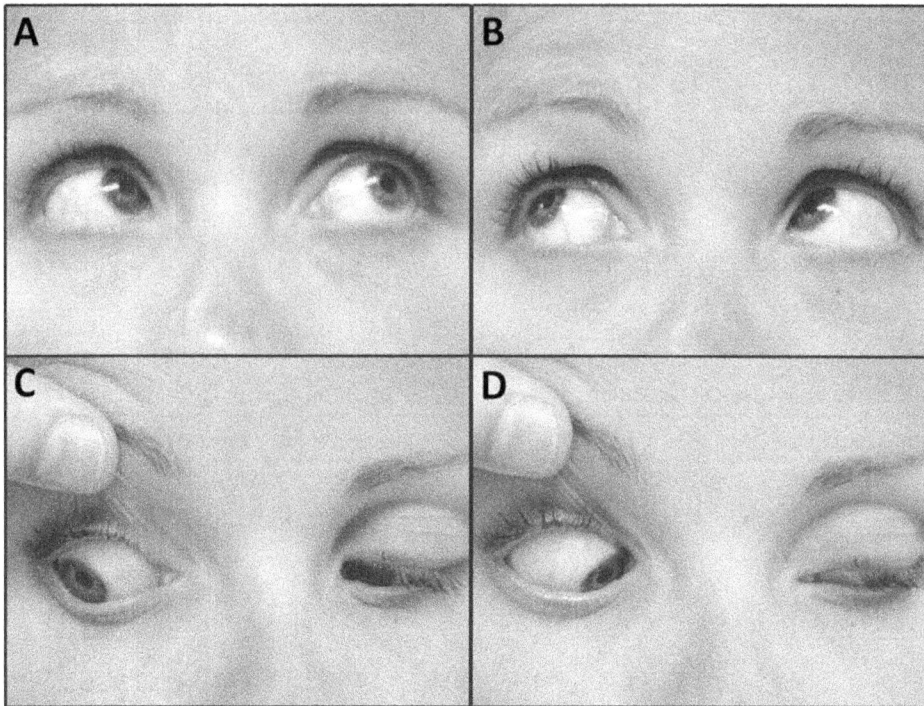

Figure 2.14 Tertiary Gazes

are not detectable by the naked eye: microsaccades, microdrift, and microtremor.[30] When something disrupts fixation, the patient may complain of *oscillopsia*, which is the perception of a moving environment. Deficits in the fixation system itself or intrusions of other motions, such as pathological nystagmus, disrupt fixation. For example, you might ask a person to stare at the point of your pen as you hold it in front of their eyes. If the patient can keep their eyes steady on the pen point, they are said to be *maintaining fixation*. This term also describes a patient who is looking at an object during certain tests. For example, if you observe nystagmus while you ask the patient to look at the pen tip (which represents a cerebellar problem) you will document that the patient demonstrated "fixation nystagmus."[31] The phrase *gaze holding* is also used to describe holding the eyes in a certain position.

Reactions to trying to fixate sometimes offer clues indicating pathology. For example, if a patient develops nystagmus when trying to fixate on a target, this is suggestive of a central pathology. If a patient has nystagmus that stops while they are visually fixating, this is suggestive of a peripheral (outside of the brain) pathology. If the patient is unable to visually fixate, you will observe the eyes moving around the visual target instead of remaining stationary. This is another sign suggestive of central pathology.

SACCADES

A saccade is a very rapid movement of the eyes in one direction to bring an object that is in your peripheral vision to the fovea in the shortest possible time. Saccades are the quickest of all eye motions, and may be triggered by the appearance of a novel object seen or heard, as part of a learned behavior, from memory, or during a visual search.[3] The intrinsic stimulus for the choice of this motion is a positional error of the object of interest's image on the retina. There are a variety of circumstances in which we need saccades. They come into play when whatever you are watching begins to move faster than you can follow by using only smooth pursuit. Another example of saccades is when you hold your head still while looking back and forth between two objects that you can see within your visual field. We use saccades when our eyes move from word to word while we are reading. Specific information on saccade motion is listed in Table 2.12.[32]

There are many causes of saccadic impairments. They are described in Table 2.13.[6]

PURSUIT

Smooth pursuit is a continuous tracking motion of the eyes, and a slow-moving visual target of interest moves across the visual field. It declines with age and is generally developed and close to an adult level of function by the age of 6 months,[33] but may be seen in infants as young as 6–8 weeks of age.[34] It then continues to fine-tune through the preschool period

Table 2.12 Saccade Latency, Duration, and Amplitude

Saccade latency	200 to 250 ms Peak velocity range: 30 degrees/sec to 800 degrees/sec
Peak Duration Range	20 to 140 ms
Amplitude Range	0.5 to 40 degrees

Table 2.13 Causes of Saccadic Impairment

Impairment	Possible Causes
Slow saccades, often with hypometria	Medications (e.g., anticonvulsants, benzodiazepines) Neurodegenerative disorders
Slow horizontal saccades	Brainstem lesions
Slow vertical saccades	Midbrain lesions Ischemic diseases Inflammatory diseases Neurodegenerative diseases (especially supranuclear palsy)
Hypermetric saccades	Cerebellar lesions
Delayed-onset saccades	Supratentorial cortical dysfunction

Table 2.14 Pursuit Latency and Velocity

Latency[30]	100 to 130 ms
Velocity[20,30]	For most of us, a smooth pursuit can compensate for head movements up to a velocity of 30 degrees per second. Higher velocities are available for large-amplitude, full-field, or self-moved target motions and for top athletes who have trained themselves to watch fast-moving objects and may generate a pursuit as fast as 130 degrees per second.

but can degrade with age in some patients around the sixth decade. Smooth pursuit allows for clear vision of objects that are moving slowly within the visual environment, with the stimulus for smooth pursuit being the relative velocity of the object being watched. An example would be watching a person walk slowly across the room while you are sitting still. As the person walks across the room, you "follow" by moving your eyes in the direction in which they are walking. You can do this if the object you are watching is moving within 0 to 0.5 Hz (1 Hz = 360 degrees of motion per second).[35] Another example of smooth pursuit is when you are holding a pen in front of a person's eyes and asking them to follow the pen (eyes only) while you slowly move it left and right of center. Interestingly, during normal eye movement, the head begins to turn after about 15 degrees of eye motion.[36]

We also use smooth pursuit for keeping a stationary target on the fovea during self-motion. For example, if you want to keep your eyes on the television screen as you walk across the room. You are moving but the TV set is not. If you are turning your head while walking and looking at the television, your vestibular ocular reflex will assist in maintaining fixation. Specific information on smooth pursuit motion is listed in Table 2.14.

Many things impact smooth pursuits, including age, alertness, medications, intoxicants, and degenerative disorders of the cerebellum or extrapyramidal systems. When pursuit is not available, saccades are used to visually track objects (called *saccadic pursuit*).

There are two types of stimulus that drive vergence eye movements: image disparity, or the difference in image location seen by each eye, and image blur.[3] When our eyes move in order to correct a visual image disparity, this is called *fusional vergence*. When the eyes move to correct a blurred image, this is called *accommodative vergence*.

ACTIVITY 2.3 SMOOTH PURSUIT

Try it! Without watching a moving object (and in a quiet room), try using smooth pursuit to look from one side of the room to the other. If you are under 60 years of age (as smooth pursuit may be impaired at or above this age) and have a camera in your phone, record your eyes as you do this. You will find that you can't generate smooth pursuit eye motions without a target. If you observe carefully (or playback your video), you will realize you are using a series of saccades.[2] Use your smartphone to videotape your eye movements as you try this and then repeat it by visually tracking an object moving left to right.

VERGENCE

ACTIVITY 2.4 PRISMS

Place a wedge prism (base out) over a colleague's eye as they focus on a distant target, and you will see it converge.

Vergence is the eye motion we use to change binocular fixation, either closer or farther away from its current point of fixation. We can do this once, as when looking at a stationary object that is either further or closer than the last object we were fixing on, or we may do it continuously, as when tracking at an object that is moving toward or away from us (depth tracking). When tracking an object that is smoothly moving toward or away from us, each eye must move in the opposite direction as

Table 2.15 Horizontal Vergence Latency

Horizontal Vergence Latency	• ~200 ms for blur-driven vergence when stimulus presentation is unpredictable. • ~160 ms when the task is to change fixation from one depth to another. • There are differences between reaction times to the onset of convergence and divergence movements.

the other simultaneously. For example, if an object is moving toward us, each eye must rotate toward the midline (nasally) as it tracks the object getting closer. These eye motions are called *convergence*. The *near point of convergence*, or NPC, is the closest point that a person can still see an object as one image. As the object moves away from us, each eye rotates outwardly simultaneously (*divergence*). These motions allow each eye to center the image of the object on the fovea that we are tracking, thus perceiving one image. Specific information on vergence motions is listed in Table 2.15.[37]

Leigh and Zee describe a "near triad": three actions that are taken to see a near object clearly while using both eyes. These actions are vergence, accommodation, and pupillary constriction.[37] Vergence moves each eye so that the image of the object of interest falls on the fovea, while accommodation changing the shape, and therefore power, of the lens to focus the image on the retina. The pupil constriction, limiting the amount of light allowed into the eye, plays a minor role in focusing on near objects.[37]

As reported by Leigh and Zee, age plays a role in vergence.[37] Neonates may have ocular misalignment that resolves as vergence develops during the first 2 months of life,[38] and by 3 months, infants can make appropriate vergence movements with appropriate accommodative responses occurring later.[39,40] Vergence responses are similar from about the age of 8 years until the mid-40s.[41] The elderly have a diminution in convergence with a given accommodative stimulus.[42,43]

OPTOKINETIC NYSTAGMUS

The optokinetic system, sometimes abbreviated OPK, provides clear visual images during sustained (constant speed) head movements, sustained environmental movements, or a combination of both. These motions trigger a jerk-type of *optokinetic nystagmus* (an involuntary reflex that moves the eye quickly in one direction and slower in the opposite

direction used to fixate allowing people to track objects moving across their visual fields). Both the smooth pursuit and optokinetic systems contribute to this response.[44] Nystagmus that is activated by the OPK system is called *optokinetic nystagmus* and may be abbreviated OKN. An example of optokinetic nystagmus is trying to watch the side of the road while riding as a passenger in an automobile or looking out of a train or subway car's window. As you watch the side of the road or scene outside of the window, objects are continuously moving across your field of vision. In the examples just used, if you are in a country where you drive on the right side of the road, the images of a passenger looking out of their passenger's window would be moving across the visual field from left to right. While the nystagmus of the vestibular ocular reflex (VOR) and OKN look the same, they differ in how and why they are activated. The VOR is activated due to head motions while trying to maintain visual fixation; the OKN is activated by objects moving across the visual field of a relatively still head. The OPK system detects the movement of an object beginning in the left peripheral visual field and across the visual field. Imagine that you see a tree while riding in the car. As you look out the passenger window, the tree first appears at the far-left edge of your visual field, drawing your eyes far left in their orbits. The image of the tree moves from far left to far right across your visual field but is too quick for you to track using smooth pursuit. You track the tree from left to right using OKN and very soon find that you are at the end range of motion with your eyes looking to the right. The tree leaves your visual field completely as the car continues to move, and your eyes quickly jerk back to the far left so that you can find a new object to view and start the process all over. The tracking motions you have made from left to right as you track the tree are slower than the quicker motions to return your eyes to the far left. If you were to watch someone's eyes while they looked out of the car window, you would observe OKN with rhythmic eye motions alternating between slower tracking motions in one direction and quicker "reset" motions in the opposite direction, returning the eyes to the starting point. If you have someone sitting in a chair that can swivel 360 degrees, and spin them for about 30 seconds, after you stop the chair you will still observe nystagmus. These nystagmus movements are called optokinetic after-nystagmus (OKAN) and occur because the velocity storage mechanism of the cerebellum is used for OKN.[44]

ACTIVITY 2.5 NYSTAGMUS

Have a colleague sit in a chair that swivels. With their eyes kept open, spin the chair rapidly in one direction for about 20 or 30 seconds, then suddenly stop the chair and observe their eyes. You will see nystagmus. While the colleague is spinning, they are using nystagmus with the quick phases in the direction of spin. Once the chair is stopped, you will observe jerk nystagmus with quick phases in the opposite direction of the spin. (The mechanics behind this phenomenon are explained in a later part of this book.) For safety, wait for the colleague's dizziness to end before allowing them to stand.

To accurately move the eyes to see clearly, one must use the integration of OKN, smooth pursuit, saccades, fixation, and the vestibular ocular reflex. As far as movement is concerned, the eyes do not provide enough information to tell you if you are moving or if the world is moving around you. An example of this is when you are sitting in a car at a stoplight and the car next to you starts to drift forward. The OPK system detects the movement of the car drifting; however, you do not know if the car next to you is moving or if your car is moving. As a result, you quickly press harder on the brake pedal. After a moment, you realize that you were sitting still the entire time. If the car next to you drifts again, you do not have the same reflexive reaction to slam on the brakes, as your brain now realizes that you are not moving. Your eyes are only one of the systems contributing to a sense of motion and balance. We need information from other systems besides vision to appropriately detect and plan useful and functional movements. Nystagmus occurring inappropriately can often be found during the examination and may represent a vestibular or central pathology. More specific information regarding the findings of nystagmus will be discussed in Chapter 11.

VESTIBULAR OCULAR REFLEX (VOR)

VOR occurs automatically to keep our eyes on a target while our heads are in motion. This reflex moves the eyes in the opposite direction of head movement. To maintain steady gaze (also called gaze stabilization) the brain primarily uses information from the vestibular labyrinths (explained in Chapter 3) and visual cues.[44] The vestibular system responds to angular (rotational) and linear (translational) movements of the head, as well as the roll/tilt of the head.

When you look at someone while shaking your head yes or no, your eyes need to stay on the target as the head moves. As your head rotates to the left and the right while you shake your head no, the eyes need to rotate in the exact opposite direction and at the same speed as the head so that the visual target remains stable. Another example is when you walk, your head moves both horizontally and vertically, but the visual field remains stable due to the VOR that moves the eyes in the opposite direction of the head motion and at the same speed. The vestibular system gathers head movement information from the labyrinths (or semicircular canals detecting rotational head movements) and the otolith organs (utricle detecting linear movements on a horizontal plane and saccule detecting linear movements on a vertical plane). The vestibular system is responsible in part for a person's static balance and stability during dynamic movements. The vestibular system will be explained further in Chapter 3.

VISUAL REFLEXES

THE PUPILLARY LIGHT REFLEX

Examiners use the acronym PERRLA when checking for a pupillary response:

P: Pupils
E: Equal
R: Round
R: Reactive
L: (Reactive to) Light
A: Accommodation

There are both sympathetic and parasympathetic neurally controlled pupillary responses. The short explanation of each is as follows:

Parasympathetic sequence

1. Light shines into the eye
2. Ciliary muscle contracts
3. Ciliary zonules relax
4. Lens bulges and focuses light on the retina
5. Pupils constrict to prevent diverging light rays from entering the eye

Sympathetic

1. Ciliary muscle relaxes
2. Zonules tighten
3. Lens flattens
4. Pupil dilates allowing more light into the eye

Looking at Figure 2.15 you can follow the more detailed explanations of the pupil light reflex.

DIRECT AND INDIRECT LIGHT REFLEXES

There are two visual light reflexes: direct and consensual light reflexes, also called the pupillary reflexes. Imagine you shine a light in the left eye only. This will cause a "direct" light reflex in the left eye, while the right eye will have a consensual light reflex.

Direct Light Reflex

Light shines directly into one eye onto the nasal retina. For our example, we will imagine this is the left eye. Information travels along the optic nerve, decussates at the optic chiasm and synapses with the contralateral pretectal nucleus, and then to each (left and right) Edinger-Westphal nucleus (EWN). The information that flows to the left EWN next travels to the ciliary ganglion and activates the sphincter pupillae and constricts the iris.

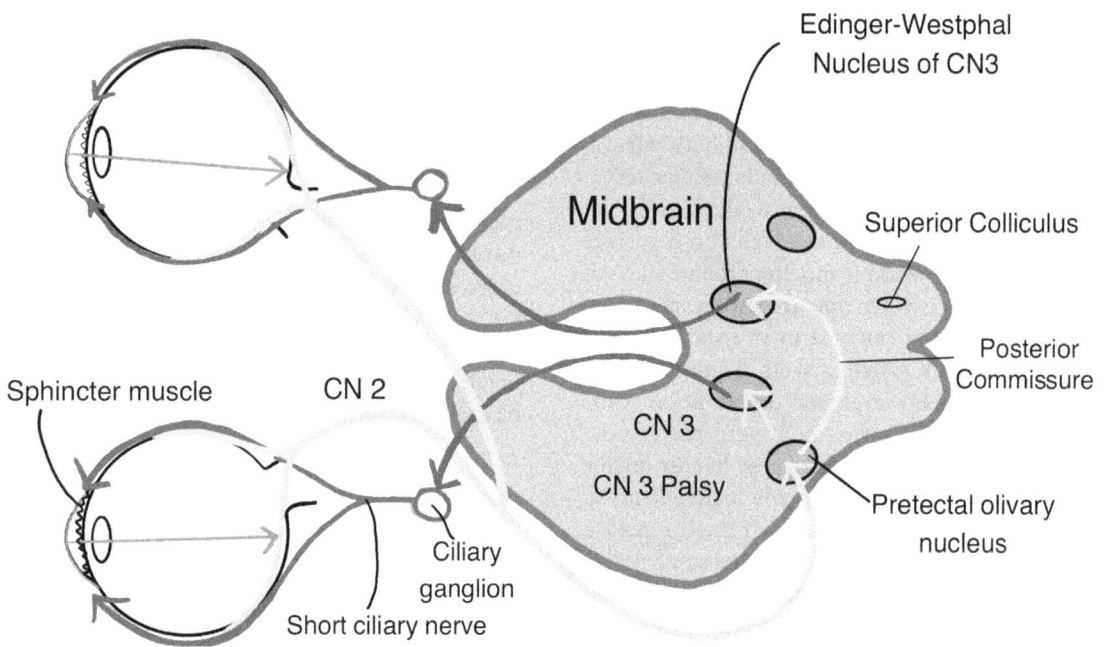

Figure 2.15 Pupillary Light Reflex

Consensual Light Reflex

As described in the direct light reflex until it reaches the contralateral EWN. Information that is sent to the right EWN, travels to the right ciliary ganglion and constricts the right pupil.

ACCOMMODATION REFLEX

This reflex responds to a change of fixation on objects that are at different distances from the eyes. It coordinates vergence, accommodation, and pupil size to allow for clear focus once fixation changes. Blur-related visual information from the eyes travels the optic pathway to the primary visual cortex. Next it is sent along the superior longitudinal fasciculus to the frontal eye fields located in the frontal cortex. Next, corticonuclear fibers of the pyramidal tract travel to the oculomotor nucleus (bilaterally) to activate CN III (oculomotor nerve) to activate the medial rectus, ciliary muscle, and sphincter pupillae.

IMPAIRMENTS WITH THE SYSTEM

EYE DISORDER CLASSIFICATIONS

Eye disorders are classified by the location of the disorder, and there are four main types:

1. *Anterior segment*: Includes everything anterior to the lens.
2. *Lenticular*: These are disorders of the lens.
3. *Posterior segment*: Includes everything posterior to the lens up to the optic nerve.
4. *Visual pathway*: Includes the visual pathway from the optic nerve to the occipital cortex.

Examples of eye disorders for each category are listed in Table 2.16.

VISUAL PATHWAY DAMAGE

The effect of visual pathway damage depends on where the damage occurs along the pathway. Based on an oculomotor examination, one may be able to speculate where the damage occurred before getting imaging results. Before getting too deep into describing the effects of damage, let us first discuss how we reference the visual fields.

First, we will discuss hemifields. A *hemifield* is "half of the eye." If you drew a line straight down the middle of the eye, you would divide the eye into a left hemifield and a right hemifield as seen in Figure 2.16. Note, we will always use the patient's perspective when describing position. So, the patient's left hemifield is on the patient's left side, not the viewer's left as they look at the patient.

If you were to draw a line across the middle of the eye from left to right horizontally, we can describe the eye as having a superior and inferior hemifield. If we draw both a horizontal line through the middle of the eye and a vertical line through the middle of the eye, we can divide the eye into four quadrants. They are named for their positions relative to the patient (upper right quadrant, upper left quadrant, lower right quadrant, lower left quadrant).

Now that we have a basic understanding of terminology to describe visual loss, we will return to the visual pathway and the effects of damage to different parts. If there is damage to the pathway before the optic chiasm, the patient will have vision loss in one eye thus affecting both hemifields of the same eye. Damage after the chiasm will affect both eyes, but only one hemifield. See Figure 2.17.

Where there is a loss of half of the visual field, i.e., when someone only has the perception of half of the full visual field, it is called a *hemianopia* (aka hemianopsia). When the patient is missing only the left hemifield, it is called a left hemianopia and is termed a right hemianopia when they are missing only the right hemifield. When they are missing the same hemifield from each eye, we use the term *homonymous* to describe this. If our patient were missing the left visual field of each eye, we would call this left homonymous hemianopia (Figure 2.18). When we read this description, we realize that the left hemifield of each eye (homonymous) is missing (hemianopia).

Heteronymous hemianopia affects different sides of each eye and is usually caused by a tumor to the pituitary gland, which is positioned directly below the optic chiasm. For example, you may only be able to see out of the nasal fields of each

Table 2.16 Eye Disorders

Lens Condition	Description
Cataract	An opacity occurring in the lens reducing visual acuity
Subluxation/dislocation	Resulting from trauma, or with a hereditary syndrome such as Marfan syndrome
Posterior Condition	**Description**
Optic nerve atrophy	Loss of nerve fibers in the optic nerve; may be congenital, acquired, or due to a variety of diseases
Optic neuritis	Inflammation of the optic nerve head
Papilledema	Edema of the optic disc due to elevated intracranial pressure
Central retinal vein occlusion	Loss of vision secondary to emboli (cardiac)
Diabetic neuropathy	Microaneurysms, retinal hemorrhage, and exudates due to disease of retinal vasculature secondary to diabetes
Retinopathy or prematurity	Secondary to use of O2; includes neovascularization, retinal dragging, scarring, and retinal detachment
Age-related macular degeneration	No. 1 cause of blindness in the US for those >60 years
Retinal detachment	Retina detaches from the choroid. Leads to loss of vision if not corrected.
Visual Pathway Condition	**Description**
Glaucoma	Visual field defects caused by damage to retinal nerve fiber bundles at the optic nerve head; deficits are paracentral, arcuate scotomas, or nasal steps
Opacities of ocular media	General depression of sensitivity due to corneal opacities, cataracts, or vitreous opacities
Optic nerve disease	Caused by monocular visual field defects, including papilledema, optic neuritis, compressive optic neuropathy, and drusen.
Optic chiasm disease	Bitemporal hemianopic defect commonly caused by a pituitary gland tumor
Retrochiasmal visual pathway disease	Hemianopic field defects

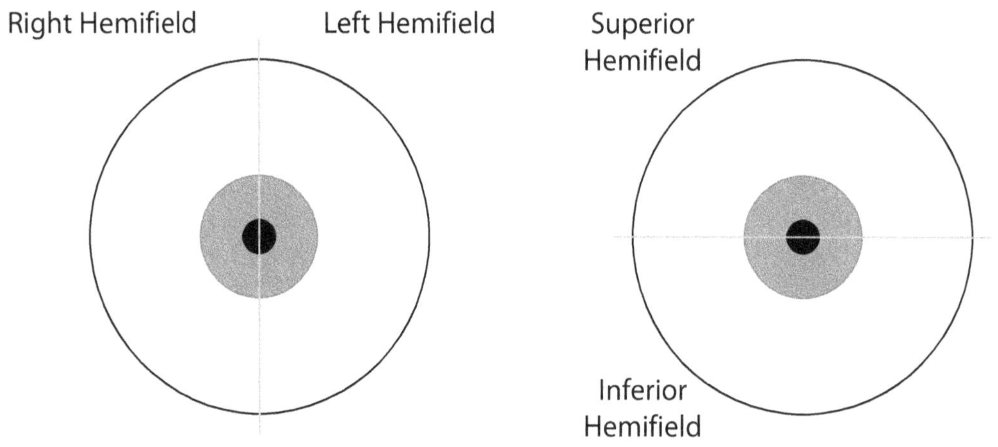

Figure 2.16 Hemifields

eye (bitemporal hemianopia) or the temporal fields of each eye (binasal hemianopia). For bitemporal hemianopia (Figure 2.19), the damage is to medial decussating nasal fibers coming from the retina crossing in the optic chiasm.[45] Binasal hemianopia is rare as a neurologic condition and is caused by optic chiasm deficits (damage to the lateral fibers of the optic nerve) (Figure 2.20). It is more likely caused by glaucoma.

When a person perceives only three of the four visual quadrants, it is called a *quadrantanopia* (Figure 2.21).

SCOTOMAS

Scotomas are blind spots in the visual field, and there are three types:

1. Scintillating scotoma
2. Paracentral scotoma
3. Central scotoma

Symptoms of a *scintillating scotoma* include a recurring sensation of luminous or arc-shaped appearance in front of the eyes. This type of scotoma does not appear as a dark spot.

Paracentral scotoma is not directly in the line of sight but is a partial or total loss of vision within 10 degrees of fixation. When accompanied by a peripheral vision loss it can lead to tunnel vision.

Central scotoma is directly in the line of sight. A person with central scotoma may have improved vision in dimly lit places, as the pupils dilate to allow in more light.

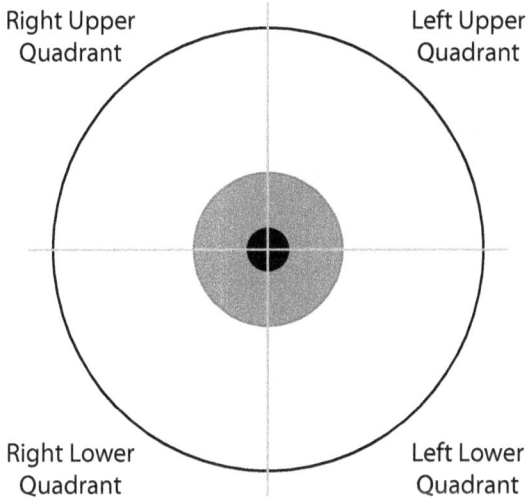

Figure 2.17 Visual Quadrants

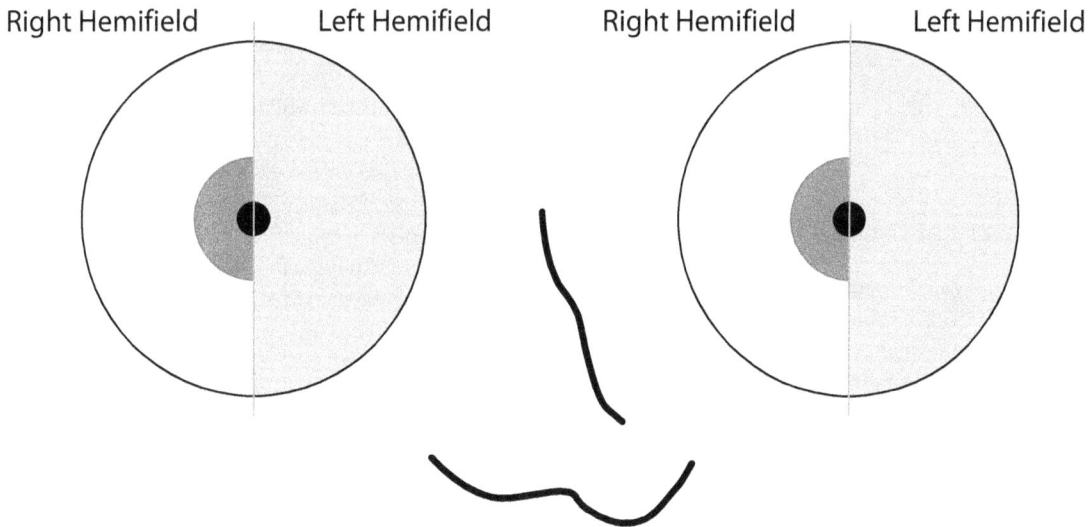

Figure 2.18 Homonymous Hemianopia

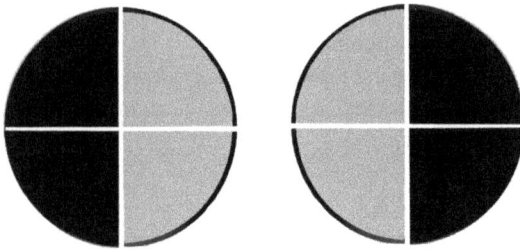

Figure 2.19 Bitemporal Hemianopia

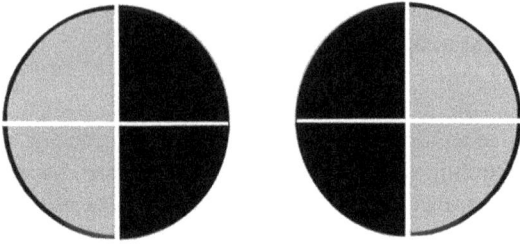

Figure 2.20 Binasal Hemianopia

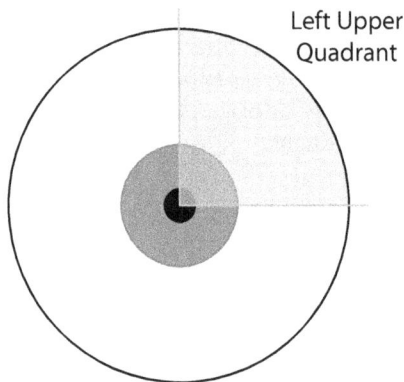

FIGURE 2.21 Left Upper Quadrantanopia

Scotomas can be caused by a combination of factors including medications, sclerotherapy, diabetic retinopathy, glaucoma, and optic neuropathy. Symptoms of scotoma include:

- Difficulty seeing details and colors
- Temporary or permanent vision loss
- A single or multiple blind spots
- Floaters or "dots"

Scotomas are diagnosed by visual field testing and dilated eye examinations. Scotomas in the center of vision cannot be corrected with surgery, glasses, or contact lenses. Treatments include controlling glare, increasing the font size for reading, and the use of magnifiers (Figure 2.22).

Visual Field Cuts

A visual field cut is when part or all of a visual field is not perceived due to damage to the visual pathway. Depending on the location of the damage, different visual field cut patterns emerge. Table 2.17 describes the visual field cut and the corresponding location of visual pathway damage.

Visual Field Defects versus Unilateral Spatial Inattention

As unilateral visual inattention often occurs with a visual field loss, clinicians often confuse the two. Recall that a visual field defect is the absence of vision in part or all of the visual field. Unilateral spatial inattention, however, is not due to a loss of the visual field but the inattention of the brain to part of the visual field. That is to say, the visual field is intact, but the person acts as if they are unaware of it. Visual inattention is more common following right hemisphere strokes affecting about 80% of people with these strokes. It usually resolves within 10 days, however, for 10% of patients, it may continue for weeks or even months.[46] For some, it can become a permanent condition. Interventions exist to treat the deficits caused by hemianopia but not the actual physical damage creating the hemianopia. Visual therapy can be employed thus training patients to visually scan. Prisms are also used by optometrists and therapists to rehabilitate these patients.

Those with visual inattention (also called "neglect") behave as if they are no longer aware of events or objects on one side. For example, they may only eat food on one side of their plates, only wash one side of their body, and shave only one side of their face. They may not use the arm or leg on the affected side as if they are unaware of it. They do not orient or notice people or objects on their affected side.

Some tests screen the visual field, such as the Line Bisection Test, Letter Cancellation, Bells Test, and Star Cancellation Test. These tests are

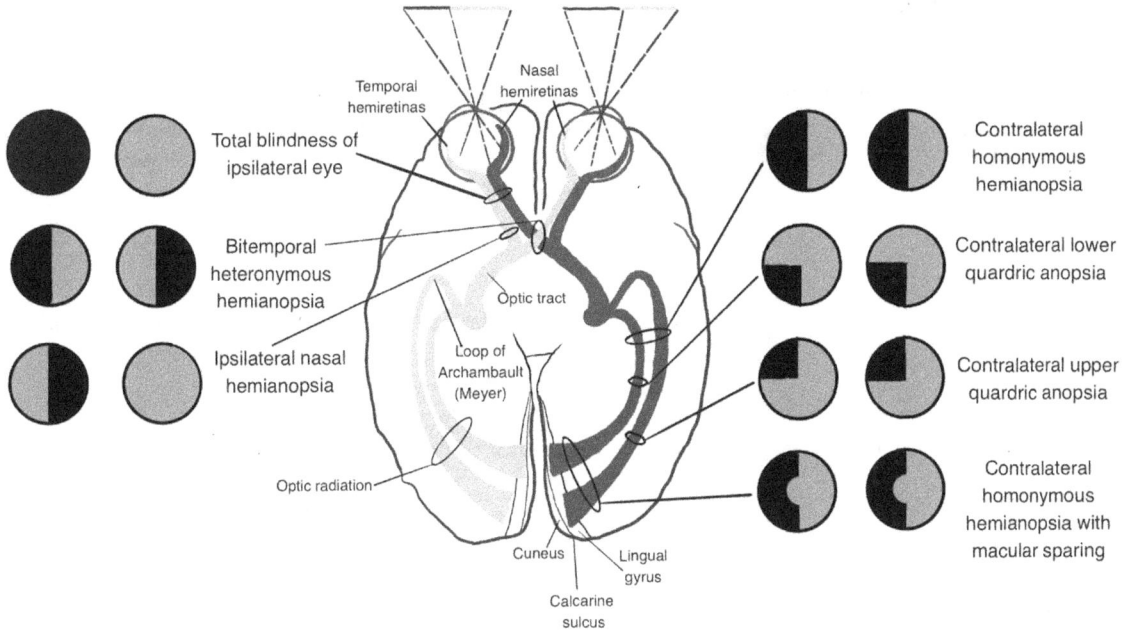

Figure 2.22 Visual Pathway Damage

not specific to inattention, however, but may also indicate a visual field loss. Instructions on how to recognize unilateral inattention will be detailed in Chapter 11.

DIPLOPIA

Diplopia is a common condition, and approximately 50,000 people each year go to the emergency department of a hospital because of it.[47] Diplopia, also known as double vision, is a condition in which an object is seen as a double image.[29] According to Jain, images can present side by side, one on top of the other, or tilted.[29] Diplopia can be monocular (in one eye only), but more typically is binocular. Binocular diplopia resolves by closing one eye, whereas when the diplopia persists after closing one eye it is termed monocular diplopia.

In the pediatric patient, signs of diplopia include squinting, covering one eye with their hand, or abnormal head postures while viewing something.[48] Binocular diplopia occurs when the lines of sight of each eye are not pointing with needed accuracy at the same object.[5] This misalignment is rarely due to a weakness of an extraocular muscle.

Vertical diplopia can be caused by skew deviations resulting from oculomotor nerve palsy, superior oblique palsy, restrictive ophthalmopathy, and myasthenia gravis. It is often seen following a stroke or head injury.

Causes of diplopia may include head trauma, stroke, alcohol intoxication, migraines, and astigmatism. Other causes may include diseases such as myasthenia gravis, Graves' disease, multiple sclerosis, and vestibular neuritis.

Monocular diplopia is associated with conditions of dry eyes, corneal scarring, cataract, retinal membranes, or non-organic causes.[29] According to Root, "There aren't really any mechanisms of monocular doubling that occur at the retina or further back in the neuro pathway." As diplopia is undesirable and intolerable, the body compensates to eliminate it by either adapting to the misalignment (until age 6) by tilting or turning the head, or by trying to restore alignment using voluntary muscular effort. Treatments of diplopia vary depending on the cause and include vision therapy, partially occluding one eye, the use of prisms, surgery, or special contact lenses.

Table 2.17 Visual Field Cuts

Visual Field Cut Description	Visual Representation	Visual Pathway Damage Location	Causes
Total blindness of one eye called an anopsia		Complete lesion in the optic nerve anterior to the optic chiasm ipsilateral to vision loss	• Papilledema secondary to increased CSF pressure • Blockage of central artery of the retina • Optic neuritis secondary to multiple sclerosis
Ipsilateral nasal hemianopia		Monocular and ipsilateral vision loss secondary to a lesion of the nerves carrying nasal field information when it occurs anterior to the optic chiasm	• Aneurysms of the internal carotid artery
Bitemporal heteronymous hemianopia		A lesion in the optic chiasm (seen with tumors to the pituitary)	• Pituitary adenoma • Aneurysm at the junction of the anterior cerebral artery and anterior communicating artery
Contralateral homonymous hemianopia		Lesions to optic tracts	• Occlusion of anterior choroidal artery • Occlusion of thalamogeniculate artery
Contralateral homonymous lower quadrantanopia		Lesions to the non-Meyer's loop of the optic radiation	• Typically, by lesions as the pathway passes through the parietal lobe
Contralateral homonymous upper quadrantanopia		Lesions to the Meyer's loop of the optic radiation	• Infarct to the inferior division of the inferior cerebral artery
Contralateral homonymous hemianopia with macular sparring		Lesions to the primary visual cortex	• Lesions to the primary visual cortex

EYE DISEASES ASSOCIATED WITH LOW VISION

The term *low vision* refers to vision loss that cannot be corrected by medical or surgical treatments, or conventional eyeglasses.[49] Persons with low vision need to learn to compensate for their condition. Vision rehabilitation teaches these patients new strategies to navigate their environments.[49] In addition, there are is an entire family of optical devices that can be prescribed by the optometrist to help patients with low vision connect with the visual world.

According to Whittaker et al., common conditions that are associated with low vision include:[50]

• Age-related macular degeneration (AMD)
• Cataract
• Diabetic retinopathy
• Glaucoma

Age-Related Macular Degeneration (AMD)

AMD is an eye disease that is caused by damage to the macula with age and results in distorted central vision. AMD usually occurs in patients over 55 years of age with the prevalence increasing with age. Thirty percent of people 75 years of age and older have AMD. Risk factors for AMD include age, smoking, genetics, gender (female), race (white people are at higher risk), high intake of fats, high cholesterol, hypertension, cardiovascular disease, ultraviolet light exposure, obesity, and cataract surgery. Symptoms of AMD are listed in Table 2.18. It is the leading cause of vision loss for older adults, and there are two types: wet AMD and dry AMD.[51]

AMD TREATMENTS

In early AMD there are no current treatments. For intermediate AMD, dietary supplements of vitamins and minerals are prescribed. There are several medical treatments for wet AMD including medications and laser treatments. While there is no medical treatment to restore vision loss, there are treatments available to assist people with AMD to use their vision. Some of these treatments include:

- Low vision rehabilitation, eccentric viewing training
- Devices to compensate for impaired visual acuity (e.g., magnifiers)
- Environmental changes, especially lighting
- Education/support groups
- Training to visually scan
- Use of Amsler grid
- Appointments every 6 months

Cataract

A cataract is an opacification of the lens that affects vision. Age-related cataracts develop in one of two ways:

1. Clumps of protein reduce the sharpness of the image reaching the retina.
2. The lens slowly changes to a yellow-brown color making the lens cloudy.

Symptoms associated with cataracts include:

- Blurry vision
- Seeing double (rare), or having a ghost image with the involved eye
- Light sensitivity (especially with oncoming headlights at night) to glare
- Difficulty seeing well at night
- Needing more light when reading
- Seeing bright colors as faded or yellow

The most common cause of cataracts is the normal physiologic changes that occur with age, as people over 60 usually start to have some clouding of their lenses. Other less common causes include genetic factors, diabetes, smoking, having had a previous eye injury or surgery, radiation treatments to the upper body, use of corticosteroids, and spending considerable time in the sun (especially without UV protective sunglasses).[52]

Cataracts can only be removed with surgery; the cloudy lens is removed, and an artificial lens is

Table 2.18 Symptoms of AMD

Early Dry AMD	No Symptoms
Intermediate dry AMD	• Some have no symptoms • Others have mild blurriness in their central vision or trouble seeing in low lighting
Late AMD (wet or dry)	• Straight lines look distorted • Distorted area near the center of your vision • Over time the blurry area gets bigger, or you see blank spots • Colors seem less bright • Trouble seeing in low lighting

implanted. Some people opt for *monovision*, where the lens of one eye is implanted to assist vision at a distance, while the other eye has an artificial lens implanted to assist near vision. Low vision rehabilitation is another treatment option that manages the impairment of contrast and light sensitivity, and visual acuity.

Diabetic Retinopathy

As the name implies, diabetic retinopathy is a complication of diabetes that threatens vision. It affects blood vessels in the light-sensitive layers of the retina that in later stages may cause dark floating spots or streaks.[53] According to Root, one in five newly diagnosed diabetics will show signs of retinopathy on examination. There are four stages:[5]

1. *Mild non-proliferative retinopathy*: Microaneurysms occur in retinal blood vessels.
2. *Moderate non-proliferative retinopathy*: Some retinal blood vessels become blocked.
3. *Severe non-proliferative retinopathy*: Many more retinal blood vessels become blocked causing the growth of new blood vessels.
4. *Proliferative retinopathy*: New fragile and abnormal blood vessels grow along the retina and the surface of the vitreous fluid inside the eye. When they leak and bleed into the vitreous fluid, they cause vision loss and blindness. Floaters and retinal tears follow. Fluid leaking into the center of the macula causes macular swelling and blurred vision.

TREATMENTS FOR DIABETIC RETINOPATHY

Treatments focus on controlling lighting and glare as well as compensating for acuity loss. Medical treatments include laser photocoagulation to shrink blood vessels, vitrectomy, and anti-VEGF drugs.

Glaucoma

Glaucoma is a group of eye diseases that cause an elevation of pressure in the eye and can cause vision loss and blindness by damaging the optic nerve. It disrupts the equilibrium between the production

Table 2.19 Fall Risk with Glaucoma

Time Frame	Probability
12 months	45% chance of falling 12% chance of an injury due to falling
24 months	61% chance of falling 40% chance of injury due to falling

and drainage of aqueous fluid, increasing intraocular pressure (IOP). As IOP increases, nerve damage in the eye occurs. Symptoms can start slowly and may not initially be noticed but are found with a comprehensive dilated eye examination. There is a slow loss of vision over time starting with the peripheral vision, especially nasally. According to Ramulu et al., people who have glaucoma are at a higher fall risk than the general population.[54] This fall risk is likely due to decreased visual function and reduced contrast sensitivity (Table 2.19).

GLAUCOMA TREATMENTS

There is no cure for glaucoma, however, early treatment can often stop damage and protect vision. Risk factors for African Americans and Hispanics include being older than 40 years of age and being older than 60 years for other ethnic groups. Treatments include:[55]

- *Medications*: Pills, ointments, and eye drops that either help drain fluid more effectively or suppress the production of aqueous fluid
- *Laser trabeculoplasty*: Stretches drainage holes; effectiveness diminishes over time
- *Surgery*: Make new openings for fluid drainage (70–80% effective)
- *Low vision rehab*: Teach visual scanning, lenses, magnification, modification of lighting and contrast

OTHER CONDITIONS IMPAIRING VISION

Retinal Detachment

Retinal detachment happens when the retina is pulled away from its normal position at the back of the eye (a separation between the sensory retina and the underlying retinal pigment epithelium [RPE] and choroid plexus).[5] It presents with several symptoms, including:

- Sudden appearance of floaters
- Flashes of light
- Gradually reduced peripheral vision
- Tunnel vision
- Blurred vision
- Curtain-like shadow over the visual field

Causes of retinal detachment include eye trauma, cataract surgery, family history, advanced diabetes, posterior vitreous detachment, aging, extreme near-sightedness, and other eye disorders/diseases.

TREATMENTS FOR RETINAL DETACHMENT

There are currently two treatments for retinal detachment. These include sealing the tear or break in the retina using laser surgery (photocoagulation) or a freezing probe (cryopexy). The other option is surgery.

Progressive Supranuclear Palsy (PSP)

PSP is a rare neurologic disorder affecting body movements, walking, balance, speech, swallowing, mood, behavior, cognition, vision, and eye movements. It is considered an "atypical Parkinsonism" and a Parkinson-plus disorder. It is a frontotemporal disorder of unknown etiology. It affects those over 50 years of age, and presents with gait difficulties and falls, with ophthalmoplegia being the hallmark of progression.[56] Eye movement abnormalities begin at a median of 4 years after diagnosis.[56] Early on, slowed vertical saccades may be the only sign, with downgaze affected before upgaze. Other oculomotor signs may include square wave jerks during fixation, loss of optokinetic nystagmus (especially vertically), loss of convergence, blepharospasm, eyelid-opening apraxia, and VOR may be lost later in the disease progression.[56] Toward the end of the disease the eyes may be immobile. Vertical gaze impairments lead to difficulty reading, spilling food while eating, and falling while walking.[57] Referral to optometry to assess the need for vision therapy and prisms may be useful. Referral to physical and occupational therapy

should be considered to address functional mobility and ADLs.

VISUAL EFFICIENCY DISORDERS

Visual efficiency disorders include accommodative disorders, binocular vision disorders, amblyopia, and other mobility disorders.

Accommodative Disorders

Remember, accommodation is when the eye is "focusing" on an object. There are several accommodative disorders, including:

- *Accommodative excess*: The amplitude of accommodation is normal, but the ciliary muscles tend to intermittently spasm, e.g., after reading, a person has blurred vision when looking at a distance.
- *Accommodative infacility*: The amplitude of accommodation is normal, but the speed of the response is reduced, e.g., when looking from near to far or far to near.
- *Accommodative insufficiency*: The amount of accommodation available is less than expected for a person's age.
- *Presbyopia*: Near visual acuity is decreased because of an age-related decline in accommodative ability. (This is why you need reading glasses as you get older!)

Refraction

The *refractive power of the eye* is its ability to change the angle of the light rays as they pass through the eye to arrive on the retina to form a focused image. This refraction is accomplished with the cornea (which provides the majority of the refraction) and the lens. The refractive power of the cornea is fixed, but the lens can change shape and thereby increase or decrease its refractive power. If there are no refractive errors, this is termed *emmetropia*. Light rays entering the eye are focused directly on the retina. A person with emmetropia can see both near and far without issue. *Ametropia*, on the other hand, is an umbrella term that indicates there is a refractive error. The term ametropia includes myopia, hyperopia, astigmatism, and presbyopia.

Myopia, also called nearsightedness, is when light rays enter the eye and focus in front of (short of) the retina. Vision is blurred at a distance but clear for near vision. People with myopia often hold things close to their eyes. The eyeball has a longer length than those with hyperopia (Figure 2.23).

Hyperopia, also called farsightedness or hypermetropia, is when the eyeball is too short from front to back, and light rays entering the eye are focused behind the retina. When muscle action cannot adjust for the degree of hyperopia, blurred vision results. A low degree of hyperopia is considered normal, however, high degrees of hyperopia may lead to amblyopia and loss of vision (Figure 2.24).

Astigmatism is when the optics of the eye is not spherically shaped but more like a cylinder. This causes light rays entering the eye to focus on two different points causing blurred and distorted vision both near and far. If not corrected, this may lead to amblyopia. Small degrees of astigmatism

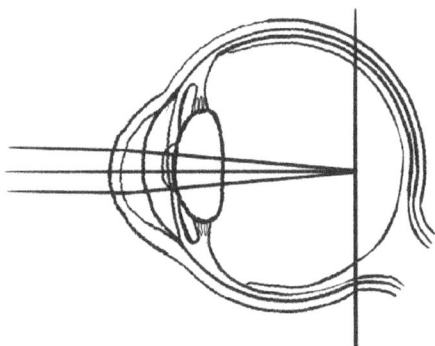

Figure 2.23 Myopia

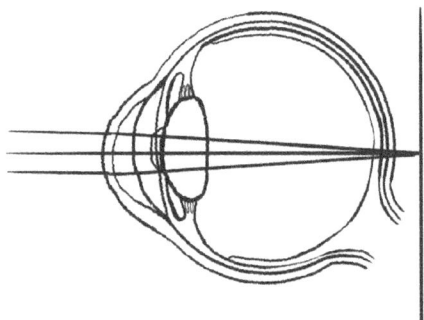

Figure 2.24 Hyperopia

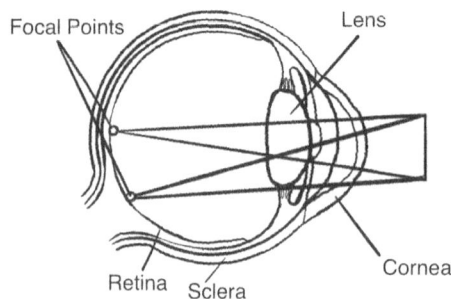

Figure 2.25 Astigmatism

are common and are generally overcome without symptoms (Figure 2.25).

Presbyopia is a normal age-related change that usually begins around age 40. The lens begins to lose flexibility and becomes more difficult to change shape when attempting to accommodate for near vision. Even those with emmetropia will eventually develop presbyopia. If the eyes have different needs or astigmatism, then prescription reading glasses may be required.

According to Rutner et al., there is a higher percentage of refractive disorders in children with special needs than in the general population. The authors report the following:[58]

- 50–80% in mental retardation
- 43–65% in Down syndrome
- 50–70% in cerebral palsy

VISION CHANGES WITH ACQUIRED BRAIN INJURIES

Visual abilities often change after a cerebrovascular accident (CVA) or a traumatic brain injury (TBI), particularly for hyperopia and presbyopia.[59] Following a TBI, patients often complain of difficulty judging the space between objects, and themselves and objects. They have problems moving their eyes to the desired location. According to Rutner et al., 90% of TBI patients experience one or more oculomotor dysfunctions, and 40% have visual dysfunction that persists more than 3 months after injury.[58]

For children who have suffered a concussion, Swanson et al. found that the majority are affected with the following visual systems affected: VOR, convergence, accommodation, saccades, and smooth pursuit. Additionally, up to 52% report light sensitivity, up to 39% report blurred vision, and up to 70% have signs of accommodative, binocular vision, or saccadic abnormalities.[60] Visual defects often seen after an acquired brain injury (ABI) include:

- Nerve palsy
- Post-trauma vision syndrome
- Visual field defects
- Unilateral spatial inattention
- Altered egocentric location (AEL)/visual midline shift syndrome (VMSS)

CRANIAL NERVE DAMAGE

CN III Oculomotor Nerve Palsy

A complete oculomotor nucleus lesion will cause an ipsilateral CN III palsy, weakness of the contralateral superior rectus, and bilateral ptosis. Lesions involving the superior rectus subnucleus impair elevation of both eyes.[61]

Causes of CN III palsy include, but are not limited to, infarction, hemorrhage, demyelination, tumors, trauma, infection, hydrocephalus, Sjögren syndrome, herpes zoster, ophthalmoplegic migraine, and nerve infarction due to diabetes.[61]

WEBER SYNDROME

Weber syndrome causes contralateral oculomotor hemiplegia,[61] with anterior damage to CN III (oculomotor nerve) and parasympathetic ipsilateral and the crux cerebri (carrying descending motor fibers to the contralateral body). This affects the actions of the:

- *Superior rectus* (eye elevation and medial rotation)
- *Inferior oblique* (lateral rotation and eye elevation)
- *Inferior rectus* (depression of the eye and medial rotation)
- *Medial rectus* (medial rotation)

Therefore, you will see the eye move down and out. Since the parasympathetic nerves normally constrict the pupil, the eye will now be fixed and dilated.

CN IV Trochlear Nerve Palsy

The trochlear nerve originates in the midbrain at the level of the inferior colliculus on the sides of the periaqueductal gray matter medial to the medial lemniscus and exits the midbrain and crosses to the contralateral eye. It has the longest course in the cranial cavity.

It innervates the superior oblique muscle, responsible for *intorsion* (internal rotation), depression of the eyeball, and lateral rotation.

CN IV palsy accounts for most cases of acquired vertical strabismus.[61] The patient presents with hypertropia of the affected eye that will increase during adduction and depression. This hypertropia is maximized as the head is tilted toward the side of the lesion and minimized on the contralateral side.[61] Often they have a head tilt away from the side of the lesion, as leaning toward the affected side will increase the diplopia. Other signs include hypometric downward saccades.

Causes of CN IV palsy include aneurysm of the posterior cerebral artery, infarction, demyelination, hemorrhage, trauma, tumors, hydrocephalus, meningitis, herpes zoster, Sjögren syndrome, dental anesthesia, aneurysm of internal carotid artery, infection of cavernous sinus, cavernous sinus thrombosis, meningitis, and trauma to the orbital cavity compressing the trochlear nerve, and microvascular ischemia associated with diabetes.

CN VI Abducens Nerve Palsy

CN VI originates in the pons. Facial nerve fibers move behind CN VI creating a facial colliculus (depression of the fourth ventricle). CN VI is located at the level of the facial colliculus and moves downward and laterally, and out at the pontomedullary junction medial to CN VIII and CN VII. The route then runs anterior to the anterior inferior cerebellar artery (AICA).

After exiting the pontomedullary junction, it moves up the clivus and over the petrous temporal bone, and into the Dorello's canal, after exiting into the cavernous sinus (between the meningeal layer and periosteal layer of the dura mater). It exits the cavity and enters the superior orbital fissure into the orbital cavity, moves through the annulus of Zinn, then supplying the lateral rectus muscle.

CN VI controls lateral rotation (abduction).

CN VI nerve palsy is the most common cranial neuropathy affecting eye movements.[61] The patient appears with abduction that is restricted or slowed, an esotropic adducted eye, or in mild cases, an esophoria that is greatest when looking to the side of the lesion. They complain of horizontal diplopia that is worse when viewing distant objects and when looking ipsilaterally.[61]

CN VI nerve palsy is caused by Duane syndrome, inflammation, tumors, infarction, abscess in pons, multiple sclerosis demyelinating nerve affecting nucleus, vasculitic issue of AICA compressing CN VI, high intracranial pressure, aneurysm or fistula of internal carotid artery, trauma to orbit, Sjögren syndrome, meningitis, and ophthalmoplegic migraine.

In children up to age 3, a head turn to the involved side is the most prominent finding, without complaints of diplopia. Other causes in children and adolescence include tumors, trauma, or in association with a virus or vaccination.[61]

MYASTHENIA GRAVIS

Myasthenia gravis is characterized by fatigable weakness and is a disorder of the postsynaptic neuromuscular junction that commonly affects eye and lid movements. Several forms have been identified, including the classic form associated with antibodies that interfere with the nicotinic acetylcholine receptors, as well as variants to antibodies directed against other neuromuscular junction components, congenital, neonatal, and juvenile forms.[61]

Classic Myasthenia Gravis

The initial presentation in about two-thirds of patients includes ptosis and diplopia. Of those who only present with oculomotor symptoms, within 2 years up to 80% develop generalized weakness.[61] Ocular manifestations of myasthenia gravis include the aforementioned ptosis and diplopia, the inability to sustain prolonged eyelid closure, hypometric large saccades, hypermetric small saccades, quivering motions during saccades, eyelid twitch, and gaze-evoked centripetal drift or nystagmus.[61]

POST-TRAUMA VISION SYNDROME (PTVS)

PTVS is a neuroprocessing disorder that is the result of head trauma that interrupts the visual processing system and can result from a degenerative process or acquired brain injury. It is sometimes referred to as ambient visual disorder. [62]

Signs and symptoms of PTVS may include convergence insufficiency, headaches, diplopia, blurred near-vision, light sensitivity, visual field loss, exotropia, exophoria, accommodative dysfunction, difficulties in concentrating and attention, difficulty reading, poor spatial judgment or depth perception, visual–spatial distortion, and abnormal egocentric location.[8,63] According to the Neuro-Optometric Rehabilitation Association, common characteristics include increased myopia, low blink rate, spatial disorientation, poor fixation ability, overfocalization, difficulty releasing fixation (focal binding), and unstable ambient vision.[63] Suter et al. point out that those with vision problems following a traumatic brain injury will demonstrate "visual deficits in terms of coordination, balance, veering during mobility, ability to concentrate for near-point tasks, inability to tolerate visually crowded places, and difficulty reading that may or may not be related to blur."[8]

Virtually all brain-injured patients have some dysfunction of the ability to simultaneously process central (foveal) and peripheral (ambient) vision. These patients have a slower visual processing speed, become anxious in crowds, get lost easily, have difficulty shopping, become overwhelmed by "too much stuff," complain of dizziness, and have poor lane control while driving.

While assessing a patient with head trauma, Padula points out that it is important to observe posture while sitting, standing, and ambulating, and to note any changes in these postures or movements if lenses and/or prisms are introduced.[64] If the patient already has prescription spectacles, the patient should be examined while wearing them, as visual acuity may change after a head injury. Therapists using prisms should only do so under the direction of the optometrist.

Treatment includes neuro-optometric rehabilitation that includes prisms and partial selective occlusion in conjunction with physical and occupational therapy.

ALTERED EGOCENTRIC LOCATION AND VISUAL MIDLINE SHIFT SYNDROME

For those patients who have had a stroke or traumatic brain injury, the individual's sense of "straight ahead" may be altered. This condition has been described by many terms, including disturbed egocentric space representation, perception of straight-ahead orientation, egocentric spatial frame of reference, perceived midline, body midline perception, and visual subjective body midline. Ciuffreda and Ludlam prefer the term abnormal egocentric localization (AEL), whereas Padula uses the term visual midline shift syndrome (VMSS).[65]

Spatial sense is "the relationship of objects in the world to the individual, and the relationship of the individual to the objects in the world," and includes the components of orientation (knowing where an individual is located with respect to objects in the environment) and localization (information regarding where the object is located with respect to the individual).[65] Ciuffreda and Ludlam explain that localization has two aspects: oculocentric and egocentric. Oculocentric localization is a foveally based location of objects and is monocularly based, whereas egocentric localization is the location of objects with reference to the center of the trunk along the midline and is a binocularly based system.[65]

According to Padula et al.,[64] the patient with VMSS (or AEL) has an altered perception of the midline of their body. The patient's perception of midline is shifted (left, right, up, or down) from its actual position along the coronal plane and may be caused by neurological dysfunctions, including cerebrovascular accidents, traumatic brain injuries, multiple sclerosis, and cerebral palsy. Given a

visual target, a person with VMSS may interpret their midpoint (i.e., a point directly in front of their face) as being deviated about an inch in the direction of the perceived shift, with most cases having a lateral deviation. Ciuffreda explains that AEL is not actually a shift along the coronal plane, but instead represents a perception of the patient's center as being rotated about the egocenter.[65] This misperception may result in poor balance and posture, spatial disorientation, lateralward bias in walking, dizziness, or a sense of being out of sync with the environment.[65] The perceived midline rotation or shift usually is away from the neurologically impaired side.[66] According to Harris, it is possible to see a combination of these factors, with a person having a shift of their egocentric locus, while not having an angular rotation in their perception of straight ahead and vice versa.[67] Whatever the cause, the patient's sense of straight ahead is altered and may be addressed by the treatment team.

AEL or VMSS is treated primarily by a neuro-optometrist with yoked prisms, but treatment may begin in acute care or rehab by a physical or occupational therapist under the direction of a physician or neuro-optometrist. Testing of AEL/VMSS is covered in Chapter 11.

NYSTAGMUS

The word *nystagmus* is used to describe one nystagmus or many. It acts as the singular and plural form of the word. It is important to remember that nystagmus may be normal (physiological) and necessary at times. It is when they occur spontaneously, inappropriately at the wrong time, or to excess that they become an impairment (pathological). When nystagmus occur in a way that does not help us position our eyes to assist in clear vision, the nystagmus are pathological.

There are many different types of nystagmus. We will discuss observations of pathologic nystagmus you may see during the oculomotor exam. You may notice nystagmus while the patient is at rest (not performing any instructed eye motion) and are spontaneous in nature. Or, you may notice nystagmus with pursuits, gazes, or post-head shake. Later, we will discuss testing optokinetic nystagmus, as it is not part of the minimal test battery listed at the beginning of this chapter. Nystagmus actions are used to assist in the diagnosis of vestibular and central conditions.

Types of Nystagmus

There are different types of nystagmus that may be observed during your oculomotor examination. Rupinder et al. listed eight different types of physiologic nystagmus and eighteen different types of pathological nystagmus, not counting the many subtypes.[68] Some common nystagmus types you may see are discussed next.

Congenital nystagmus is observed during pursuit testing and usually occurs as the eye passes the primary gaze position during the excursion. The eye "jiggles" horizontally and then continues pursuit. The patient may or may not complain of oscillopsia, and this nystagmus is not physiological. That is to say, it does not help us keep our eyes on a target.

Jerk nystagmus is a term that describes an involuntary, reflexive movement of the eye that usually has a fast and a slow phase in opposite directions. The fast phase (which is used to name the direction of the nystagmus) is a quick resetting motion that allows the patient to quickly reposition the eye so that it may track again. The saccadic system mediates the fast phase of the nystagmus. The slow phase is a visual tracking motion run by the smooth pursuit system. Jerk nystagmus may be either physiological or pathological. This type of nystagmus is often observed due to vestibular imbalance.

Gaze-evoked nystagmus, which are movements elicited by eccentric gazes, are the most common type of nystagmus. They are a type of jerk nystagmus and may be seen in healthy individuals near ocular end-ranges (typically up to 3 beats or less), and also with pathology before end-ranges and at end-ranges (typically more than 3 beats).

Positional nystagmus occur when patients are moved into a provocative position, and may be secondary to the push/pull of endolymph or otoconia on the cupula, or be a central positional nystagmus due to cerebellar and/or brainstem dysfunction.[69]

Pendular nystagmus are rhythmic and sinusoidal, and do not have a fast phase. The nystagmus motions are of equal speed in each direction. They may move in any direction: horizontal, vertical, torsional, elliptical, and may even be dissociated (each eye moving in different directions).

Congenital nystagmus usually appear at 6 weeks to 3 months of age and are lifelong. They are conjugate and horizontal and often have a pendular waveform but may develop into a jerk type of nystagmus. Even though the eyes are constantly moving, the patient does not report oscillopsia.

Direction-changing nystagmus, as the name implies, change the direction of the fast phases depending on the direction of gaze. When observed, the patient should be referred to neurology.

Periodic alternating nystagmus (PAN) are rhythmic, horizontal jerk nystagmus movements that have a fast phase in one direction, and last for up to about 2 minutes and then pause and reverse direction for another 1–2 minutes. When observed, the patient should be referred to neurology.

Vertical (up-/downbeat) nystagmus are vertical nystagmus movements with quick phases up for upbeating nystagmus and down for downbeating nystagmus. When observed, the patient should be referred to neurology.

See-saw nystagmus are pendular-type nystagmus movements in which one eye elevates and intorts, while the contralateral eye depresses and extorts. When observed, the patient should be referred to neurology.

Torsional nystagmus describes a torsional movement of the eye(s) like a car's steering wheel turning. When observed, the patient should be referred to neurology.

During the oculomotor examination, you should note the type of nystagmus and direction of fast phases. If you have the equipment, you may be able to observe nystagmus under fixation (such as room light) versus when fixation is removed (darkness) using Frenzel goggles or infrared (IR) goggles.

This is helpful to stage pathologies such as labyrinthitis and neuritis, as well as assist in the differentiation of central versus peripheral (vestibular) pathologies.

Grading Nystagmus

When peripheral ear pathology is suspected, gaze-evoked jerk nystagmus are graded using the following scale:

- *Grade I*: Unidirectional gaze nystagmus is seen only when the eyes are directed toward the fast phase component of the nystagmus. An easy way to remember this is that Grade I is only seen in one position.
- *Grade II*: Unidirectional nystagmus is seen in the primary position of the eyes and also when gaze is directed toward the fast phases of the nystagmus. An easy way to remember this is that Grade II is seen in two eye positions.
- *Grade III*: Unidirectional gaze nystagmus is seen when gazes are directed toward the slow phase component, in primary gaze, and toward the quick phase components of the nystagmus. An easy way to remember this is that nystagmus is seen in three eye positions.

It is important to remember that these are unidirectional nystagmus and not direction changing.

Vertical Nystagmus

Vertical nystagmus is typically an indication of central pathology.

Downbeating nystagmus (DBN) may be categorized as structural versus nonstructural using an MRI to differentiate.[70] Nonstructural causes include gluten ataxia, nutritional deficiencies, and paraneoplastic syndromes.[70] DBN is also seen in intoxication and diffuse diseases (encephalitis, etc.), but its main causes include cerebellar atrophy and craniocervical abnormalities.[71] "Common etiological diagnoses include cerebellar degenerative diseases, stroke, vestibular migraine, Chiari malformation, spinocerebellar ataxia type 6, parataxia type 2, Meniere's disease, sub-vestibular neuritis, etc."[72] Other clear etiologies include acoustic neuroma, Hunt syndrome, light cupula, and vestibular paroxysmia.[72]

Upbeating nystagmus (fixation-induced) is the result of damage to the cerebellum, pons, or caudal medulla.[71] The main etiologies of these brainstem lesions are ischemia, tumors, Wernicke encephalopathy, cerebellar degeneration, and intoxication.

Important Points Regarding Nystagmus

- Medications such as sedatives, tranquilizers, anticonvulsants, and alcohol may cause gaze-evoked nystagmus.
- Peripheral dysfunction/infection or central dysfunction/lesion may cause spontaneous nystagmus (aka resting nystagmus) or gaze-evoked nystagmus.
- Direction-changing nystagmus (e.g., quick phases beating left with leftward gaze and right with rightward gaze) is an indication of central pathology.
- Nystagmus brought on by gaze fixation is an indication of central pathology.
- Rebound nystagmus (which occurs after bringing the eyes back to center following lateral gaze of at least 10 seconds, and with quick phases in the opposite direction of the held gaze) generally indicates cerebellar dysfunction or damage.[73]
- Signs of a peripheral vestibular loss include nystagmus that is suppressed by fixing the gaze. Nystagmus that begins or increases with gaze in one horizontal direction but decreases or stops with gaze in the opposite direction is most often an indication of peripheral pathology. While peripheral issues are more likely to be the cause of unilateral gaze nystagmus, there are central issues that may cause this, such as brainstem or cerebellar lesions.

Pursuit

Testing pursuit has its challenges. The patient must have central vision to pursue, and performance may be affected by attention, and inattentive or uncooperative subjects can perform poorly without having any significant central lesion. The ability to pursue is also affected by the velocity, acceleration, and frequency of the target. There is a lack of a standard pursuit paradigm associated with a well-defined normal data set. Because of all of these issues, and the fact that disturbances of pursuit are usually nonspecific, pursuit is of minor diagnostic utility.[74]

Disorders of smooth pursuit include:

- Advanced age
- Brainstem disorders
- Cerebellar disorders
- Cerebral cortical disturbances
- Congenital nystagmus
- Drug ingestion
- Inattention
- Visual disorders

REFERENCES

1. DeRemer S. Function of Rods and Cones. Discovery Eye Foundation; 2014. Accessed 8/28/2022. https://discoveryeye.org/rods -and-cones-they-give-us-color-and-night -vision/.
2. Merriam-Webster. *Vision.* Merriam-Webster; 2023. https://www.merriam-webster.com/ dictionary/vision.
3. Leigh RJ, Zee DS. A survey of eye movements characteristics and teleology. *The Neurology of Eye Movements.* Oxford University Press; 2015:chap 1.
4. Scheiman M. *Understanding and Managing Vision Deficits: A Guide for Occupational Therapists.* 3rd ed. Slack Incorporated; 2011.
5. Root T. *OphthoBook.* Vol 1. CreateSpace Independent Publishing Platform; 2009.
6. Brandt T, Dieterich M, Strupp M. *Vertigo and Dizziness: Common Complaints.* 2nd ed. Springer; 2014.
7. Kaur K, Gurnani B. Contrast Sensitivity. *StatPearls.* StatPearls Publishing; Updated 2023. https://www.ncbi.nlm.nih.gov/books/ NBK580542/.
8. Suter P, Hellerstein L, Harvey L, Gutcher K. What is vision rehabilitation following brain injury? In: Suter P, Harvey L, eds. *Vision Rehabilitation—Multidisciplinary Care of the Patient Following Brain Injury.* CRC Press; 2011:1–30:chap 1.
9. Bron AJ, Tripathi RC, Triapthi BJ. *Wolff's Anatomy of the Eye and Orbit.* Taylor & Francis; 1998.
10. Snell R, Lemp M. *Clinical Anatomy of the Eye.* 2nd ed. Wiley India Exclusive; 2016.
11. Bron A, Tripathi R, Triapthi B. The eyeball and its dimensions. *Wolff's Anatomy of the Eye and Orbit.* 8th ed. Taylor & Francis; 1998.
12. Caleb L, Shumway C, Motlagh M, Wade M. *Anatomy, Head and Neck, Eye Superior Rectus Muscle.* StatPearls Publishing; 2021. https://www.ncbi.nlm.nih.gov/books/ NBK526067/.
13. Caleb L, Shumway C, Motlagh M, Wade M. *Anatomy, Head and Neck, Eye Inferior Rectus Muscle.* StatPearls Publishing; 2021. 2023. https://www.ncbi.nlm.nih.gov/books/ NBK518978/.
14. Caleb L, Shumway C, Motlagh M, Wade M. *Anatomy, Head and Neck, Eye Medial Rectus Muscles.* StatPearls Publishing; 2021. https://www.ncbi.nlm.nih.gov/books/ NBK519026/.
15. Cabrera AF, Suarez-Quintanilla J. *Anatomy, Head and Neck, Eye Lateral Rectus Muscle.* StatPearls Publishing; 2021. https://www .ncbi.nlm.nih.gov/books/NBK539721/.
16. Adbelhady A, Patel B, Aslam S, Aboud DA. *Anatomy, Head and Neck, Eye Superior Oblique Muscle.* StatPearls Publishing; 2021. https://www.ncbi.nlm.nih.gov/books/ NBK537152/.
17. Gupta N, Patel B. *Anatomy, Head and Neck, Eye Inferior Oblique Muscles.* StatPearls Publishing; 2021. https://www.ncbi.nlm.nih .gov/books/NBK545253/.
18. Merriam-Webster. *Tropia.* 2022. https:// www.merriam-webster.com/medical/tropia.
19. Clinic M. Lazy Eye (amblyopia). Accessed 9/15/2022, 2022. https://www.mayoclinic .org/diseases-conditions/lazy-eye/symp- toms-causes/syc-20352391.
20. Ciuffreda K. Personal communication via phone. Subject: Amblyopia. 01/05/2022.

21. Institute NE. Amblyopia. Updated 22/09/2022. Accessed 10/29/2022, https://www.nei.nih.gov/learn-about-eye-health/eye-conditions-and-diseases/amblyopia-lazy-eye.

22. Merriam-Webster. *Phoria*. https://www.merriam-webster.com/medical/phoria.

23. Suleiman A, Lithgow B, Anssari N, Ashiri M, Moussavi Z, Mansouri B. Correlation between ocular and vestibular abnormalities and convergence insufficiency in post-concussion syndrome. *Neuroophthalmology*. Jun 2020;44(3):157–167. doi:10.1080/01658107.2019.1653325.

24. Jang JU, Jang JY, Tai-Hyung K, Moon HW. Effectiveness of vision therapy in school children with symptomatic convergence insufficiency. *J Ophthalmic Vis Res*. Apr–Jun 2017;12(2):187–192. doi:10.4103/jovr.jovr_249_15.

25. Shahid s. *Parietal Lobe*. Ken Hub; Updated 07/20/2023. Accessed 10/07/2023. https://www.kenhub.com/en/library/anatomy/parietal-lobe.

26. Huff T, Mahabadi N, Tadi P. Neuroanatomy, Visual Cortex. *StatPearls*. StatPearls Publishing Copyright © 2022, StatPearls Publishing LLC.; 2022.

27. Sceleanu A. Arteries of visual cortex. *Oftalmologia*. 2002;54(3):87–90. Arterele cortexului vizual occipital.

28. Gandhi NJ, Katnani HA. Motor functions of the superior colliculus. *Annu Rev Neurosci*. 2011;34:205–231. doi:10.1146/annurev-neuro-061010-113728.

29. Jain S. Diplopia: diagnosis and management. *Clin Med (Lond)*. Mar 2022;22(2):104–106. doi:10.7861/clinmed.2022-0045.

30. Wong A. *Eye Movement Disorders*. 2008, Oxford University Press.

31. Lee SU, Kim HJ, Choi JY, Choi JH, Zee DS, Kim JS. Nystagmus only with fixation in the light: a rare central sign due to cerebellar malfunction. *J Neurol*. Jul 2022;269(7):3879–3890. doi:10.1007/s00415-022-11108-9.

32. Dell'Osso L, Daroff R. Eye movement characteristics and recording techniques. *Neuro-Ophthalmology*, 2006;20:237–343.

33. Rine R, Wiener-Vacher S. Evaluation and treatment of vestibular dysfunction in children. *NeuroRehabilitation*. 2013;32(3):507–518. doi:10.3233/nre-130873.

34. Ciuffreda K, Tannen B. *Eye Movement Basics for the Clinician*. Mosby; 1995.

35. Martins A, Kowler E, Palmer C. Smooth pursuit of small-amplitude sinusoidal motion. *J Opt Soc Am A*. Feb 1985;2(2):234–242. doi:10.1364/josaa.2.000234.

36. Shumway C, Motlagh M, Wade M. Anatomy, head and neck, eye inferior rectus muscle. *StatPearls*. StatPearls Publishing Copyright © 2022, StatPearls Publishing LLC.; 2022.

37. Leigh R, Zee D. Vergence eye movements. *The Neurology of Eye Movements*. 5 ed. Oxford University Press; 2015:chap 9.

38. Horwood A. Neonatal misalignments reflect vergence development but rarely become esotropia. *Br J Ophthalmol*. 2003;87:1146–1150.

39. Hainline L, Riddell PM. Binocular alignment and vergence in early infancy. *Vision Res*. 1995;35:3229–3236.

40. Thorn F, Gwiazda J, Cruz A, et al. The development of eye alignment, convergence, and sensory binocularity in young infants. *Invest Ophthalmol Vis Sci*. 1994;35:544–553.

41. Qing Y, Kapoula Z. Saccade-vergence dynamics and interaction in children and in adults. *Exp Brain Res*. 2004;156:212–223.

42. Heron G, Charman W, Schor C. Dynamics of the accommodation response to abrupt changes in target vergence as a function of age. *Vision Res*. 2001;41:507–519.

43. Heron G, Charman W, Schor C. Age changes in the interactions between the accommodation and vergence systems. *Optom Vis Sci*. 2001;78:754–762.

44. Leigh R, Zee D. *The Vestibular-Optokinetic System*. 5 ed. Oxford University Press; 2015:chap 3.

45. Ruddy J, Asuncion RMD, Cardenas AC. Hemianopsia. *StatPearls*. StatPearls Publishing; 2024. https://www.ncbi.nlm.nih.gov/books/NBK562262/.

46. Kent Clinical Neuropsychology Service. Visual inattention and visual field loss. 2020. https://www.bing.com/ck/a?!&&p=8f69f3f

f1cb1eb4e7e1df2e84637c331436295f8234
0d94f84cc4bbe9500f9bcJmltdHM9MTY
1Mzc2NjE4NiZpZ3VpZD0xZDVhY2M3ZS0
1MTczLTRkOTktOTc4Yi02NjNmMWEwYjV
iMTYmaW5zaWQ9NTE5MQ&ptn=3&fclid
=884a5baf-debc-11ec-b084-ead7f9e8eb51
&u=a1aHR0cHM6Ly93d3cuZWdodWZ0L
m5ocy51ay9FYXN5U2l0ZVdlYi9HYXRld2F5T
Gluay5hc3B4P2FsSWQ9Mjl4OTUw&ntb=1.

47. Clinic C. *Diplopia* (Double vision). Cleveland Clinic. Accessed 9/15/2022, 2022.

48. K D. Approach to the pediatric patient with acute vision change. Uptodate.com; 2022. Accessed 8/28/2022. https://www.uptodate.com/contents/approach-to-the-pediatric-patient-with-acute-vision-change#!.

49. Turbert D, Gudgel D. What is Low Vision? 2021. 9/23/2021. Accessed 9/15/2022.

50. Whittaker S, Scheiman M, Sokol-McKay D. *Low Vision Rehabilitation: A Practical Guide for Occupational Therapists*. 2 ed. Slack Incorporated; 2015.

51. Armstrong R. Overview of risk factors for age-related macular degeneration (AMD). *J Stem Cells*. 2015;10(3):171–191.

52. Boyd K. What are Cataracts? American Academy of Opthalmology. 9/6/2022.

53. Institute NE. Diabetic Retinopathy. National Institues of Health. Updated 8/07/2022. Accessed 10/30/2022, https://www.nei.nih.gov/.

54. Ramulu P, Mihailovic A, West S, Friedman D, Gitlin L. What is a fall risk factor? Factors associated with falls per time or per step in individuals with glaucoma. *J Am Geriatr Soc*. 2019;67(1):87–92. doi:10.1111/jgs.15609.

55. Institute NE. Glaucoma. NIH. Accessed 9/15/2022, 2022. read://https_www.nei.nih.gov/?url=https%3A%2F%2Fwww.nei.nih.gov%2Flearn-about-eye-health%2Feye-conditions-and-diseases%2Fglaucoma.

56. Agarwal S, Gilbert R. Progressive Supranuclear Palsy. *StatPearls*. StatPearls Publishing; Updated 2023. https://www.ncbi.nlm.nih.gov/books/NBK526098/.

57. Boeve BF. Progressive supranuclear palsy. *Parkinsonism Relat Disord*. Jan 2012;18 Suppl 1:S192–S194. doi:10.1016/s1353-8020(11)70060-8.

58. Rutner D, Kapoor N, Ciuffreda KJ, Shoshana C, Han ME, Suchoff I. Occurrence of ocular disease in traumatic brain injury in a selected sample: a retrospective analysis. *Brain Injury*. 2006;20(10):1079–1086. doi:10.1080/02699050600909904.

59. Ciuffreda KJ, Kapoor N, Rutner D, Suchoff IB, Han ME, Craig S. Occurrence of oculomotor dysfunctions in acquired brain injury: a retrospective analysis. *Optometry*. Apr 2007;78(4):155–161. doi:10.1016/j.optm.2006.11.011.

60. Swanson M, Weise K, Dreer L, et al. Academic difficulty and vision symptoms children with concussion. *Optom Vis Sci*. 2018;94(1):60–67.

61. Leigh R, Zee D. Peripheral ocular motor palsies and strabismus. *The Neurology of Eye Movements*. 5 ed. Oxford University Press; 2015:chap 10.

62. Padula WV, Capo-Aponte JE, Padula WV, Singman EL, Jenness J. The consequence of spatial visual processing dysfunction caused by traumatic brain injury (TBI). *Brain Inj*. 2017;31(5):589–600. doi:10.1080/02699052.2017.1291991.

63. International N-ORA. Post-Trauma Vision Syndrome & Visual Midline Shift Syndrome. A Rehabilitation Professional's Guide. https://noravisionrehab.org/uploads/media/NORA_VMSS_PDF_9-16-18_FINAL.pdf.

64. Padula W, Munitz R, Margrun WM. *Neuro-Visual Processing Rehabilitation: An Interdisciplinary Approach*. Optometric Extension Program Foundation, Inc.; 2012.

65. KJ C, DP L. Egocentric localization - normal and abnormal aspects. In: Suter PS, Harvey LH, eds. *Vision Rehabilitation - Multidisciplinary Care of the Patient Following Brain Injury*. CRC Press; 2011:193–211:chap 6.

66. Letheren C. *Neuro-Optometric Rehabilitation of Neuroprocessing Disorders*. Presentation at NORA Conference, Buffalo, NY, 2017.

67. Harris PA. The use of lenses to improve quality of life following brain injury. In: Sutter P, Harvey L, eds. *Vision*

Rehabilitation - Multidisciplinary Care of the Patient Following Brain Injury. CRC Press; 2011:chap 7.

68. Sekhon RK, Rocha Cabrero F, Deibel JP. Nystagmus Types. *StatPearls*. StatPearls Publishing; Updated 2023. https://www.ncbi.nlm.nih.gov/books/NBK539711/.

69. Lemos J, Strupp M. Central positional nystagmus: an update. *J Neurol*. Apr 2022;269(4):1851–1860. doi:10.1007/s00415-021-10852-8.

70. Tran TM, Lee MS, McClelland CM. Downbeat nystagmus: a clinical review of diagnosis and management. *Curr Opin Ophthalmol*. Nov 1 2021;32(6):504–514. doi:10.1097/icu.0000000000000802.

71. Pierrot-Deseilligny C, Milea D. Vertical nystagmus: clinical facts and hypotheses. *Brain*. Jun 2005;128(Pt 6):1237–1246. doi:10.1093/brain/awh532.

72. Zhang S, Lang Y, Wang W, et al. Analysis of etiology and clinical features of spontaneous downbeat nystagmus: a retrospective study. *Front Neurol*. 2024;15:1326879. doi:10.3389/fneur.2024.1326879.

73. Lin CY, Young YH. Rebound nystagmus. *Laryngoscope*. 1999;109(11):1803–1805.

74. Hain TC. Tracking Test (Smooth Pursuit). Dizziness-and-balance.com. Updated 26/10/2023. Accessed 12/02/23, 2023. https://dizziness-and-balance.com/practice/tracking_test.htm.

3

Ear Anatomy and Vestibular Anatomy

Chapter Goals

1. Describe the ear anatomy
2. Describe vestibular anatomy
3. List the vestibular laws
4. List the vestibular reflexes

EAR ANATOMY

Figure 3.1 shows a cross-section of the ear. As depicted, the ear can be divided into three sections: the Outer ear, the middle ear, and the inner ear. The ear holds organs for hearing as well as balance.

OUTER EAR

The outer ear consists of the pinna (the part of your ear you can see in a mirror) and the ear canal that ends at the tympanic membrane (eardrum). The pinna directs sound waves to the ear canal where they vibrate the tympanic membrane.

MIDDLE EAR

The middle ear has been extensively described[1, 2] and extends from the tympanic membrane (part of the *lateral wall*) to the medial wall of the inner ear (which is also the lateral wall of the inner ear). The *superior wall* (roof) is formed by a thin bone from the petrous portion of the temporal bone and separates the middle ear with the *middle cranial fossa*

that houses the temporal lobe of the brain. The middle ear is air-filled and contains three small bones that conduct vibrations from the tympanic membrane to the inner ear. These bones, called *auditory ossicles*, are named the malleus, incus, and the stapes (the smallest bone in the human body). Along the *medial wall* (which is formed by the lateral wall of the *inner ear*) there are two areas called "windows" that separate the middle and inner ear. These windows are the *oval window* and *round window*. The oval window is comprised of a connective tissue membrane, while the round window is covered by a secondary tympanic membrane (also called the *round window membrane*). The malleus is connected to the tympanic membrane (eardrum), while the stapes is connected to the oval window, with the incus acting as a bridge between these two bones.

GEEK STUFF

You can remember the difference between the oval and round windows by remembering you can hear "**Oh** my, the **O**val window carries sound."

The round window membrane is inferior to the oval window and separates the middle ear from the cochlea of the inner ear. As the oval window is depressed by the stapes, the round window moves outward toward the middle ear, allowing for movement of the endolymph in the cochlea of the inner

DOI: 10.1201/9781003524441-3

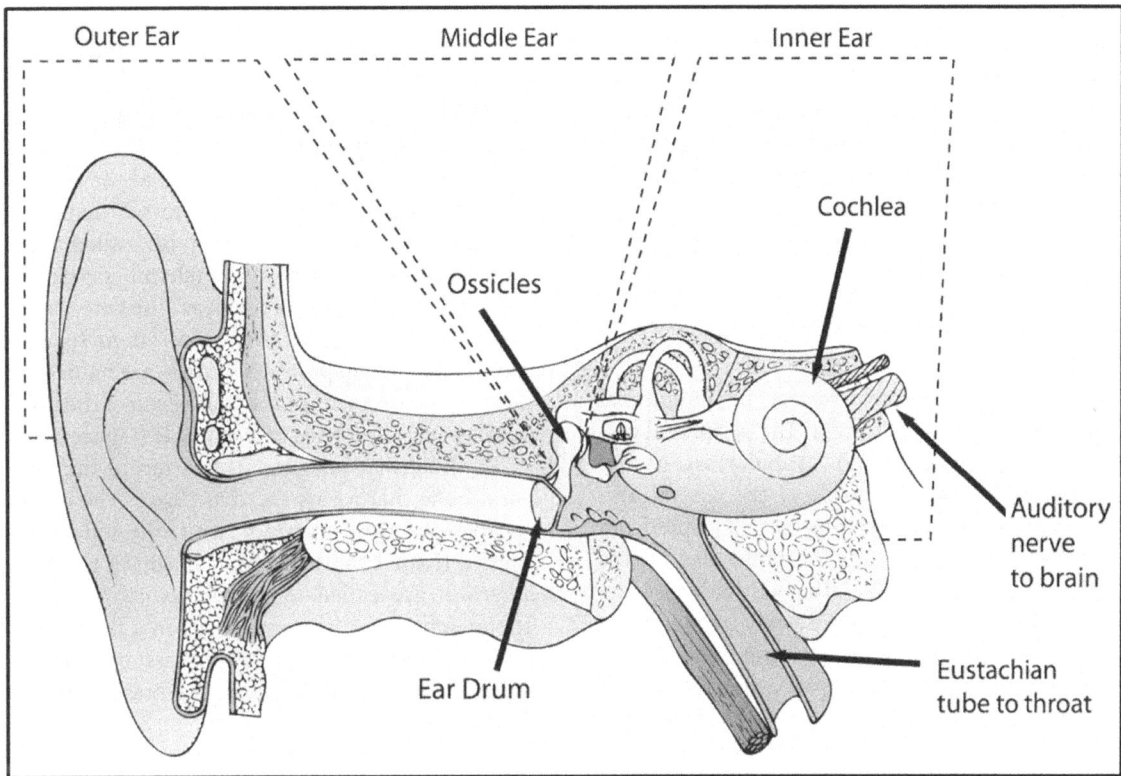

Figure 3.1 Ear Diagram

ear. Also contained on the medial wall is the tympanic plexus (CN IX), supplying the middle ear and a bulge that is due to the facial nerve.

The *anterior wall* of the middle ear is a thin bony plate that separates the middle ear from the internal carotid artery, and superiorly along the anterior wall has an opening of the eustachian tube that connects the middle ear to the nasopharynx (in the back of the throat). The eustachian tubes help to drain fluid from the middle ear and equalize pressure inside of the ears. •

GEEK STUFF

When there are external pressure changes, such as when you are in an airplane that is taking off or landing, the reason you yawn is to try to open the eustachian tubes to equalize pressure on the eardrum.

The *inferior wall* (floor) separates the middle ear from the superior bulb of the internal jugular vein and has a canal for the tympanic part of CN IX (glossopharyngeal nerve).

The *posterior wall* (mastoid wall) of the middle ear is comprised of the temporal bone at the level of the mastoid process (and air cells) and lateral vestibular semicircular canal. There is a hole in the posterior wall (called the mastoid antrum) allowing air from the air cells of the mastoid to communicate with the middle ear when pressure is too low.

There are two muscles in the middle ear called the tensor tympani muscle and stapedius muscle. These muscles contract in response to loud noises and inhibit the vibrations along the bones to reduce the transmission of sound to protect the cochlea. This action is called the *acoustic reflex*.

INNER EAR

The inner ear can be divided into two parts: the cochlear component and the vestibular component. While the cochlear component is responsible for hearing, the vestibular component deals with balance, head motion, gaze stabilization of the eyes, and posture. Let's look closer at each of these components.

VESTIBULAR COMPONENT: VESTIBULAR ANATOMY

Figure 3.1 depicts a cross-section in the coronal plane (frontal plane) of the ear. The peripheral vestibular system includes the vestibular organs and the nerves, which are outside of the central nervous system, that conduct information to and from these organs (Figure 3.2). The vestibular organs share cranial nerve VIII (the vestibulocochlear nerve) with the cochlea and assist in maintaining posture, regulating muscle tone, maintaining equilibrium, and stabilizing gaze when the head is in motion. The vestibular system also assists in the perception of self-motion, spatial navigation, and spatial memory.

The entire peripheral vestibular system is about the size of your thumbnail, and you have a vestibular organ in each ear. A closer look at the peripheral vestibular system allows us to see that there are three semicircular canals (also called *labyrinths*), and two otolith organs (chambers) named the *utricle* and *saccule* in each ear. The three semicircular canals—the *anterior* canal, *lateral* (or horizontal) canal, and *posterior* canal—are named for their orientation within the head. Each of the three canals begins and ends in the utricle (Figure 3.3).

The hollowed-out petrous portion of the temporal bone that forms the structure of the canals is called the bony labyrinth, while the softer connective tissue canals that float inside of the *bony labyrinth* are called the *membranous labyrinth*. The membranous labyrinth floats in a fluid called *perilymph* (which has a low potassium concentration) in a similar way as the brain floats in

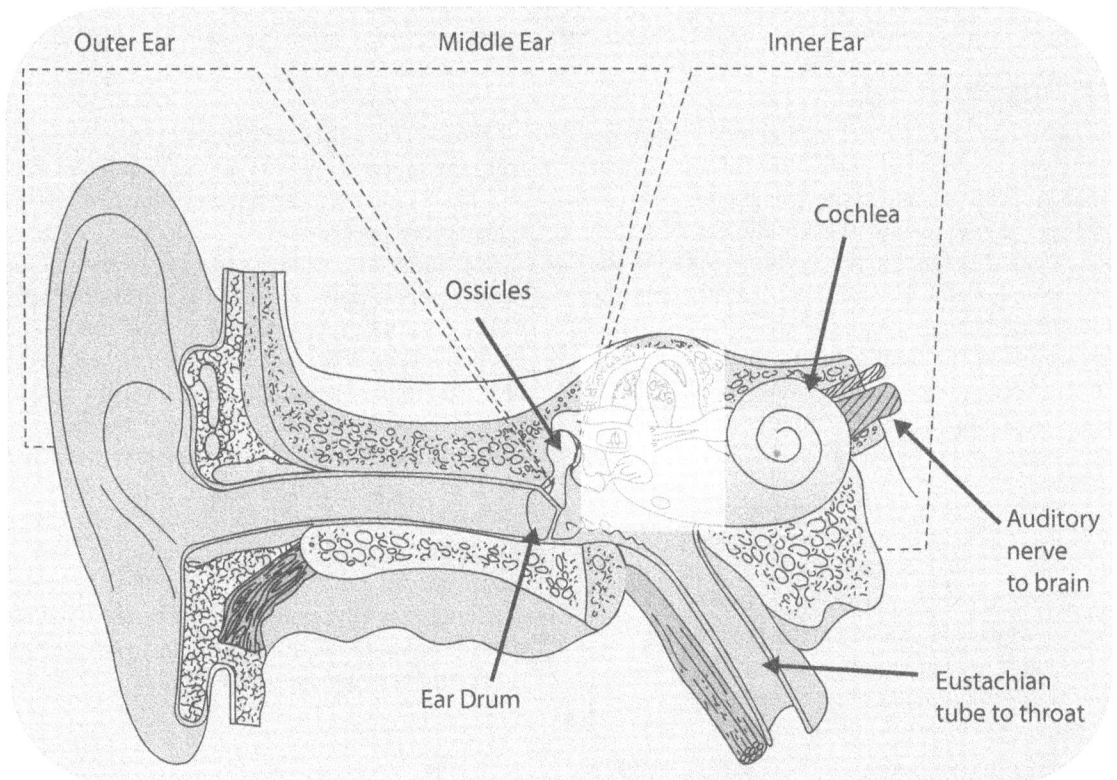

Figure 3.2 Ear Diagram with Highlighted Vestibular System

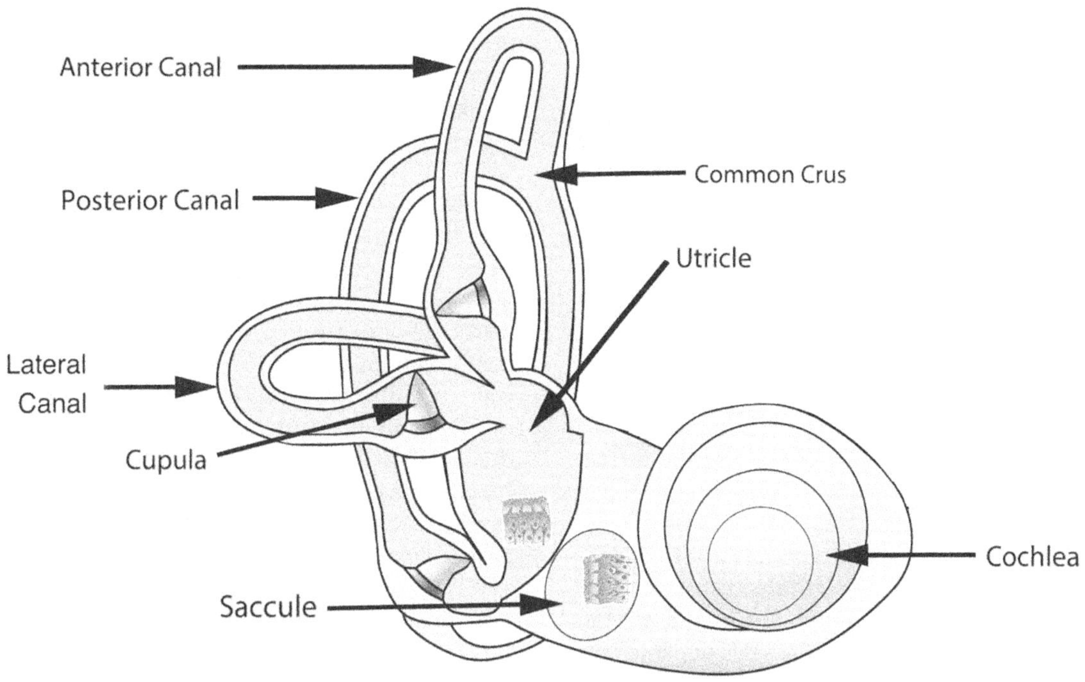

Figure 3.3 Vestibular System

cerebrospinal fluid inside the skull. The membranous labyrinth canals and otoliths contain a fluid called *endolymph* (which has a high concentration of potassium).

The anterior and posterior canals are oriented closer to the vertical plane, while the lateral canal is oriented roughly (~30-degree tilt) to the horizontal plane. The canals are responsible for detecting *angular velocity changes of motion* and do not normally detect the pull of gravity. The otolith organs are responsible for detecting *changes in linear velocity* (e.g., up/down, front/back, and side to side), as well as the pull of gravity to detect tilting of the head. The system in the left ear is the mirror image of the system in the right. Between functions of the chambers and canals, you are aware of any motion of your head.

The concept of neutral buoyancy is important to the understanding of the function of the inner ear. Before continuing to review vestibular anatomy and physiology, consider the following concept. For a moment, imagine that you have a large glass of water sitting on a table. Above the glass, you hold a rock. If you drop the rock it will fall through the air toward the glass of water. This happens

because the rock is heavier than the air surrounding it. Once the rock hits the water, it will sink through it until it hits the bottom of the glass. This happens because the rock is heavier than the water surrounding it. If you were to tilt the glass, the rock would fall toward the lowest point of the glass that is closest to the ground. Now imagine that you are holding a cube of ice. If you drop it while holding it over the glass of water, it will fall through the air until it hits the water. This happens because the ice cube is heavier than the air surrounding it. However, once it is in the water, the ice cube will float because the ice is lighter than the water. In fact, if you were to reach down to the bottom of the glass while holding the ice cube and then let go of it, the ice would rise until it reached the surface of the water. Finally, imagine that you had an object the size of an ice cube, but it weighed exactly the same as water. If you reached halfway down into the glass of water and let go, it would not rise since it is not lighter than the water around it. It would not sink since it is not heavier than the water around it. Instead, it would stay wherever you let go of it since it is *neutrally buoyant,* weighing the same as the water around it. Parts of the inner ear that only detect motion (the cupulae of the canals) are neutrally buoyant, weighing the same as the endolymph, and detect only velocity changes do to a lag of the endolymph pushing against the cupulae, while other parts (the otoconia crystals of the otolithic membranes, which we will review later) are not neutrally buoyant and are heavier than the endolymph, therefore causing the otoliths to shift toward the ground detecting tilt due to the pull of gravity. The otoliths, therefore, detect motion as well as the pull of gravity.

Semicircular Canals

As mentioned, all three canals (anterior, lateral, and posterior) begin and end in the utricle. The anterior and posterior canals begin with a common canal (called the *common crus*), which divides to become these canals. They are sometimes referred to as the *vertical canals* since they are oriented (roughly) vertically to the ground and about 45 degrees from the sagittal plane. The lateral canal is oriented roughly horizontally to the ground but with a 30-degree angle upward (cephalad) as it travels anteriorly to reconnect to the utricle. All three canals leave the utricle and then bend back to reattach to it, forming a semicircle (hence, the name semicircular canal). Just before it reconnects to the utricle, the end of each canal widens into an area called an *ampulla*. Inside each ampulla are groups of hair cells contained in a gelatinous matrix structure called a *cupula* (Figure 3.4). The cupula in each of the canals completely blocks off the canal space, and endolymph cannot move past it. The hair cells inside the cupula connect to nerves leading to the brain. The movement

of the cupula (and hair cells within it) due to the pressure of the endolymph against of side of the cupula during angular head motions changes the firing rates of these nerves compared to their resting rates. Recall, the cupula is neutrally buoyant weighing the same as the endolymph that surrounds it and is not affected by gravity. If you tilt your head, the cupula will not sink or bend in the endolymph toward the ground. Being neutrally buoyant, the cupula of each canal cannot normally detect gravity; therefore, you cannot use the information coming from the semicircular canals to tell you where the ground is or whether you are tilting. For example, if you move from sitting to lying, the cupula will not be "pulled down" by gravity. As you move your head, the fluid inside the system lags a bit behind the motion of the skull and pushes against the cupula. This pressure will push against the cupula making it billow toward or away from the utricle (think of a sail filling with wind) depending on the direction of the fluid lag. These cupulae will detect the velocity and direction of the head's movement but not the ultimate position of your head with respect to gravity.

ACTIVITY 3.1 FLUID INERTIAL LAG

To gain a better understanding of the inertial fluid lag, take a half-full clear bottle of water and hold it sideways (make sure the lid is tight!). If you quickly move the bottle to your left, you will see the water collecting on the right side of the bottle. Why does this happen? Initially, as you move the bottle, it is moving faster than the water inside of it. As a result, fluid builds on the right side of the bottle as it moves left.

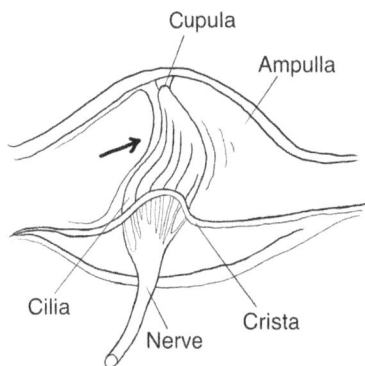

Figure 3.4 Cupula

As you quickly turn your head to the left, the motion of the endolymph inside the lateral canals of each ear lags behind the head motion—called *inertial lag*—and puts pressure on the cupula. Recall that the peripheral vestibular organs are mirror images of each other. So, as you turn your head, the endolymph in the lateral canal of one ear will push the cupula inward toward the utricle, thus increasing the nerve firing rates, while in the other ear the endolymph will move away from the cupula, deflecting it away from the utricle, thus slowing the firing rates of that ear. This push–pull relationship holds true for each coplanar canal pair.

The nerves attached to the peripheral vestibular organs are constantly sending signals, even while sitting still, that change the firing rates during velocity or position changes of the head. At rest, the hairs of each group are standing up in a neutral position and the nerves fire at a relatively constant rate, called the *resting rate*. According to Goebel and Sumer,[3] the resting rate of the vestibular neurons is about 90 spikes per second with a range of 10 to 200 spikes per second. However, if you move, the fluid presses or pulls against the cupula and makes the hairs bend. When the hairs bend, the nerves change their firing rates. In each group of hair cells there are rows of hairs, with each row taller than the one preceding it in a stepwise fashion. We refer to these rows of hairs collectively as *stereocilia*. Ultimately you reach one very tall hair cell, called the *kinocilium*, which is the tallest in the group. The hair cells in each group connect to each other, and if one bends, they will all bend. If the group of hairs bends in the direction of the tall kinocilium, the associated nerve increases its firing rate. The farther the hairs bend toward the kinocilium, the faster the nerve will fire. Conversely, if the group of hairs bends toward the shortest row of hairs, the nerve will slow its firing rate. The farther the hairs bend toward the shorter rows, the more slowly the nerve will fire. Once movement stops, the hairs return to their upright neutral position and the nerve returns to the resting firing rate. It is important to understand that the bending of hair cells in the ampullae of each canal normally only occurs with changes of head velocity, and signals from the canals will remain at the resting firing rate whenever the head is either still or moving at a constant velocity.

During angular head motions, the vestibular organ that is ipsilateral to the direction of motion can increase the firing rates up to 400 spikes per second.[4] The brain compares nerve firing rates of the cupulae and otoliths of each ear to determine in which direction and how quickly the head is moving. It is the change from the resting firing

rate that indicates how you are moving or turning, in which direction, and how quickly. Because the canals are semicircular, under normal conditions, only angular head motions will create endolymph flow deflecting the cupulae.

GEEK STUFF

There are tiny thread-like connections from the tip of each cilium to a non-specific cation channel on the side of the taller neighboring cilium. The tip links function like a string connected to a hinged hatch. When the cilia are bent toward the tallest one, the channels are opened, much like a trap door. According to Gray (2020), opening these channels allows an influx of potassium, which in turn opens calcium channels that initiate the receptor potential. This mechanism transduces mechanical energy into neural impulses. An inward K^+ current depolarizes the cell and opens voltage-dependent calcium channels. This in turn causes neurotransmitter release at the basal end of the hair cell, eliciting an action potential in the dendrites of the VIIIth cranial nerve.[2]

Another common everyday analogy may help to clarify this process. Imagine you have a tire that you fill with water and then lay flat on the ground. How could you get the water inside the tire to move around the inside of it in a circular fashion? If you were to lift the tire up and down, the water would not move around in a circle. If you wanted to get the water flowing in a circular motion, you would have to move or spin the tire in a circular motion. Once you had it moving in a circle, the water inside the tire would begin to flow around either clockwise or counterclockwise, depending on the way you turn it. Now that you have this picture in mind, imagine that you are in an upright position and that each canal (anterior, lateral, and

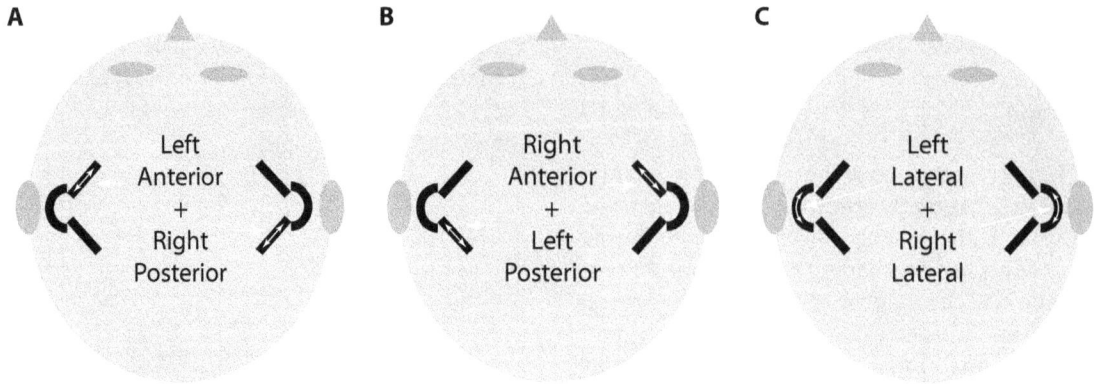

Figure 3.5 Coplanar Pairs

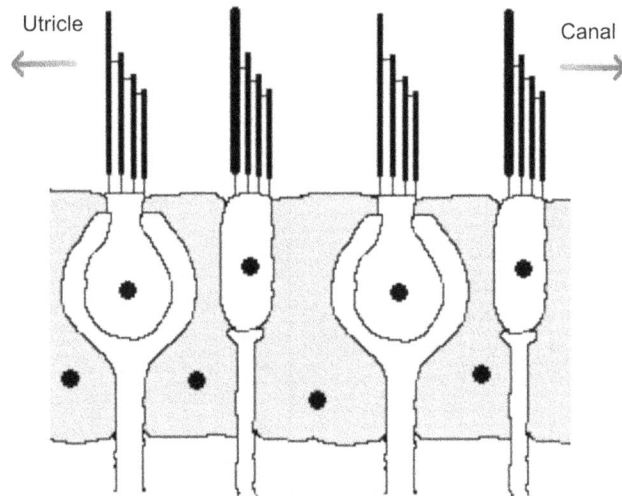

Figure 3.6 Cilia Arrangement in the Lateral Canal Cupulae

posterior), being almost a complete circle, is filled with fluid. The only way to get the cupulae blocking off these canals to bend, and thereby bend the groups of hairs within them, is to get endolymph moving in a circular fashion around the canal. If you simply moved up and down (as in an elevator), front/back, or side to side, the endolymph would not push against the cupula.

How do you know in which direction you are moving? The canals of one ear work in a push–pull system with those of the other ear. Canals that are in the same plane of motion work together; they are called *coplanar pairs*. The pairs that work together are as follows:

- Left **a**nterior canal and **r**ight **p**osterior canal. This pair is often referred to as the *LARP* (Figure 3.5A).
- **R**ight **a**nterior canal and **l**eft **p**osterior canal. This pair is often referred to as the *RALP* (Figure 3.5B).
- Left lateral canal and right lateral canal (Figure 3.5C).

Taking a closer look at the lateral canals, you can see that each ear has groups of hairs in the lateral canal that are arranged from short to tall rows as you move in a lateral-to-medial direction (Figure 3.6).

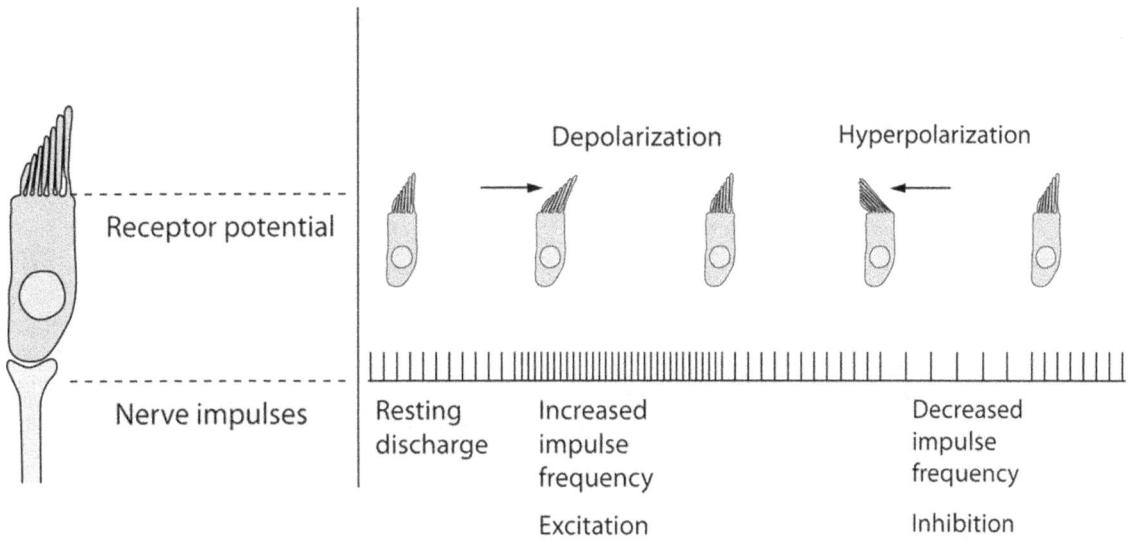

Figure 3.7 Vestibular Nerve Activation

Just like a tug-of-war, each coplanar pair works as a push–pull system. If each ear is sending the same resting-rate signal, the brain senses no motion from the vestibular system. If you turn your head to the left, the left lateral canal will increase its firing rate while at the same time the right lateral canal will decrease its firing rate. If you were to rotate your head to the right, the right lateral canal would increase its firing rate while the coplanar pair (the left lateral canal) would at the same time decrease its firing rate. The hairs in the canals will normally bend only if there is a change of velocity. The brain compares the firing rate coming from each pair. So, if you are turning continuously at a constant velocity, the vestibular system would not detect the motion.

When there is a difference between the firing rates of the coplanar pairs, the brain interprets that change in firing rates as motion. This is possible because of the arrangement of the groups of hair cells.

Refer to Figure 3.7. Recall that each group of hairs is spring-like and prefers standing in its neutral position. In this example, a person sits still. The hash-marked lines indicate the firing rates of the nerves, with each hash mark indicating a discharge of the nerve. If you turn your head to the right, there is a lag in the fluid, which bends the hairs. For the right lateral canal, this means you are bending the hairs toward the tall hair cell, and this increases the nerves' firing rate. If you stay still, the hair cells return to their preferred position, and the nerve returns to its resting firing rate. If you turn your head to the left, there is a lag of the fluid within the canal, and the hairs bend toward the small hair, slowing the nerve's firing rate. When you stop moving, the hairs once again return to their preferred resting position, and the nerve returns to its resting rate.

Using Figure 3.8, you can see that when all hair groups bend owing to motion of the head, one ear would increase the nerve's firing rate while the other ear would slow its firing rate. The image is of the head as viewed from above. The canals involved are also depicted.

Otolith Organs

Like the groups of hair cells located in the cupulae of the canals, the otolith organs (utricle and saccule) each also have groups of hair cells on a kidney-shaped area called the *macula*. There are some differences between the arrangements of these groups of hairs compared with those at the end of the canals in the ampullae. As you have learned, the canals work as pairs during inertial lag owing to the push–pull system created by the mirror-image arrangements of the hair cells of each ear. This is not the case for the utricles and saccules of each ear. The hair cells in each otolith organ are not all arranged in the same orientation (such as each group arranged short to tall). Instead, each macula has some groups arranged short to tall while other groups are tall to short. Imagine two football teams facing each other. Each utricle and saccule has a macula that is roughly divided along the middle of the kidney shape—half of the macula having groups of hairs arranged short to tall while the other half has groups arranged tall to short (Figure 3.14).

When this one macula is moved, the nerves associated with it will not all send the same message, as is the case in the canals. Instead, it will send some nerve signals that are faster than the resting rate and some that are slower. When you compare the signals of the utricle or saccule of one ear with those of the other ear, you will not get a push–pull system. As a result, the otoliths do not work in pairs, since they are each sending the same types of information. Refer to Figures 3.15 and 3.16 for a cross section of an otolith organ (utricle or saccule).

Another difference between the maculae of the otolith organs and the cupulae of the canals is the shape of the matrix that contains the groups of hair cells. In the otolith organs, this matrix is the *otolithic membrane*, and it is not shaped like a sail that blocks off an area, as the cupulae do in the canals. Instead, the matrices are like kidney-shaped pans

The Effect of Left Posterior Head Motion on Vestibular Nerve Activity		
Motion: Left posteriorly 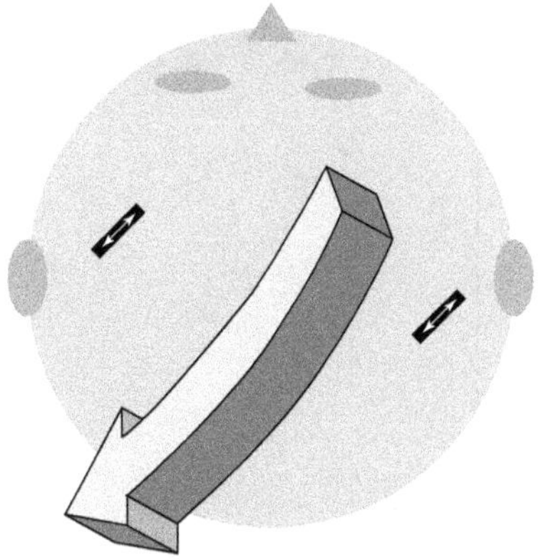	Increased firing rate of the left posterior canal's vestibular nerve	Decreased firing rate of the right anterior canal's vestibular nerve

Figure 3.8 Left Posterior Head Motion | | |

The Effect of Right Anterior Head Motion on Vestibular Nerve Activity		
Motion: Right anteriorly 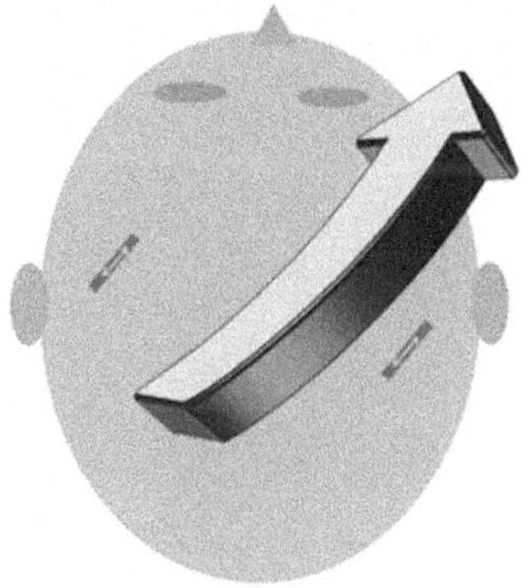	Increased firing rate of the right anterior canal's vestibular nerve	Decreased firing rate of the left posterior canal's vestibular nerve

Figure 3.9 Right Anterior Head Motion | | |

The Effect of Right Posterior Head Motion on Vestibular Nerve Activity		
Motion: Right posteriorly 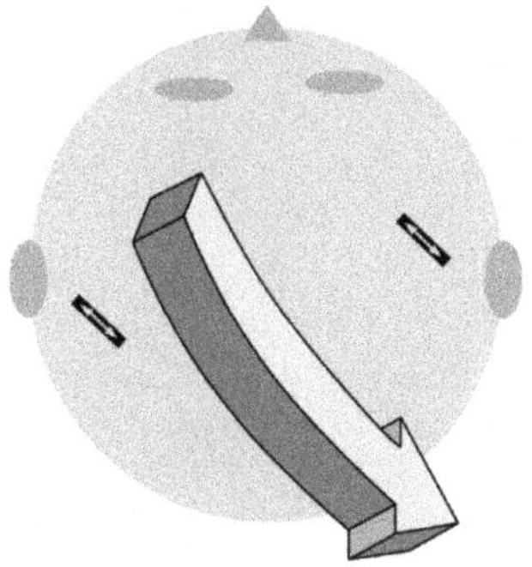	Increased firing rate of the right posterior canal's vestibular nerve	Decreased firing rate of the left anterior canal's vestibular nerve

Figure 3.10 Right Posterior Head Motion | | |

The Effect of Left Anterior Head Motion on Vestibular Nerve Activity		
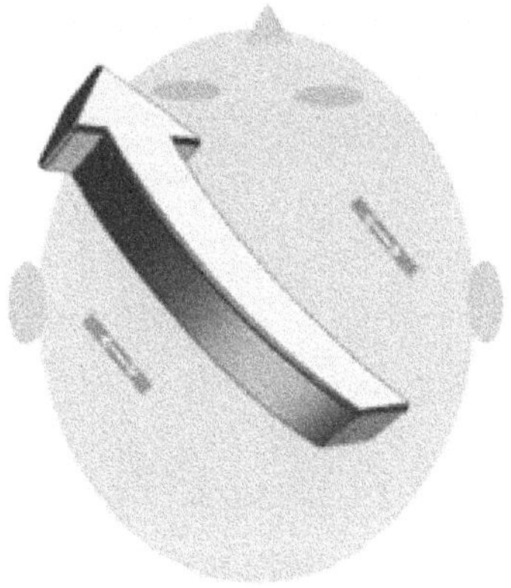 Motion: Left anteriorly	Increased firing rate of the left anterior canal's vestibular nerve	Decreased firing rate of the right posterior canal's vestibular nerve
Figure 3.11 Left Anterior Head Motion		

The Effect of Right Head Rotation Motion on Vestibular Nerve Activity		
Motion: Right rotation	Increased firing rate of the right lateral canal's vestibular nerve	Decreased firing rate of the left lateral canal's vestibular nerve
Figure 3.12 Right Head Rotation		

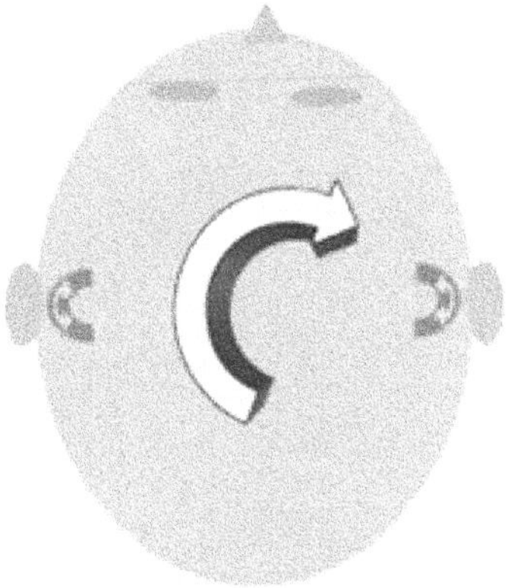

The Effect of Left Head Rotation on Vestibular Nerve Activity		
Motion: Left rotation	Increased firing rate of the left lateral canal's vestibular nerve activity	Decreased firing rate of the right lateral canal's vestibular nerve activity
Figure 3.13 Left Head Rotation		

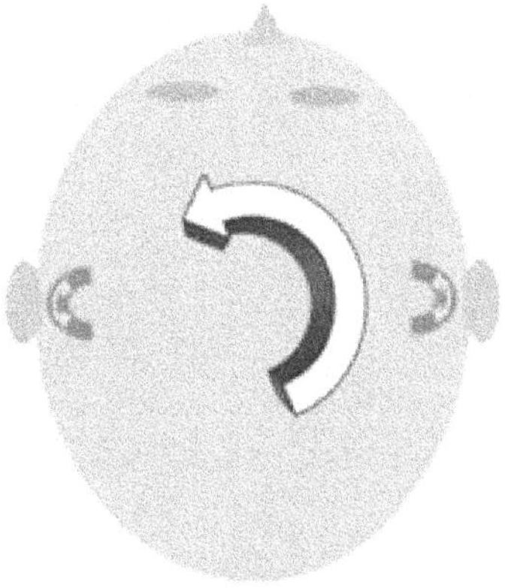

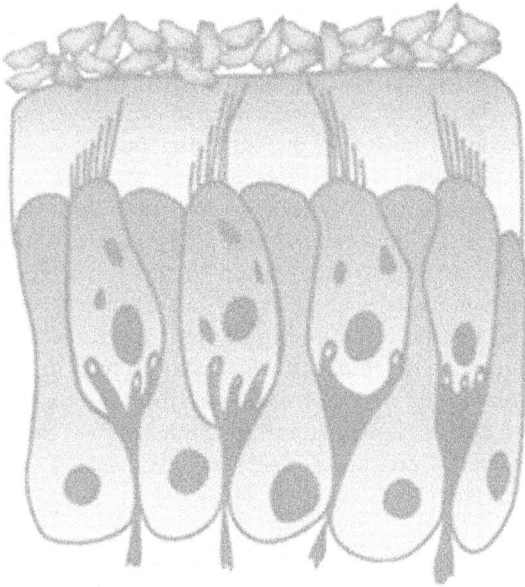

Figure 3.14 Utricle

Figure 3.15 Saccule

Figure 3.16 Otolith Cross Section

that sit on the otolith's floor in the case of the utricle, and on the anterior wall edge in the case of the saccule. These otolithic membranes do not block off part of the chamber.

Finally, the utricles and saccules have *otoconia*, or calcium carbonate crystals, anchored on top of each otolithic membrane, making it sensitive to the pull of gravity as they are heavier than the endolymph. Since these crystals are heavier than the endolymph, the otolithic membrane is no longer neutrally buoyant. If you tilt, the otoconia pull on the matrix and shift it toward the ground. The shifting otolithic membrane bends the groups of hairs contained within, changing the firing rates of the nerves, and alerting the person to head tilting. Besides detecting gravity, the utricle and saccule also detect changes in velocity, like the cupulae.

- *Utricle* The macula of the utricle is oriented horizontally, with the groups of hairs coming up like grass growing from the ground. As you move front to back or side to side (any horizontal-plane movement), the hair cells bend and detect the motion. When you press your foot on the gas pedal, you *feel* the acceleration of the car. When you see the police waiting behind the billboard to catch speeders, you *feel* the sudden deceleration as you slam on your brakes! The utricle is responsible for these sensations. Since it also detects the pull of gravity, it can also detect tilt.

- *Saccule* The macula of the saccule is located on its medial wall. This anatomy is like that of the utricle, but owing to the positioning within the chamber, its hairs come out laterally as if growing out of a wall. When you move vertically, the force of this motion causes these hair cell groups to bend and give you sensations and information about these motions. When you are in an elevator, you can't see anything moving, but you *feel* yourself-rising or falling. The saccule is responsible for these sensations.

An easy way to remember which otolith detects which motion is to think of the *U* in utricle and the *S* in saccule. Imagine the ends of the letters are hair cells. If you were to hold the *U* in the palm of your hand, how could you get the hair cells (ends of the letter) to wiggle? If you moved your hand up and down, would they move? No. If you were to move your hand horizontally in any direction would they wiggle? Yes! So, the utricle detects horizontal movements.

Vestibular Fluids

We have mentioned both endolymph and perilymph as part of the vestibular anatomy.

- *Perilymph*   Perilymph is the extracellular fluid inside the bony labyrinth that surrounds the membranes of the vestibular system. The vestibular organs "float" in the perilymph. Perilymph contains both potassium and sodium with sodium having the higher concentration.
- *Endolymph*   This extracellular fluid is contained inside the vestibular system (semicircular canals, utricle, and saccule) as well as the cochlea. It contains high levels of potassium and lower levels of sodium. It is produced and absorbed by the endolymphatic sac, which the utricle and saccule connect to via the endolymphatic duct.

VESTIBULAR NEURAL CONNECTIONS

Recall that cranial nerve VIII (vestibulocochlear nerve) carries information from the ear to the brain. The vestibulocochlear nerve carries information to the vestibular nuclei, which also receives some information from vision and somatosensory inputs. It ascends to areas of the cortex for perception, while descending pathways carry vestibular input to the spinal cord for control of head and body in space.[5] The central vestibular paths extend from the vestibular nuclei via the midbrain and thalamus to multiple areas in the cortex including the insular–opercular cortex, ventrolateral prefrontal cortex, parietal lobe, cingulum, and cerebellar vermis and hemispheres.[5]

Let's trace it from the brain to the ear. CN VIII leaves the vestibular nuclei at the junction of the pons and medulla, travels through the cerebellopontine angle and enters the internal auditory canal (which is a passage through the skull), then divides into the auditory nerve and the vestibular nerve. The vestibular nerve further divides into the superior and inferior vestibular nerves with the superior vestibular nerve innervating the anterior canal, lateral canal, and utricle. The inferior vestibular nerve innervates the posterior canal and saccule. An easy way to remember this is to associate the vestibular anatomical relationships of the posterior canal (which sits the lowest in the head) and the saccule (which is smaller than the utricle) as being "inferior."

There are four main vestibular nuclei that process information. They are the superior nucleus, lateral nucleus, the medial nucleus, and inferior nucleus (Tables 3.1 to 3.4).[6]

Table 3.1 Superior Vestibular Nucleus Connections and Jobs

Superior Vestibular Nucleus (SVN)	
Connections	**Jobs**
Afferent: From the superior and posterior semicircular canals. Another major group of afferent nerves comes from the cerebellum. There are also some connections from the otolith organs.	Aids in coordination and postural adjustments.
Efferent connections travel to oculomotor nuclei.	*Mediates:* VOR with the MVN.

GEEK STUFF

Information leaving the vestibular nuclei have four destinations:[7]

1. Down the vestibulospinal tract to the extensor muscles (for the vestibulospinal and vestibulocollic reflexes). From the lateral vestibular nucleus to the trunk and limbs, and from the medial vestibular nucleus to the head and neck.
2. Information travels to/from the cerebellum. From all vestibular nuclei, information travels through the inferior cerebellar peduncle to synapse with the vestigial nucleus in the flocculonodular lobe of the cerebellum (aka vestibular cerebellum). Information also flows back to the vestibular nucleus to influence the descending tracks.
3. Up the medial longitudinal fasciculus (MLF) to cranial nerves III, IV, and VI (those that control eye movement, and thus the vestibular ocular reflex). From the medial vestibular nucleus, information flows to the contralateral abducens nucleus (CN IV). From CN IV, information then travels up the MLF and crosses over to stimulate contralateral lateral rectus muscle and cranial nerves III (oculomotor) and IV (trochlear).
4. A fourth pathway is suggested to go to the thalamus (ventral posterior medial nucleus), and then to the internal capsule, and exits through the corona radiata to the lateral postcentral gyrus (primary somatosensory cortex), the insular cortex, and temporoparietal cortex. This pathway is believed to bring conscious awareness of vestibular sensations.

VESTIBULAR BLOOD SUPPLY

The inner ear is supplied by the labyrinthine artery (from the anterior inferior cerebellar artery). This artery gives off two main branches:

1. *Common cochlear artery*: Divides into the main cochlear artery and vestibulocochlear artery. The vestibulocochlear artery forms the posterior vestibular and cochlear arteries. The apical three-fourths of the cochlea is supplied by the main cochlear artery, while the basal cochlea is supplied by the cochlear ramus.[8]
2. *Anterior vestibular arteries*: Supplies the utricle, superior saccule, and ampullae of the superior and lateral semicircular canals. The posterior vestibular artery supplies the inferior saccule and ampulla of the posterior semicircular canal.[8,9]

Vestibular Laws

There are a few laws governing the vestibular system. The first three are named after a German researcher named Arnold Ewald, who created them in 1882. The other vestibular law is Alexander's law, which was created in 1912 by Gustav Alexander, an Austrian otolaryngologist.

EWALD'S LAWS

Ewald's laws are as follows:

1. A stimulation of the semicircular canal causes a movement of the eyes in the plane of the stimulated canal.
   - (For example, if you stimulated the right lateral vestibular canal, you would expect to see lateral eye motions.)

2. In the horizontal semicircular canals, an ampullopetal endolymph movement causes a greater stimulation than an ampullofugal one.
   - (The terms ampullopetal and ampullofugal describe the direction of endolymph flow within the canal. *Ampullo-* refers to the ampulla, while *-petal* indicates "moving toward." Therefore, an ampullopetal motion is one that describes motion toward the ampulla. By contrast, ampullofugal indicates movement away from the ampulla. Ewald's second law tells us that the force of endolymph moving toward the ampulla will cause vestibular excitement. In the vertical semicircular canals, the reverse is true.)

Table 3.2 Lateral Vestibular Nucleus Connections and Jobs

Lateral Vestibular Nucleus (Deiter's Nucleus) (LVN)	
Connections	**Job**
Afferent: Major afferent contributions are from the entire vestibular apparatus and flocculonodular lobe of the cerebellum, with some components from the spine and other areas.	It is important for the control of the vestibulospinal reflex.
Efferent: Most efferent fibers from this nucleus go to the spinal cord, although it also connects to oculomotor neurons.	

Table 3.3 Medial Vestibular Nucleus Connections and Jobs

Medial Vestibular Nucleus (Nucleus of Schwalbe or the Triangular Nucleus) (MVN)	
Connections	**Jobs**
Afferent connections: This nucleus receives afferent fibers from lateral semicircular canals and the contralateral medial vestibular nucleus and other areas of the brain. Specific sections of this nucleus contain different afferent connections. • Superior section: Contributing afferent fibers come from the semicircular canals and cerebellum. • Middle section: Contributing afferents from the utricle and saccule. • Caudal section: Contributing afferents come from the cerebellum.	• It is important for coordinating eye, head, and neck movements. • Mediates the VCR. • Mediates the VOR with the superior vestibular nucleus.
Efferent connections run to the cervical and upper thoracic spinal levels, the oculomotor nerves, the cerebellum, and contralateral vestibular nuclei.	

Table 3.4 Inferior Vestibular Nucleus Connections and Jobs

Inferior Vestibular Nucleus (Descending or Spinal Nucleus) (IVN)	
Connections	**Job**
Afferent connections: from the otolith organs and cerebellum. Receives information regarding head tilt and gravity.	Integrates vestibular signals from each side (left and right ears and vestibular nuclei) with the cerebellum and reticular formation.
Efferent connections: contralateral vestibular nuclei.	

3. The third law states that ampullopetal endolymph flow in the vertical canals (movement toward the ampulla) causes less vestibular excitement than endolymph flow away from it (anterior and posterior semicircular canals).

Laws 2 and 3 are explained by the arrangements of hair cells within the lateral canals versus the vertical canals.

ALEXANDER'S LAW

Another commonly referred to law is Alexander's law. This law states that:

1. After an acute vestibular loss, fast phases of nystagmus beat toward the healthy ear.
2. Spontaneous nystagmus of a patient with a vestibular lesion is more intense when the patient looks in the direction of the fast phase.

Vestibular Reflexes

The vestibular system mediates a number of reflexes whose names indicate the systems that are working together to produce the reflex. These include the VOR, VSR, and VCR (Figure 3.17):

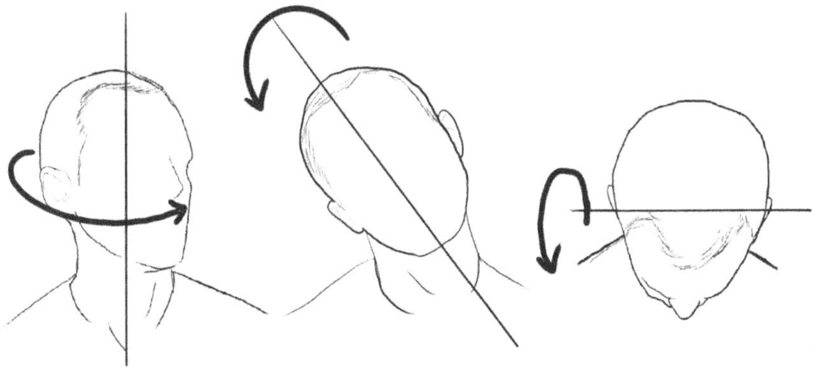

Figure 3.17 Vestibular Reflex Motions

- *VOR*: Vestibulo-ocular reflex (the vestibular system working with the eyes)
- *VSR*: Vestibulospinal reflex (the vestibular system working with the spinal muscles)
- *VCR*: Vestibulocollic reflex (the vestibular system working with the neck muscles)

These reflexes keep vision stable during head motions, assist in balance control, and help to right the head if the body tilts. As explained earlier, nystagmus is an involuntary, rhythmic movement of the eye. Jerk nystagmus moves quickly in one direction and slowly in the opposite direction. The slow phase of this movement is for visual tracking, while the quick (fast) phase is to reset the eye to prepare to track again. Nystagmus are named for the quick phases of motion. They may be linear (left-right, up-down, or in the planes of the stimulated canals) or rotational. The rotational variety, *rotary* (or torsional) *nystagmus*, turns (rotates) the eye (a motion like that of the turning of a car's steering wheel).

You can use observed nystagmus to help diagnose a variety of conditions. While nystagmus are helpful for maintaining clear vision during head motions, they may also add to a feeling of vertigo (a sensation of motion) when they occur at the wrong times owing to pathology.

There are cervical reflexes that supplement the vestibular reflex information. These cervical reflexes are weak and are difficult to illicit even in a lab. However, when they are impaired, the conflict between information of the vestibular system and the neck can add to a sense of dizziness and disequilibrium. These reflexes include the cervico-ocular reflex (COR), cervico-spinal reflex (CSR), and cervico-collic reflex (CCR). These reflexes arise from stretch reflexes in the neck and their actions mimic those of their vestibular matches.

THE VESTIBULO-OCULAR REFLEX

The VOR is responsible for maintaining stable visual images during head motions by moving the eyes at the appropriate speed and direction (the same speed but opposite the direction of head motion). The VOR works between head motions (frequencies) of 0.5 and 5 Hz; 1 Hz of motion is equal to 360 degrees of motion per second. Most head motions during the day are between 0.5 and 4 Hz, so you use the VOR throughout the day. The latency of the VOR in one study was found to be 8.6 ms.[10] This is much faster than eye motions generated by the smooth pursuit system, which are less than 70 degrees/sec,[11] with latencies between 118.04 and 144.75 ms.[12]

The VOR works in three motion planes: yaw, roll, and pitch. Yaw is the "no" motion of the head, pitch is the "yes" motion, and roll is the ear-to-shoulder motion. For example, pick out one letter on this page and keep your eyes on it while you shake your head no quickly. If your eyes do not move and instead move with the head as it turns, as you shake your head you will see whatever is directly in front of you at each moment during the head turn and not on the letter on the page (blurring vision). To keep your eyes on a target while your head is in motion, the VOR turns your eyes in the *opposite direction* of your head motion and at *exactly the same speed*. In this way, your eyes always stay pointed at the target, even if your head moves. The VOR "turns on" to help you keep your eyes pointing at the visual target. As you shake your head, the inner ear detects the speed and direction of your head and relays the information to the oculomotor nuclei, which will activate the eye muscles to move the eyes so that they stay on the target. When everything is working correctly, you will be able to keep the image of your target clear (within the speeds of motion in which the reflex works).

VESTIBULOSPINAL REFLEX

The VSR helps to maintain balance. If you tilt too far and are in danger of falling, the muscles on the side of the body ipsilateral to the tilt will go into extension, and the arm and leg on that side will quickly come out to prevent you from falling. At the same time the muscles on the other side of the body will decrease tone or relax. This causes a righting reaction.

VESTIBULOCOLLIC REFLEX

The VCR is similar to the VSR, only it works on the neck muscles alone, not the entire body. It helps to right the head against gravity to maintain an "eyes level" (horizontal to the ground) posture. As your body tilts, this reflex is used to right your head so that you see the world in a level fashion.

To summarize, the vestibular system provides information about your head motion as well as your position and allows you to use reflexes to move your eyes appropriately. It also adjusts muscle tone to keep you balanced and positioned upright against gravity.

VESTIBULAR CHANGES WITH AGE

According to Furman et al., age-associated changes in the vestibular system include degeneration of the otoconia (crystals), degeneration of hair cells, loss of vestibular afferents, and a reduction in the number of cells in the vestibular nuclei.[13]

Benign paroxysmal positional vertigo (BPPV) is more common with advancing age, which suggests there may be an age-related component. In a retrospective review of 53 patients diagnosed with BPPV, the incidence of BPPV increased 38% with each decade of life.[14] The peak incidence of idiopathic BPPV occurs between the ages of 50 and 70. It may occur at any age; however, in those under 35 years of age it is rare without a history of head trauma.[15]

Vestibular function seems to decline with age. There has been one longitudinal study that looked at the VOR over a 5-year period ($n = 57$, mean age 82). In the study, there was a significant amplitude-dependent decrease in gain and an increase in phase lead of the VOR. There was a decrease in gain of the visual-vestibular responses at low-frequency sinusoidal stimulation.[16]

Cochlear Component

The cochlea is shaped like a spiral (osseous spiral lamina) with the conical central bony axis called the modiolus. The cochlea consists of three canals that travel together in this spiral that turns about 2.75 times around the modiolus and contains the cochlear nerve and spiral ganglion. These canals are called the vestibular duct (or *scala vestibuli*), the tympanic duct (or *scala tympani*), and the cochlear duct (or *scala media*). You may also think of these canals as being in a spiral tube that is divided into three compartments with the membranes that separate them connecting from the outer wall of the canal to one point on the inner wall called the spiral limbus.

After sound waves enter the ear canal and vibrate the tympanic membrane, the vibrations travel via the auditory ossicles to the oval window. The vibrations travel through the perilymph, which is behind the oval window up the spiral of the cochlea via the vestibular canal (scala vestibuli) until it reaches the apex (called the *helicotrema*), at which point the canal changes names and is now called the tympanic canal (scala tympani). The vibrations travel back down the spiral through the tympanic canal and push against (and moves) the round window. Between these canals (the vestibular and tympanic canals) is the triangular or wedge-shaped cochlear duct (scala media) that is filled with endolymph. It is separated from the vestibular duct above by the vestibular membrane (also called Reissner's membrane) and from the tympanic duct below by the basilar membrane.

The cochlear duct contains the *organ of Corti*, which has rows of hair cells located on the floor of the cochlear duct (on top of the basilar membrane). Just like the groups of hair cells in the vestibular system, there are rows of stereocilia moving from shorter to taller hair cells until they reach one tall kinocilia. Also like the hair cells of the vestibular system, there are cross-links that while the hairs are bending toward the kinocilia open channels that allow the influx of (primarily) potassium and calcium. The hair cells are covered by a gelatinous *tectorial membrane.* As sound waves travel toward the cochlear apex, they will cause the basilar membrane to vibrate. At the base of the spiral, the basilar membrane is comprised of short and stiff fibers. As the ducts move toward the cochlear apex, the fibers of the basilar membrane become longer and less stiff. High-frequency sounds stimulate hair cells closer to the base of the cochlea, while low-frequency sounds stimulate the hair cells near the apex. As the basilar membrane vibrates, it causes movement of the endolymph that bends the hair cells causing depolarization of the nerves, releasing the neurotransmitter glutamate that increases the action potential of the nerve, and we detect sound. Humans can detect sounds between ~20 Hz and 20,000 Hz. Normal conversation is typically between 1,500 and 4,000 Hz.

GEEK STUFF

One theory why high-frequency hearing loss is common for older adults is that all sound waves (both low and high frequencies) must pass through the base of the cochlea, thus wearing it out like a carpet that has high foot traffic.

REFERENCES

1. Jones O. The Middle Ear. Updated 12/22/2022. Accessed 9/30/2023. https://teachmeanatomy.info/head/organs/ear/middle-ear/.

2. Gray L. *Neuroscience Online.* University of Texas Health Science Center of Houston, McGovern Medical School; Reviewed 2020. Accessed 2024. https://nba.uth.tmc.edu/neuroscience/m/s2/chapter12.html.

3. Goebel JA, Sumer B. Ento Key, Fastest Otolaryngology & Opthalmology Insight Engine. *Otolaryngology.* Accessed 3/10/2024. https://entokey.com/vestibular-physiology/.

4. Fernandez C, Goldberg J. Physiology of peripheral neurons innervating semicircular canals of the squirrel monkey. II. Response to sinusoidal stimulation and dynamics of peripheral vestibular system. *J Neurophysiol.* 1971;34(4):661–675. doi:10.1152/jn.1971.34.4.661.

5. Dieterich M, Brandt T. Central vestibular networking for sensorimotor control, cognition, and emotion. *Curr Opin Neurol.* 2024;37(1):74–82. doi:10.1097/WCO.0000000000001233.

6. Hernandez E, Das JM. Neuroanatomy, Nucleus Vestibular. *StatPearls.* StatPearls Publishing; Updated 2022. Accessed 2024. https://www.ncbi.nlm.nih.gov/books/NBK562261/.

7. Yoo H, Mihalia D. Neuroanatomy, Vestibular Pathways. *StatPearls.* StatPearls Publishing; 2022. Updated 01/2023. Accessed 1/06/2024. https://www.ncbi.nlm.nih.gov/books/NBK557380/.

8. Simões J, Vlaminck S, Seiça R, Acke F, Miguéis A. Vascular mechanisms in acute unilateral peripheral vestibulopathy: a systematic review. *Acta Otorhinolaryngologica Italica.* 2021;41(5):401–409. doi:10.14639/0392-100X-N1543.

9. Kim JS, Lee H. Inner ear dysfunction due to vertebrobasilar ischemic stroke. *Semin Neurol.* 2009;29:534–540. doi:10.1055/s-0029-1241037.

10. Collewijn H, Smeets JB. Early components of the human vestibulo-ocular response to head rotation: latency and gain. *J Neurophysiol.* 2000;84(1):376–389. doi:10.1152/jn.2000.84.1.376.

11. Wong A. *Eye Movement Disorders.* Oxford University Press; 2008.

12. Hirota M, Kato K, Fukushima M, Ikeda Y, Hayashi T, Mizota A. Analysis of smooth pursuit eye movements in a clinical context by tracking the target and eyes. *Sci Rep.* 2022;12(1):8501. doi:10.1038/s41598-022-12630-6.

13. Furman JM, Raz Y, Whitney SL. Geriatric vestibulopathy assessment and management. *Curr Opin Otolaryngol Head Neck Surg.* 2010;18(5):386–389. doi:10.1097/MOO.0b013e32833ce5a6.

14. Froehling DA, Silverstein MD, Mohr DN, Beatty CW, Offord KP, Ballard DJ. Benign positional vertigo: incidence and prognosis in a population-based study in Olmsted County, Minnesota. *Mayo Clin Proc.* 1991;66(6):596–601. doi:10.1016/s0025-6196(12)60518-7.

15. Palmeri R, Kumar A. Benign Paroxysmal Positional Vertigo. *StatPearls.* StatPearls Publishing; Updated 2022. https://www.ncbi.nlm.nih.gov/books/NBK470308/.

16. Enrietto JA, Jacobson KM, Baloh RW. Aging effects on auditory and vestibular responses: a longitudinal study. *J Otolaryngol.* 1999;20(6):371–378. doi:10.1016/s0196-0709(99)90076-5.

4

Musculoskeletal and Somatosensory Anatomy

Chapter Goals

1. Describe posture
2. Describe how the spine affects balance
3. Describe the skeleton
4. List muscles involved in balance and posture
5. Describe the anatomy and function of the somatosensory system

This chapter discusses only the musculoskeletal and somatosensory components that contribute to a sense and control of balance, as well as illustrating important bones of the cranium, spine, and limbs. Musculoskeletal components of balance include the muscle groups that hold us up against gravity and those used reflexively to maintain balance. Limitations of these muscles or the joints they move may affect information collected from the somatosensory system and impair balance. Weaknesses or loss of normal range of motion in the presence of a good balance strategy may also impair balance.

MUSCULOSKELETAL SYSTEM

POSTURE

Ideal posture provides a body position in which all body segments are balanced around the center

of gravity and provides mechanical advantages for movement. If the body segments are not sufficiently supported by the base of support, the patient may have compromised balance. As with the example of stacking boxes, if each box is stacked directly on top of the one below, the stack is more stable. In terms of the human, consider the following body regions to be "boxes": the head, shoulders, hips, and feet. When looking at a patient, are the "boxes" lined up? When patients lean or bend, they shift their center of gravity. If the shape of the spine, or muscle weakness or tightness causes postural changes, the center of gravity may be moved away from the base of support. As an example, a study of healthy computer-based workers ($n = 30$) versus controls ($n = 30$) found that subjects with a forward head posture (found in the computer-based workers) had postural imbalance and impaired ability to regulate movements in forward and backward directions.[10]

Examine your patient's posture from the front, back, and side. Do postural changes place the patient at risk? If so, will stretching contracted muscles and strengthening weaker, overstretched muscles help?

THE SKELETAL SYSTEM

The bones of the skeletal system provide the structure that shapes our bodies and provide an anchor from which muscles pull to move our bodies. It also acts as a storage for minerals and manufactures blood cells.[1] The bones form joints where they

DOI: 10.1201/9781003524441-4

articulate and are supported by muscle, articular cartilage, and ligaments.

The Spine and Balance

The shape of the spine and the available trunk range of motion (ROM) affect balance. If patients have weak back extensors, tight hip flexors, and a forward head posture, their center of gravity (COG) will be forward and maybe even outside of the limits of stability.

Radiologists use a tool called the C7 plumb line. The C7 plumb line describes a vertical line from the midpoint of the C7 vertebral body to the ground. The relation of this plumb line to other anatomical markers is used to discuss the relationship between the spine and pelvis. If the line is too far anterior, the spine is not well balanced. If the line is too far posterior, patients often complain of back pain. The line of gravity (LOG) from the COG of a standing patient to the ground is not the same as the C7 plumb line, as the LOG runs through the body's center of gravity, while the C7 plumb line is a vertical line from C7 to the ground.[2] According to Kim et al.:

> The C7 plumb line is a radiographic reference to determine the sagittal vertical axis, the most traditional measurement of sagittal balance of the spine. A vertical line is drawn from the center of the C7 vertebral body in a caudal direction. The line should connect with, or be within 5 mm of, the superior–posterior endplate of S1. This is considered within the tolerable range for health-related quality of life outcomes. However, as patients age, they lean forward and tolerate slightly more positive sagittal alignment.[3]

There is much more radiologically speaking when discussing balance, including pelvic incidence, pelvic tilt, and lumbar lordosis. But for our discussion, we will stick with the C7 plumb line and line of gravity, and the realization that the shape of the spine can have a profound impact on a patient's ability to balance.

The position of the C7 plumb line can be positive, neutral, or negative:[4]

- *Positive balance*: The plumb line passes more than 2 cm in front of the posterosuperior corner of the S1 vertebral body (Spine A in Figure 4.1).
- *Neutral balance*: The plumb line passes within 2 cm of the posterosuperior corner of the S1 vertebral body (Spine B in Figure 4.1).
- *Negative balance*: The plumb line passes more than 2 cm behind the posterosuperior corner of the S1 vertebral body (Spine C in Figure 4.1).

According to Le Huec et al., "In most pathological settings, the centre of gravity is too far forward with a mechanical axis located in front of the femoral heads."[5] Using Figure 4.2, imagine an elderly patient with a flexed posture. The C7 plumb line and the COG are anterior to the base of support. Having a constant awareness (consciously or unconsciously) of the COG helps in the decision-making process that keeps them balanced. Being able to sense the COG makes it easier to plan strategies to make successful movements or to prevent falls.

Skull

The human skull, which is comprised of 22 bones, may be divided into two regions. The first is the

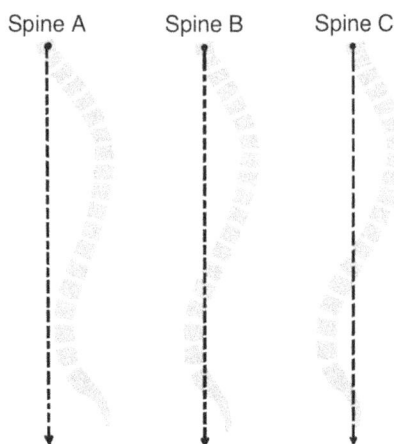

Spine A   Spine B   Spine C

Figure 4.1 Sagittal Spine with C7 Plumb Line Flexed

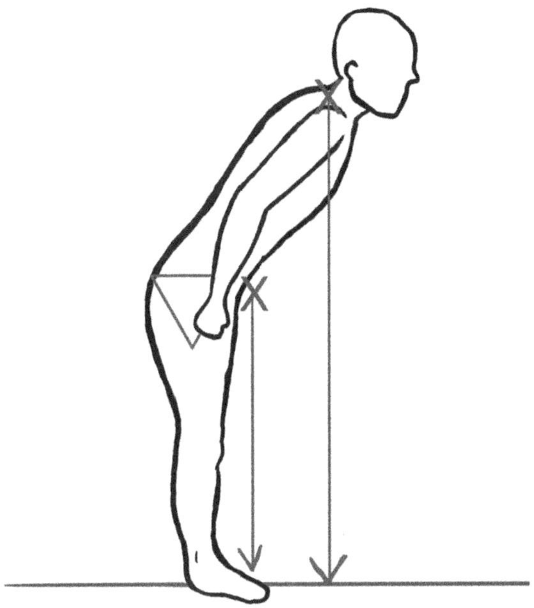

Figure 4.2 COG and C7 Plumb Line

neurocranium that protects the brain, and the second is the viscerocranium, which forms the face.[6] There are three cranial fossae (depression or hollow):

- *Anterior cranial fossa:* Contains the frontal lobe of the brain. It is formed from the frontal, sphenoid, and ethmoid bones.
- *Middle cranial fossa:* Contains the temporal lobe of the brain. It is formed from the sphenoid and two temporal bones.
- *Posterior cranial fossa:* Contains the cerebellum. It is formed from the occipital bone and two temporal bones.

There are fourteen facial bones, including two nasal conchae (bony plates on the lateral nasal cavity wall), "two nasal bones, two maxilla bones, two palatine bones, two lacrimal bones, two zygomatic bones, the mandible, and the vomer" (Figure 4.3).[6]

Atlantoaxial Joint

The first two vertebrae, C1 (atlas) and C2 (axis), of the spinal column form the atlantoaxial joint and are specifically designed to allow head on neck motions (Figure 4.4). The first segment, C1 (atlas), is ring shaped and rotates on C2 (axis). You may remember C1 as the atlas, as it is holding the head just as the Greek Titan Atlas is said to hold the world. C2 (axis) has a bony process anteriorly that sticks up (cephalad) called the odontoid process (or dens). There is no vertebral disc between C1 and C2.

There are ligaments that should be tested for integrity before any testing or treatment of the neck (or vestibular system, as these tests often involve head/neck movements). These are the *transverse* ligament and *alar* ligaments (Figure 4.5). The transverse ligament attaches to each mediolateral surface of the atlas and holds the dens of the axis against the anterior arch of the atlas. When the transverse ligament is lax or not intact, the atlantoaxial joint is allowed to sublux and may compress the spinal cord, causing symptoms that may include headache, nausea, dizziness, abnormal pupil response, nystagmus, neck pain, respiratory failure, paraplegia, quadriplegia, and even death. Conditions and disorders that are associated with atlantoaxial instability include Down syndrome, rheumatoid arthritis, and trauma.

There are two alar ligaments, each attaching to one side of the dens to a prominence on the ipsilateral medial underside of the occipital bone called the occipital condyle. These ligaments limit the amount of rotation of the head and contralateral lateral flexion of the head. Injuries to these ligaments are rare and usually caused by trauma. Symptoms may be subtle and may include neck pain and tenderness,[7] feeling like the head is too heavy, headache, cervical radiculopathy and/or myopathy, paraspinal muscle spasm, and hypermobility with a passive motion test.[8]

Vertebral Column

The vertebral column (spine) protects the spinal cord, acts as a shock absorber, acts as an attachment for muscles, transmits body weight while standing

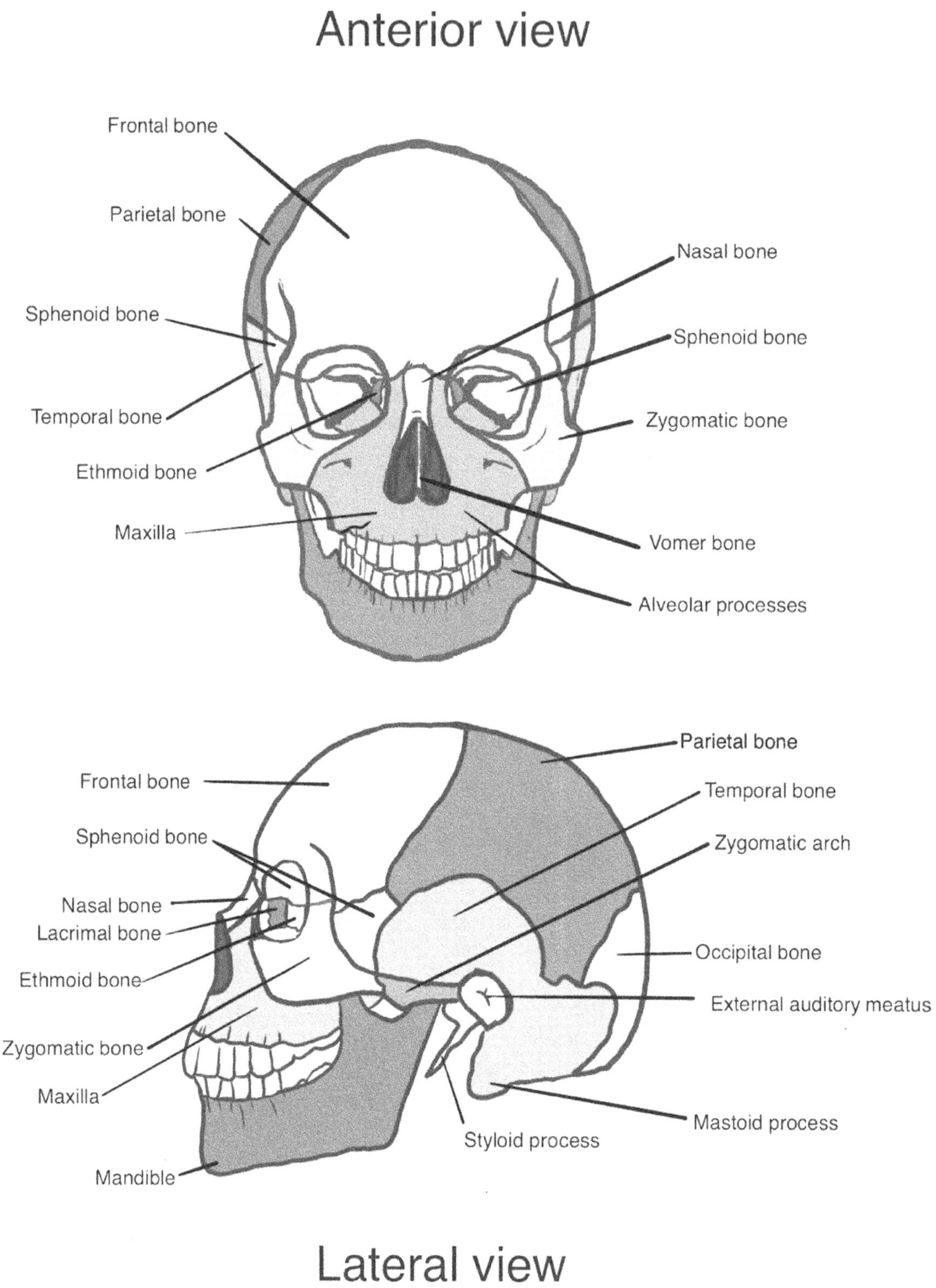

Anterior view

Frontal bone

Parietal bone

Nasal bone

Sphenoid bone

Sphenoid bone

Temporal bone

Zygomatic bone

Ethmoid bone

Maxilla

Vomer bone

Alveolar processes

Parietal bone

Frontal bone

Temporal bone

Sphenoid bone

Zygomatic arch

Nasal bone

Lacrimal bone

Ethmoid bone

Occipital bone

External auditory meatus

Zygomatic bone

Maxilla

Mastoid process

Mandible

Styloid process

Lateral view

Figure 4.3 Skeletal Cranium

Figure 4.4 Atlantoaxial Joint

Figure 4.5 Transverse and Alar Ligaments

Figure 4.6 Vertebral Column

and walking, and is composed of 33 vertebrae that are divided into 7 cervical, 12 thoracic, 5 lumbar, 5 sacral, and 4 coccygeal bone segments. These segments are separated by cartilaginous intervertebral discs (IVD). The spine has four normal curves: The cervical spine is lordotic (convex anteriorly), the thoracic spine has a kyphotic curve (concave anteriorly), the lumbar spine has a lordotic curve, and the sacrum has a kyphotic curve. These spinal segments allow for flexion, extension, lateral flexion, and torsional movements. Motions are limited depending on the specific region of the spine based on the shape and orientation of the zygapophyseal joints (facets), articular capsule tension of the facet joints, attachment to the rib cage, resistance of muscles and ligaments, and soft tissue bulk (Figure 4.6).[9]

Joints of the vertebral column are listed in Table 4.1.[10–12]

Major ligaments of the spine are listed in Table 4.2.[10,13]

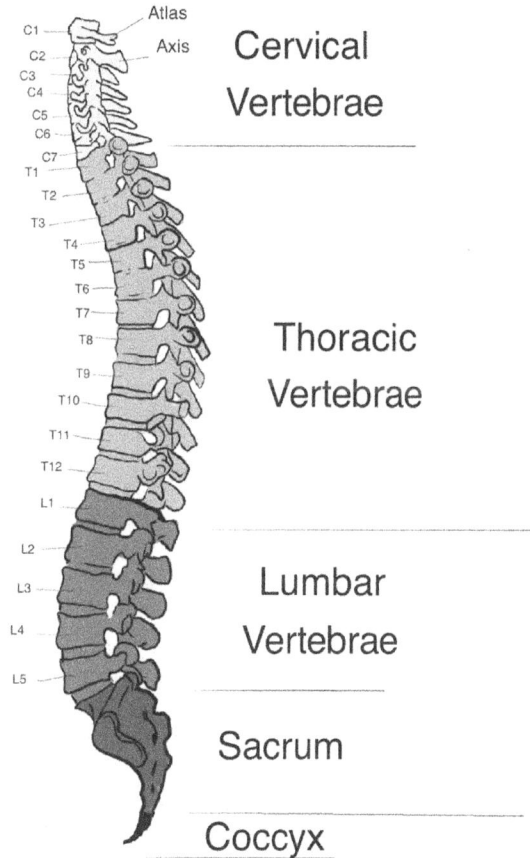

The spinal cord is within the spinal column extending from the brainstem to the level of L1–L2 where it forms the conus medullaris. Distally, the vertebral canal contains a bundle of nerve roots called the *cauda equina* (horse's tail) because of its appearance.

Table 4.1 Joints of the Vertebral Column

Vertebral Joints	Location	Jobs/Motions
Cartilaginous (symphyses)	• Between the vertebral bodies and IVD from C2 to S1	• Holds the vertebrae together
Uncovertebral	• Between the uncinate processes on the superolateral surface of a vertebral body and the inferolateral surfaces of the vertebral bodies of the vertebral bodies that are superior to them from C3–C7	• Control cervical spine movements • Stabilizes the neck
Zygapophyseal (facet)	• Between the superior and inferior articular processes of adjoining vertebrae and are enclosed by a joint capsules	• *Cervical*: Slope inferiorly from anterior to posterior allowing flexion, extension, lateral flexion, and rotation • *Thoracic*: Joints are oriented vertically permitting rotation but limiting flexion–extension • *Lumbar*: Oriented in the sagittal plane with adjacent processes interlocked allowing only limited flexion–extension and lateral flexion • *Thoracic*: Joints are vertically oriented, allowing for rotation while restricting flexion and extension
Atlanto-occipital	• A pair of condyloid synovial joints between the superior articular surfaces of the atlas and the occipital bone condyles	• Permits flexion-extension of the head (the nodding yes motion) • Permits slight lateral flexion and rotation
Atlanto-axial	• *Lateral* (2): Between inferior facts of lateral C1 and the superior articular facets of C2 • *Median*: A synovial pivot joint between the dens and the anterior arch of the atlas	• Permits head rotation
Costovertebral (head of ribs)	• Superior and Inferior facets at the head of the ribs articulate • Ribs 2–9 articulate with the bodies of two adjacent vertebrae • Ribs 1, 11, and 12 have one facet on the corresponding thoracic vertebrae	• Allows ribs to lift up (anteriorly) and outward (laterally) during breathing • Allows a small degree of gliding and rotation
Costotransverse	• Between articular facets on the tubercle of the rib and the transverse process of its numerically equivalent vertebra (ribs 1–10)	
Sacroiliac (SI)	• Between the spine and pelvis	• A stiff synovial joint with only a few degrees of motion • Provides stability to the trunk • Offsets the load of the trunk to the lower limbs

Table 4.2 Major Ligaments of the Spine

Spinal Ligament	Location	Provides
Posterior longitudinal	• Along the posterior surface of vertebral bodies within the vertebral canal between C2 and the sacrum	• Weakly resists hyperflexion • Prevents posterior herniation of intervertebral discs
Anterior longitudinal	• Anterolateral surfaces of the vertebral bodies and IVD from the occipital bone and C1 to the sacrum	• Prevents hyperextension of the spine
Ligamenta flava	• Connect laminae of adjacent vertebral arches on each side	• Resists separation of the laminae during flexion to aid in a return of the vertebral column to its erect anatomical posture
Supraspinous ligament	• Connects the tips of the spinous processes from C7 to the sacrum	• Prevents separation of the spinous processes during flexion • Resists hyperflexion
Nuchal	• Triangular band of the posterior neck (posterior border of foramen magnum) extending between the base of the skull and C7	• Resists flexion and restores head to its anatomical position • Acts as an attachment for muscles of the posterior neck and shoulder
Interspinous	• Connect adjacent vertebral spine processes	• Limits flexion • Limits hyperflexion • Stabilizes lumbar vertebrae
Intertransverse	• Connect the transverse process of adjoining vertebrae	• Limits lateral flexion of the vertebral column

Thoracic Cage

Men and women each have 12 pairs of curved, flat bones that form the thoracic cage (rib cage) (Figure 4.7). Seven pairs articulate directly with the sternum (which is the bone in the anterior midline of the chest), while three other pairs indirectly attach by costal cartilage. In adults, the sternum is comprised of three fused bones (cephalad to caudal): manubrium, body of the sternum, and xiphoid. The ribs provide protection to the heart, lungs, and thoracic blood vessels.

Most ribs have the following features: a head with two articular facets, tubercle (a knobby prominence), neck, shaft, and costal groove. The exceptions to these include:[14]

- The first rib is short, has two costal grooves, and one articular facet.
- The second rib has a tuberosity (a large tubercle) on the superior surface for the serratus anterior muscle attachment.
- The tenth rib has only one articular facet.

- The eleventh rib has one articular facet and no neck.
- The twelfth rib has one articular facet and no neck

Upper Extremity

The upper extremity has three sections—the upper arm, forearm, and hand—and extends from the shoulder and contains 30 bones, 27 of which are in the hand.[15,16]

SHOULDER GIRDLE

Joints of the shoulder girdle include the glenohumeral joint (GHJ), sternoclavicular joint (SCJ), acromioclavicular joint (ACJ), and scapulothoracic joints.

Scapula and Glenohumeral Joint

Scapula The scapula is a flat and triangular-shaped bone on the posterior aspect of the thoracic cage and has two processes: the coracoid and acromion (Figure 4.8). It has a ridge (spine of the

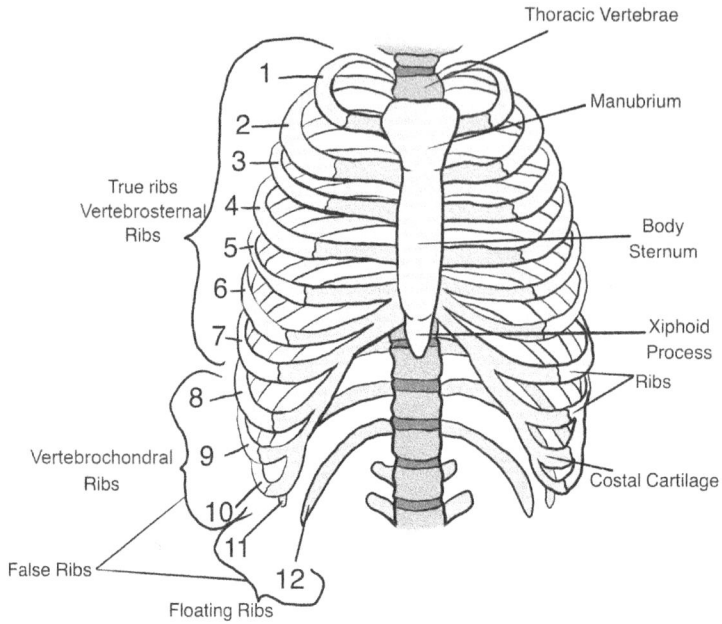

Figure 4.7 Thoracic Cage

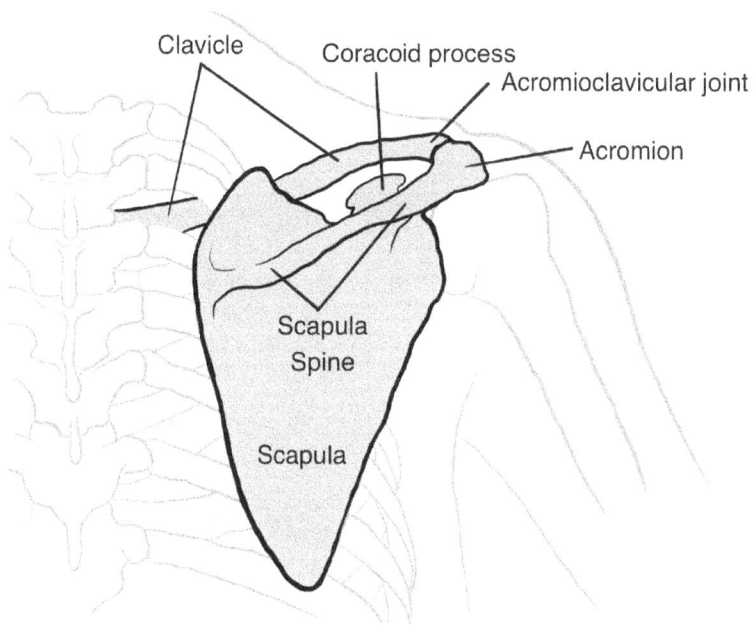

Figure 4.8 Scapula/GHJ

scapula) on the posterior surface that separates it unevenly into a superior fossa (supraspinous fossa) and a larger inferior infraspinous fossa.[17] The scapulothoracic joint is not a true joint but slides between the medial scapular border and ribs 2–7. Motions occurring at the scapulothoracic joint include primary motion of elevation/depression; secondary motions of protraction/retraction, upward/downward rotation, internal (IR)/external rotation (ER), anterior/posterior tipping; and shoulder abduction (60 degrees of abduction after GH does 120 degrees).[18]

Several muscles originate on the scapula (aka shoulder blade) and attach to (insert on) the scapula.[17]

There are many ligaments involved with the GHJ, but those of the scapula are listed in Table 4.3.[19]

GHJ The humerus bone is the only bone of the upper arm, and it articulates proximally with the glenoid fossa of the scapula. It is considered a synovial ball-and-socket joint and is the most mobile joint of the body.[20] It is enclosed by a joint capsule that wraps around the anatomic neck of the humerus to the rim of the glenoid fossa, and is stabilized by the joint congruity, glenoid labrum (fibrocartilaginous ring that lines the articular cartilage of the glenoid fossa), glenohumeral ligaments, and negative intraarticular pressure.[21] Motions of the GHJ include flexion, extension, internal/external rotation, and abduction/adduction. Due to the available motions and loose joint capsule, this joint is the most common to dislocate.[22] Synovial fluid and several bursae reduce friction of the joint (subacromial/subdeltoid bursa, subcoracoid bursa, subscapular bursa).

ELBOW

The humerus connects distally with the proximal ulna and radius bones, forming a synovial hinge joint. The proximal ulna and radius (which is not as long) also articulate with each other in a "pivot

Table 4.3 Ligaments of the Scapula

Ligament	Supports/Stabilizes
Coracohumeral	• Reinforces upper part of the GHJ capsule • Protects the humeral head
Coracoclavicular	• Attaches the scapula to the clavicle • Provides vertical stability at the ACJ • Transmits weight from the upper limb to the axial skeleton
Coracoacromial	• Protects the humeral head • Prevents superior dislocation of the humeral head • Transmits loads across the scapula
Acromioclavicular	• Reinforces upper part of the GHJ capsule • Stabilizes the AC joint
Superior glenohumeral	• Stabilizes the biceps brachii tendon • Reinforces the GHJ capsule • Improves anterior joint stability
Medial glenohumeral	• Reinforces the GHJ capsule • Improves anterior joint stability • Present in 88% of the population
Inferior glenohumeral	• Reinforces the GHJ capsule • Improves anterior joint stability • Strongest of the GHJ ligaments • Main stabilizer of the shoulder when abducted • Present in 94% of the population
Spiral glenohumeral	• Reinforces the GHJ capsule • Improves anterior joint stability • Present in 45% of the population

joint" that allows pronation–supination,[15] while wide and rectangular distal end radius articulates with the ulna as well as the scaphoid and lunate carpal bones of the hand forming a condyloid-type "wrist joint."

The bones of the elbow create two joints, the humeroulnar and humeroradial joints, both of which allow flexion–extension of the joint (Figure 4.9). Ligaments of the elbow are listed in Table 4.4.

HAND

The hand consists of two rows of carpal bones (scaphoid, lunate, triquetrum, pisiform, trapezium, trapezoid, capitate, and hamate), five metacarpal bones, and fourteen phalanges (forming the fingers) (Figure 4.10). Joints of the hand are listed in Table 4.5.

Ligaments of the wrist and hand are listed in Table 4.6.

Pelvis

Joints of the pelvis include the sacroiliac joint, pubic symphysis, sacrococcygeal joint, and the Hip joint. The pelvis is formed by the bony pelvis (two hip bones that are jointed to the sacrum [sacroiliac joint]) and coccyx of the vertebral column, the pelvic cavity, the pelvic floor, and perineum.[23] It supports the weight of the upper body and acts as an attachment for the lower limbs and trunk muscles. The bony pelvis may be divided into an anterior and posterior part. The anterior part, called the pelvic girdle, is composed of two innominate (latin for 'not named') bones formed by the pubis, ischium, and ilium, and connects posteriorly to the coccyx and sacrum (spine).[23] The pubis curves medially where it meets the contralateral pubis to form the cartilaginous pubic symphysis. The top of the iliac bone forms the palpable "hip bone" and

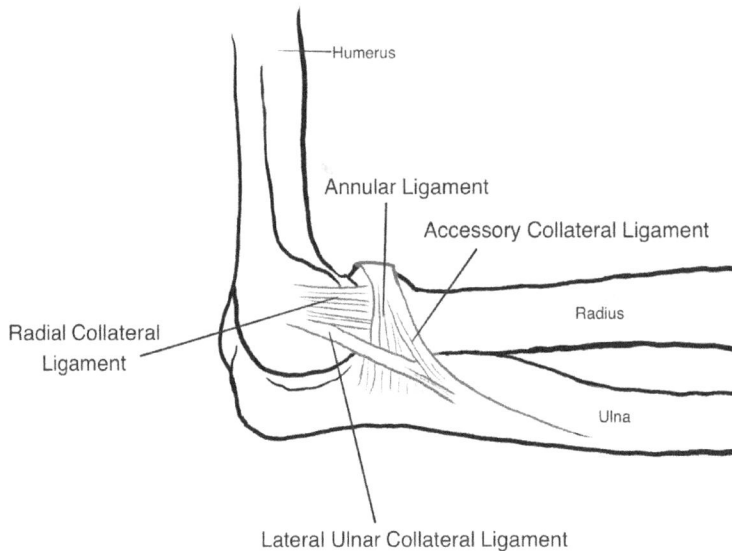

Figure 4.9 Elbow

Table 4.4 Ligaments of the Elbow

Elbow Ligament	Stabilizes/Supports
Ulnar collateral	Stabilizes the elbow during overhead activities and throwing Resists valgus forces
Radial collateral	Stabilizes the lateral elbow and resists varus forces
Annular	Stabilizes proximal radioulnar joint
Quadrate	Stabilizes the joint

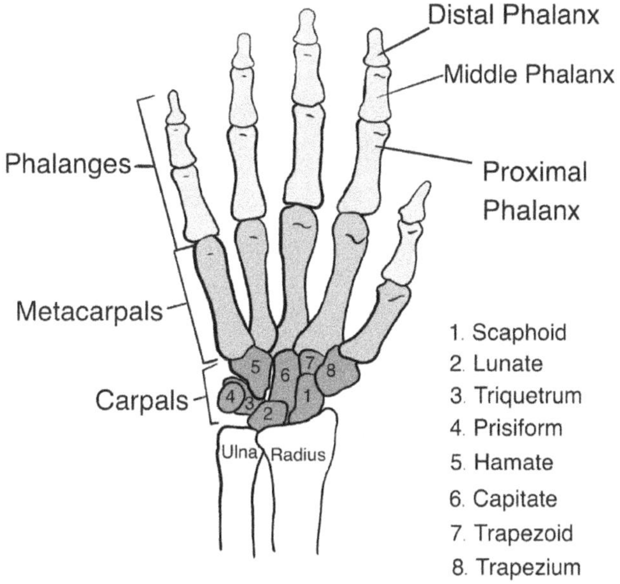

Figure 4.10 Hand

Table 4.5 Joints of the Hand

Hand Joint	Motions
Radiocarpal	Flexion/extension Abduction/adduction
Midcarpal	Flexion/extension Abduction/adduction
Carpometacarpal (CMC) (thumb)	Flexion/extension Abduction/adduction Circumduction Opposition
Carpometacarpal (CMC) (fingers)	Flexion–extension
Metacarpophalangeal (MCP)	Flexion/extension Abduction/adduction Circumduction
Interphalangeal (IP) (thumb)	Flexion Minimal extension
Proximal interphalangeal joint (PIP)	Flexion/extension
Distal interphalangeal joint (DIP)	Flexion/extension

Table 4.6 Ligaments of the Wrist and Hand

Ligaments	Supports/Stabilizes
Collateral	Prevents sideways (finger/thumb) movement of joint
Volar plate	Prevents backward bending of PIP joint during straightening of the fingers
Radial and ulnar collateral	Stability to wrist
Volar radiocarpal	Supports palm side of wrist
Dorsal radiocarpal	Supports back of wrist
Ulnocarpal and radioulnar	Main support of wrist

is called an ala (wing) (Figure 4.11). Joints of the pelvis are listed in Table 4.7.

Ligaments of the pelvis lend flexible strength to the pelvic cavity and support some of the internal pelvic structures of the pelvis, and are listed in Table 4.8.

HIP JOINT

The ilium, pubis, and ischium create a cup-shaped *acetabulum* on the lateral side of the hip bone where the femur articulates (hip joint) and covers ~40% of the femoral head. The movements and functions of the hip joint are listed in Table 4.7. It is a ball-and-socket synovial joint connecting the

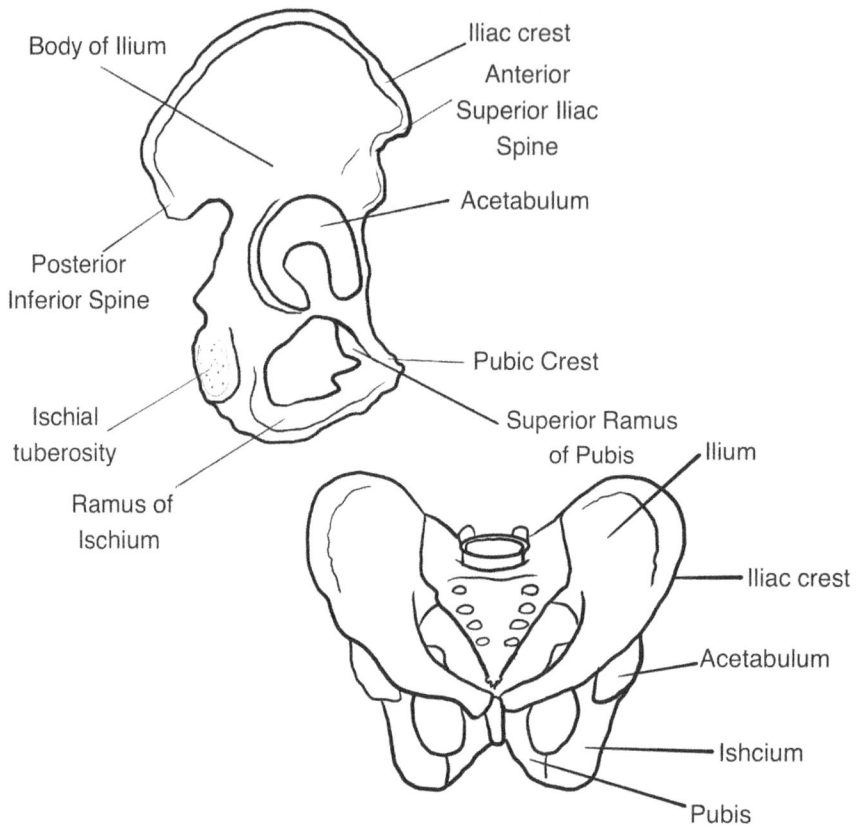

Figure 4.11 Pelvis

Table 4.7 Joints of the Pelvis

Joints of the Pelvis	Jobs/Movements
Sacroiliac	• Slight gliding and rotation
Pubic symphysis[24]	• Keeps the pelvic bones together during activity • Allows 2 mm of movement and 1 degree of rotation • Absorbs shock when walking/running • Becomes more flexible in pregnancy for giving birth
Sacrococcygeal	• Stability of the joint via cartilage
Hip joint	• Provides dynamic support of body weight • Facilitates force transmission from axial skeleton to the lower extremities • Allows flexion/extension, IR/ER, abduction/adduction

Table 4.8 Ligaments of the Pelvis

Ligament	Supports/Stabilizes
Iliolumbar[25]	• Superior and inferior bands extend from the transverse processes in a V-shape with superior bands inserting on the iliac crest and inferior bands blending with the anterior sacroiliac ligament • Stabilizes and strengthens the lumbosacral (LS) joint • Restricts the rotation at the LS joint
Sacroiliac (SI), anterior[25,26]	• Forms the anteroinferior part of the joint capsule • Supports the SI joint
Sacroiliac, interosseous	• Fills the gaps between the ilium and sacrum in the posterosuperior part of the joint
Sacroiliac, posterior	• Runs between the posterior superior iliac spine (PSIS), part of the iliac crest and sacral crests
Sacrospinous[25–27]	• Triangular extending from the coccyx and sacrum to the ischial spine • Separates the greater sciatic foramen form the lesser sciatic foramen
Sacrotuberous[25–27]	• Fan-shaped and attached to the SI ligaments, posterior superior iliac spine (PSIS), proximal coccyx, and sacrum • Forms the inferior part of the lesser sciatic foramen • Is the posteromedial part of the greater sciatic foramen • Provides stability to the posterior pelvis
Pubic, superior[26]	• Extends between pubic tubercles • Supports the pubic symphysis
Pubic, (inferior) arcuate	• Supports the pubic symphysis
Obturator membrane[26]	• Not officially a ligament • Spans the inner margin of the obturator foramen • Acts as the origin for the obturator externus and internus muscles
Inguinal[28]	• Runs between the ASIS and pubic tubercle • Forms the inguinal canal floor • Has extensions: Lacunar ligament, pectinate ligament

lower limb to the pelvic girdle and is stabilized by "bony and ligamentous restraints,"[29] a labrum (collagen fibers surrounding the acetabulum), and a joint capsule.

Ligaments of the hip joint are listed in Table 4.9.

Lower Extremity

The lower extremity may be divided into three sections: the thigh, leg, and foot. It extends from the hip and has 30 bones: the femur, patella, tibia, fibula, tarsal bones, metatarsals, and phalanges. The femur bone is the largest bone of the body and the only bone of the thigh and has a rounded proximal head that articulates with the hip as a ball-and-socket joint,[32] a greater trochanter that projects upward above the base of the neck,

is located laterally, and acts as a muscle attachment. Superomedially, the lesser trochanter acts as a muscle attachment. The distal end of the bone articulates with the patella anteriorly and the tibia distally and along with the fibula, ligaments, and muscles form the knee joint. Articulating surfaces include the lateral and medial condylar femur and tibia, and the anteroposterior articulation between the patella and femur (Figure 4.12).[33]

KNEE

The knee is the largest joint in the body and is primarily a hinge joint. It is a bicondylar compound synovial joint that allows flexion–extension and a small amount of medial–lateral rotation.[33] The knee joint has three compartments: the medial tibiofemoral compartment, the lateral tibiofemoral

Table 4.9 Ligaments of the Hip Joint

Ligaments[29]	Supports/Stabilizes
Ischiofemoral	• Attaches the posterior acetabular rim/labrum, courses circumferentially to insert on the anterior femur • Limits hip IR • Limits hip abduction with flexion
Iliofemoral	• Triangular shaped attaching the intertrochanteric line of the femur and the anterior inferior iliac spine (AIIS) • Strongest ligament in the body • Limits hip extension • Limits hip ER • Assists static erect posture • Due to its strength, 90% of hip dislocations are posterior (not anterior)
Pubofemoral	• Extends from anterior pubic ramus to anterior intertrochanteric fossa • Limits hip abduction • Limits hip extension
Annular (zona orbicularis)	• Encircles the femoral neck • Acts as a locking ring resisting hip distraction
Ligamentum teres	• Pyramid shaped from the transverse acetabular ligament attaching an anterior and stronger posterior bundle to the ischial and pubic bases • Before puberty provides secondary blood supply to femoral head • After puberty is a secondary stabilizer of the capsular ligaments[30]
Acetabular labrum	• Limits extreme ROM • Deepens the acetabulum • Dissipates large forces with stride in athletics • Provides a sealing rim around the joint • Resists hip distraction[31]

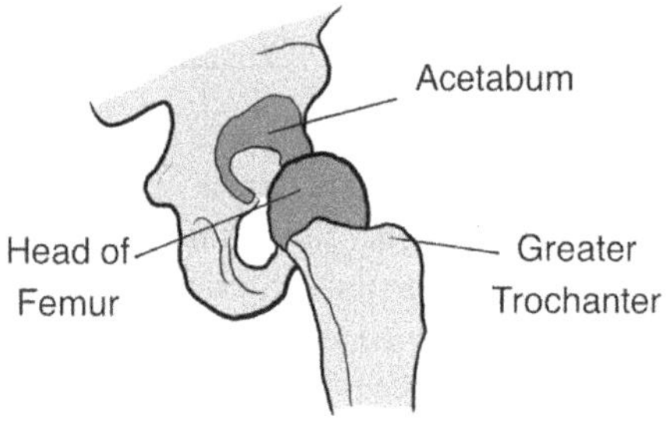

Figure 4.12 Hip Joint and Femur

compartment, and the patellofemoral compartment. It is stabilized by the quadriceps, a joint capsule, extracapsular ligaments, and intraarticular ligaments. Extracapsular ligaments include the patellar ligament, lateral collateral ligament (LCL), medial collateral ligament (MCL), oblique popliteal ligament, and the arcuate popliteal ligament. Intraarticular ligaments include the anterior cruciate ligament (ACL) that prevents knee hyperextension, posterior femoral displacement, and anterior tibial displacement in the flexed knee; the posterior cruciate ligament (PCL) that prevents hyperflexion and posterior tibial displacement and tightens the knee joint; and the lateral and medial menisci that reduces friction during articulation, acts as a shock absorber, and is a static stabilizer.[33] The ACL, PCL, LCL, and MCL all attach the tibia to the femur (Figure 4.13).

Patella

Commonly known as the kneecap, the patella is a sesamoid bone that is anterior to the knee joint in the femoral sulcus and lies inside the quadriceps tendon. It protects the knee joint from damage and gives a mechanical advantage to the quadriceps femoris muscle to pull on the tibia during knee extension. The patellar tendon runs from the apex of the patella to the tibial tuberosity of the femur. The infrapatellar bursa separates the

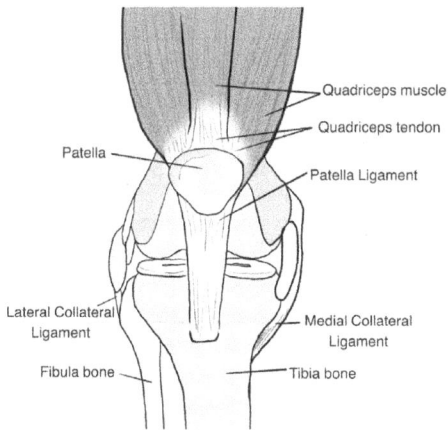

Figure 4.13 Knee and Patella

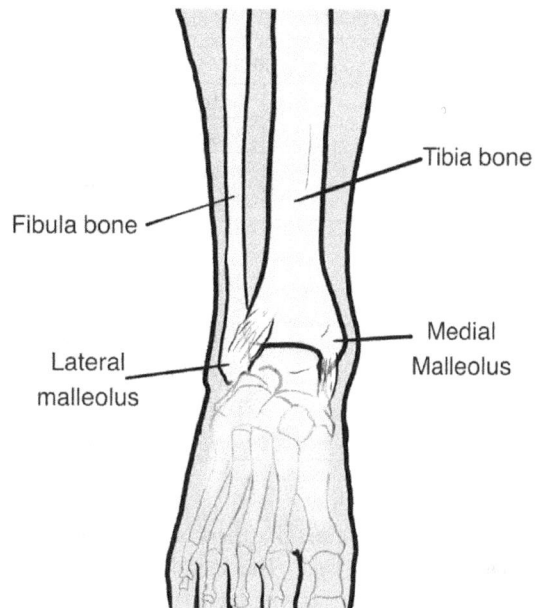

Figure 4.14 Ankle

patellar ligament from the tibia. The patella and femur form the patellofemoral joint between the posterior surface of the patella and the trochlear surface of the distal anterior femur.[34] The average dimensions of the patella are 4–4.5 cm long, 5–5.5 cm wide, and 2–2.5 cm thick, and it has a layer of cartilage on the articular side. The anterior side is concave, while the divided articular side has a medial and lateral half.

The patella provides 31% of total knee extension torque when the knee is fully extended, but only 13% between 90 degrees and 120 degrees of flexion.[34] It moves in multiple planes and movements include superior–inferior, medial–lateral, medial–lateral tilt, and medial–lateral rotation.

LEG

The leg is comprised of the tibia, which is the second largest bone in the body, and the fibula, which is lateral to the tibia. The proximal tibia has medial and lateral plateaus each with a meniscus (cartilage). The fibula is connected to the tibia proximally by the tibiofibular joint and via the interosseous membrane distally. The distal tibia (called the medial malleolus) forms the medial border of the ankle, while the distal fibula (lateral malleolus) forms the lateral ankle.

ANKLE

The ankle joint (also called the talocrural joint) is a complex, hinged synovial joint and is formed by

Table 4.10 Motions of the Ankle Joint

Joint	Motions
Subtalar	• Inversion/eversion • Abduction/adduction • Plantarflexion/dorsiflexion
Tibiotalar	• Dorsiflexion • Plantarflexion
Transverse tarsal	• Inversion/eversion • Abduction/adduction • Plantarflexion/dorsiflexion

the distal tibia, distal fibula, and talus bones as well as ligaments. There are three joints in the ankle including the talocalcaneal (subtalar) joint, tibiotalar joint, and talocalcaneonavicular (transverse-tarsal) joint (Figure 4.14). Motions occurring at these joints are listed in Table 4.10.

Important ligaments of the ankle to know are listed in Table 4.11.

FOOT

The foot provides a platform for stance, shock absorption during gait, and a lever to propel the body forward.[35] It is subdivided into the hindfoot,

Table 4.11 Ligaments of the Ankle

Ligaments		Activity That Causes Damage
Syndesmotic	Anterior tibiofibular	Extreme twisting or forceful blows
	Posterior tibiofibular	
	Interosseous	
	Transverse tibiofibular	
Lateral collateral	Posterior talofibular	Inversion ankle sprain
	Calcaneofibular	
	Anterior talofibular	
Deltoid (medial collateral)	Posterior tibiotalar	Eversion ankle sprain
	Tibiocalcaneal	
	Tibionavicular	
	Anterior tibiotalar	

midfoot, and forefoot, and has 26 bones: tarsals (there are 7), metatarsals (there are 5), and phalanges (there are 14).[35] The tarsal bones include the talus, calcaneus, navicular, medial cuneiform, intermediate cuneiform, lateral cuneiform, and cuboid. You may remember them using the mnemonic "Tiger cubs need MILC." The hindfoot (posterior aspect of foot) is comprised of the talus, calcaneus, and two tarsal bones, and is referred to as the subtalar joint.[35] The midfoot is comprised of the navicular; cuboid; and medial, middle, and lateral cuneiform bones (five of the seven tarsal bones); and allows for inversion/eversion of the foot. The forefoot (anterior aspect of the foot) is comprised of the metatarsals, phalanges (forming the toes), and sesamoid bones, and can be further divided into medial and lateral columns.[35] Rays (a metatarsal and the associated phalanges) one through three make up the medial column, while rays four and five comprise the lateral column. Rays one and two are crucial for balance, weight bearing, and gait (Figure 4.15).[35]

THE MUSCULAR SYSTEM

A list of muscles involved in balance and their innervations is in Chapter 16. There are three types of muscle tissue: cardiac muscle forming the heart, smooth muscle forming the walls of blood vessels and hollow organs, and skeletal muscle that attaches to bones to provide voluntary movement.[1] There are over 600 muscles in the human body, and they can be categorized into four groups:[1]

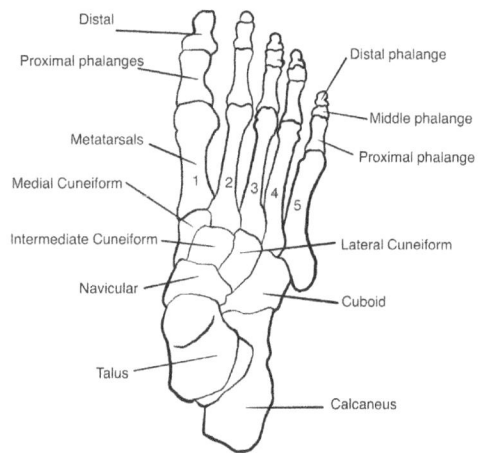

Figure 4.15 Foot

1. Muscles of the head and neck
2. Muscles of the trunk
3. Muscles of the upper limbs
4. Muscles of the lower limbs

All conscious body movements are produced by the activation of striated skeletal muscles that are attached to bones of the skeletal system (providing structural support) via tendons. Each individual muscle fiber (comprised of myofibrils containing the myofilaments of actin and myosin forming the fundamental unit of contraction called a sarcomere) is covered by a connective tissue sheath called an endomysium, with bundles of muscle fibers called fasciculi, and the tissue sheath covering each fasciculus is known as the perimysium.[36,37] The tissue sheath surrounding the entire muscle group is called the epimysium.[36,37]

The primary artery supplying blood to a muscle generally is parallel to the longitudinal axis of the muscle fiber and gives off tributaries that run perpendicular to the primary artery.[38] These tributaries then branch into arterioles and then terminal arterioles.[36,38,39]

Muscles used to aid in balance generally include core muscles (pelvic floor, internal/external obliques, transverse abdominis, rectus abdominis, and erector spinae), and hip and lower extremity muscles.

There are a number of deficits affecting the musculoskeletal system that may impair balance with common deficits including weakness to hip muscles, reduced ankle range of motion (ROM), and kyphotic postures displacing the center of gravity. Neural components needed for balance may delay muscle activation and place a person at risk of falling.

A study by Kim and Jang looked at the effect of ankle ROM in elderly individuals and found an immediate improvement in balance post-ankle mobilization.[40] In a systematic review with meta-analysis of core strengthening and performance, Rodríguez-Perea et al. observed that core training improved balance outcomes and certain aspects of sports performance.[41]

As we walk over various terrains, precise and dynamic coordination of multiple muscles, including those of the lower limbs and trunk, is required.[42] During standing balance control as well as walking, perturbations can elicit long-latency (~100 ms) muscle responses to return the body to postural equilibrium.[42] Chvatal and Ting studied muscle synergies in standing, walking, and during perturbations during both, and suggest that a common set of muscle synergies forms a motor repertoire for both locomotion and reactive balance control.[42] These synergies "appear to be modified during voluntary movements and walking to support the return of the body to the desired trajectory"[42-44] and can be recruited by a variety of neural pathways for voluntary, rhythmic, and reactive motor behaviors.[45]

A study of the effects of shoe insoles in subjects (n = 45) older than 65 years of age found that use of a heel cup with an arch support worn for at least 4 hours a day for 8 weeks enhanced standing balance.[7]

Muscle Actions

Muscles and their actions on joints are listed in Tables 4.12–4.39.

Muscle Tone

Muscle tone has been defined as "a residual tension in a muscle at rest" and is a continuous partial contraction of the muscles, which maintains posture.[47] Muscle tone is classified as either "postural" or "phasic." Postural muscle tone occurs in axial muscles where gravity is the most important inciting factor, whereas phasic muscle tone occurs in the extremities as rapid and short-duration responses and results from rapid stretching of a tendon and muscle spindle.[48,49]

To assess muscle tone, a patient's muscle is passively stretched, or a joint is passively moved. The examiner should also note any muscle atrophy

Table 4.12 Muscles of Cervical Rotation

Muscles of Cervical Rotation
• Sternocleidomastoid (contralateral rotation)
• Anterior scalene (contralateral rotation)
• Longus capitis (ipsilateral rotation)
• Longus colli (contralateral rotation by unilateral contraction)
• Suboccipital muscles (ipsilateral head rotation at C1–C2 by unilateral contraction)
• Semispinalis capitis (contralateral head and neck by unilateral contraction)
• Semispinalis cervicis (contralateral head and neck by unilateral contraction)
• Multifidus (contralateral by unilateral contraction)

Table 4.13 Muscles of Cervical Lateral Flexion

Muscles of Cervical Lateral Flexion
• Sternocleidomastoid (ipsilateral) • Scalene muscles (anterior, lateral, and posterior) (ipsilateral) • Rectus capitis lateralis (ipsilateral at C1–C2) • Longus colli (ipsilateral by bilateral contraction) • Splenius capitis (head ipsilateral rotation + lateral flexion by unilateral contraction) • Splenius cervicis (neck ipsilateral rotation + lateral flexion by unilateral contraction) • Semispinalis capitis (ipsilateral head and neck by unilateral contraction) • Semispinalis cervicis (ipsilateral head and neck by unilateral contraction) • Rotatores cervicis (rotate and laterally flex ipsilaterally by unilateral contraction) • Intertransversarii • Trapezius (ipsilateral by unilateral contraction of superior fibers) • Multifidus (ipsilateral by unilateral contraction)

Table 4.14 Muscles of Cervical/Capital Flexion–Extension

Muscles of cervical/head flexion	• Sternocleidomastoid muscles (at inferior C-spine) • Anterior scalene • Rectus capitis anterior (at C1–C2) • Longus capitis (bilateral contraction) • Longus colli
Muscles of cervical/head extension	• Sternocleidomastoid (at C1–C2 and superior C-spine) • Splenius capitis (head and neck by bilateral contraction) • Splenius cervicis (neck by bilateral contraction) • Suboccipital muscles (head at C1–C2 by unilateral contraction) • Semispinalis capitis (head and neck by bilateral contraction) • Semispinalis cervicis (head and neck by bilateral contraction) • Rotatores cervicis (bilateral contraction) • Interspinales • Trapezius (bilateral contraction of superior fibers) • Iliocostalis (neck by bilateral contraction) • Longissimus (neck by bilateral contraction) • Multifidus (neck by bilateral contraction)

when documenting muscle tone. Terms used when documenting muscle tone include:

- *Hypertonia:* An increase in resting muscle tension secondary to a communication error in the central nervous system.
- *Lead pipe:* Refers to a type of rigidity in which increased resistance is noted throughout the entire movement when the limb is passively and slowly moved.
- *Rigidity (dystonic hypertonia):* A type of hypertonicity, it refers to stiffness of the muscle. It includes cogwheel and lead pipe variations.

- *Spasticity (spastic hypertonia):* A type of hypertonia in which a velocity-dependent increase in muscle tone is noted when the limb is passively moved in a quick manner. The patient exhibits exaggerated reflexes and muscle spasms with movement.
- *Clonus:* Defined as "regular, repetitive, rhythmic contractions of a muscle subjected to sudden, maintained stretch."[50]
- *Clasp-knife phenomenon:* During a passive stretch, more resistance is felt in the initial part of movement, then a sudden release occurs.

Table 4.15 Muscles of Trunk Flexion, Extension, Side Flexion, and Rotation

Muscles of trunk flexion	• Internal abdominal oblique (bilateral contraction) • External abdominal oblique (bilateral contraction) • Rectus abdominis
Muscles of trunk extension	• Interspinales (lumbar) • Longissimus • Spinalis (T-spine by bilateral contraction) • Multifidus (bilateral contraction)
Muscles of trunk side flexion	• Semispinalis (T-spine by bilateral contraction) • Intertransversarii • Internal abdominal oblique (ipsilateral by unilateral contraction) • External abdominal oblique (ipsilateral by unilateral contraction) • Multifidus (ipsilateral by unilateral contraction)
Muscles of trunk rotation	• Semispinalis (contralateral T-spine trunk by unilateral contraction) • Internal abdominal oblique (ipsilateral by unilateral contraction) • External abdominal oblique (contralateral by unilateral contraction) • Transversus abdominis (ipsilateral by unilateral contraction) • Multifidus (contralateral by unilateral contraction)

Table 4.16 Muscles of Rib Elevation and Depression

Muscles of rib elevation	• External intercostals • Serratus posterior superior (ribs 2–5)
Muscles of rib Elevation or depression	• Internal intercostals • Innermost intercostals
Muscles of rib depression	• Serratus posterior inferior (ribs 9–12) • Rectus abdominis (abdominal muscle used while ambulating) • Pyramidalis (abdominal muscle used while ambulating)

Table 4.17 Muscles of the Core

Muscles of the Core
• Hip stabilizers • Trunk (torso) muscles • Shoulder stabilizers • Abdominal muscles • Gluteal muscles • Diaphragm • Pelvic floor

Table 4.18 Muscles of the Rotator Cuff

Muscles that originate from the scapula	• *Rotator cuff muscles:* **S**upraspinatus, infraspinatus, teres minor, **s**ubscapularis (SITS) • *Other muscles:* Deltoid, triceps brachii (long head), teres major, latissimus dorsi, coracobrachialis, biceps brachii, omohyoid muscles
Muscles that attach to (insert onto) the scapula	• Trapezius, levator scapulae, rhomboid major, rhomboid minor, serratus anterior, pectoralis minor muscle

Table 4.19 Muscles of Scapular Motion

Muscles of scapular protraction	• Serratus anterior • Assisting muscle: Pectoralis minor (draws scapula anteroinferiorly)
Muscles of scapular retraction	• Rhomboid major • Rhomboid minor • Trapezius (middle fibers)
Muscles of scapular elevation	• Levator scapulae • Trapezius (upper fibers)
Muscles of scapular depression	• Latissimus dorsi • Trapezius (lower fibers) • Assisting muscle: Pectoralis minor
Muscles of scapular medial rotation	• Rhomboid major • Rhomboid minor • Levator scapulae
Muscles of scapular lateral rotation	• Serratus anterior (lower five digitations) • Trapezius (lower fibers) • Trapezius (upper fibers)

Table 4.20 Muscles of Shoulder Flexion/Extension

Muscles of Shoulder Flexion	Muscles of Shoulder Extension
• Coracobrachialis • Anterior deltoid • Biceps brachii • Pectoralis major clavicular head when acting alone	• Latissimus dorsi • Assisting muscles: • Teres major, posterior deltoid, triceps brachii (long head)

Table 4.21 Muscles of Shoulder Abduction/Adduction

Muscles of Shoulder Abduction	Muscles of Shoulder Adduction
• Supraspinatus (0°–15°) • Lateral deltoid	• Subscapularis • Latissimus dorsi • Pectoralis major (clavicular and sternocostal heads) • Assisting muscles: • Teres minor, teres major

Table 4.22 Muscles of Shoulder Internal/External Rotation

Muscles of Shoulder IR	Muscles of Shoulder ER
• Subscapularis • Teres major • Latissimus dorsi • Pectoralis major (clavicular and sternocostal heads) • Assisting muscle: • Anterior deltoid	• Infraspinatus • Teres minor

Table 4.23 Muscle of Shoulder Scaption

Muscle of Shoulder Scaption
• Deltoid

- *Cogwheel:* Refers to a type of rigidity in which the limb moves as if it is using gears, moving in small increments with passive motion.
- *Hypotonia:* A decrease in resting muscle tension secondary to a communication error in the central nervous system.
- *Flaccid:* The muscle lacks tension at rest.
- *Normal:* Normal muscle tone refers to balanced tension of muscles at rest.

Table 4.24 Muscles of Wrist Flexion/Extension

Muscles of Wrist Flexion	Muscles of Wrist Extension
• Flexor digitorum superficialis (humeral and radial heads) • Flexor digitorum profundus • Flexor carpi ulnaris • Flexor carpi radialis • Flexor pollicis longus (weak wrist flexor) • Palmaris longus (weak wrist flexor) • Assisting muscle: Flexor digitorum superficialis	• Extensor carpi radialis longus • Extensor carpi radialis brevis • Extensor carpi ulnaris • Assisting muscle: Extensor digitorum (weak wrist extensor)

Table 4.25 Muscles of Wrist/Forearm Pronation/Supination

Muscles of Wrist/Forearm Pronation	Muscles of Wrist/Forearm Supination
• Pronator teres • Pronator quadratus • Brachioradialis (pronates to neutral when the forearm is in supination)	• Supinator • Assisting muscles: Biceps brachii (short and long heads)

Table 4.26 Muscles of Wrist Ulnar/Radial Deviation

Muscles of Wrist Ulnar Deviation (Adduction)	Muscles of Wrist Radial Deviation (Abduction)
• Extensor carpi ulnaris • Flexor carpi ulnaris	• Flexor carpi radialis • Extensor carpi radialis longus • Extensor carpi radialis brevis

THE SOMATOSENSORY SYSTEM

The somatosensory system provides information about body movement and position as well as sensations of touch, pain, temperature, pressure, and vibration. It has three main functions that mediate (1) our perception and reaction to stimuli from outside the body, (2) our perception and reaction to stimuli from inside the body, and (3) proprioceptive functions for perception and control of body position and balance.[51]

There are several types of somatosensory receptors, including *mechanoreceptors* that are stimulated by mechanical displacement of body tissues and mediate tactile and proprioceptive sensations, *thermoreceptors* that detect temperature, *nociceptors* that detect pain, and *chemoreceptors* that detect changes in the chemical composition of the blood.

Mechanoreceptors are the most numerous, and convey and process information from muscles, tendons, joints, and connective tissues of the musculoskeletal system. Information from these receptors allows for a sense of the position of body parts called *proprioception* and also of body movement called *kinesthesia*. The four main tactile mechanoreceptor groups are Merkel's disks, Meissner's corpuscles, Ruffini endings, and Pacinian corpuscles.[51]

SOMATOSENSORY NEURAL PATHWAYS

Each pathway of this cortex has a three-ordered neuronal series from the sensory receptor to the primary somatosensory cortex. The pathway (dorsal column medial lemniscus pathway [DCML]) is:[52]

Sensory receptor → dorsal root ganglion fibers → dorsal column of spinal cord → dorsal column white matter fasciculus gracilis below T6, and fasciculus cuneatus T6 and above) → nucleus gracilis and cuneatus respectively → decussate at the lower medulla and continue along the medial lemniscus to the ventral posterolateral nucleus of the thalamus→ through the internal capsule to reach the primary somatosensory cortex

The primary somatosensory cortex is located behind the central sulcus (postcentral gyrus) and receives information from the ventral posterolateral

Table 4.27 Muscles of Finger Flexion/Extension

Muscles of finger flexion	• Dorsalis interossei (MCP joints) • Palmar interossei (2nd, 4th, and 5th MCP joints) • Lumbricals (MCP joints) • Flexor digitorum profundus (MCP, PIP, and DIP) • Flexor pollicis longus (thumb MCP and IP joints) • Flexor digitorum superficialis (MCP and PIP joints) • Flexor pollicis brevis (thumb MC and MCP joints) • Opponens pollicis (thumb CMC joints)
Muscles of finger extension	• Doral interossei (IP joints) • Extensor indicis (MCP and IP joints) • Extensor pollicis brevis (thumb CMC and MCP joints) • Extensor pollicis longus (CMC, MCP, and IP joints) • Extensor digiti minimi (5th finger MCP and IP joints) • Extensor digitorum (2nd–5th MCP and IP joints) • Assisting muscles: Palmar interossei (assists IP joint), lumbricals (assists IP joint)

Table 4.28 Muscles of Finger Abduction/Adduction

Muscles of finger abduction	• Dorsal interossei (MCP joints) • Abductor digiti minimi (5th finger MCP joint) • Abductor pollicis longus (thumb CMC joint) • Abductor pollicis brevis (thumb CMC and MCP joints)
Muscles of finger adduction	• Adductor pollicis (oblique and transverse heads of thumb CMC and MCP joints) • Assisting muscles: Palmar interossei (thumb CMC and MCP joints)

Table 4.29 Muscles of Finger Opposition

Muscles of Finger Opposition
• Opponens digiti minimi (opposes 5th finger to thumb)   • Opponens pollicis (opposes thumb to the other fingers)   • Palmaris brevis (tenses skin of the ulnar side to aid grip)

Table 4.30 Muscles of Hip Flexion/Extension

Flexion	Extension
• Psoas major • Iliacus • Rectus femoris • Assisting muscles: • Pectineus, tensor fasciae latae (TFL), sartorius	• Gluteus maximus • Biceps femoris • Semitendinosus • Semimembranosus • Adductor magnus

Table 4.31 Muscles of Hip Abduction/Adduction

Abduction	Adduction

• Gluteus medius
 • Gluteus minimus
 • Assisting muscles:
   • TFL, piriformis, sartorius
	• Adductor longus
	 • Adductor brevis
	 • Adductor magnus
	 • Gracilis
	 • Assisting muscles:
	   • Pectineus, quadratus femoris, gluteus maximus

nucleus (VPL) of the thalamus via the internal capsule and corona radiata.[52] Ascending pathways of the somatosensory receptors for fine touch, pressure, vibration, and position sense project into the dorsal (posterior) column (fasciculus gracilis) and terminate in the caudal medulla at the nucleus gracilis. From there the medial lemniscus originates and projects to the VPL of the thalamus. VPL fibers connect to the primary sensory cortex and

Table 4.32 Muscles of Hip Internal/External Rotation

IR	ER
• Gluteus minimus • Gluteus medius • Assisting muscles: TFL, most adductor muscles	• Gluteus maximus • Obturator internus • Superior gemellus • Inferior gemellus • Quadratus femoris • Piriformis • Assisting muscles: Obturator externus, sartorius

Table 4.33 Muscles of the Superficial/Deep Pelvic Floor

Muscle Group	Muscle	Action
Superficial muscles	• Transverse perineal	• Fixates the perineal body • Supports the pelvic floor • Expulsion of semen in men • Expulsion of last drops of urine
	• Bulbospongiosus	• Males: Empties the urethra, assists in ejaculation and erection • Females: Erection of the clitoris, empties the greater vestibular glands • Both sexes: Supports the perineal body
	• Ischiocavernosus	• Helps to maintain the erections (penile/clitoral)
Deep muscles	• Coccygeus	• Supports pelvic viscera
	• Iliococcygeus (levator ani)	• Supports pelvic viscera
	• Pubococcygeus (levator ani)	• Supports pelvic viscera • Elevates the pelvic floor
	• Puborectalis	• Maintains fecal continence

Note: Pelvic floor muscles support the abdominal viscera and rectum by acting as a "floor" and a constrictor to the urethra, anus, and vaginal orifices.[46]

Table 4.34 Muscles of Knee Flexion/Extension

Muscles of Knee Flexion	Muscles of Knee Extension

• Semitendinosus (hamstring)
• Semimembranosus (hamstring)
• Biceps femoris (hamstring)
• Weak flexors:
  • Gracilis, sartorius, gastrocnemius, plantaris, popliteus
	• Rectus femoris (quads)
	• Vastus lateralis (quads)
	• Vastus medialis (quads)
	• Vastus intermedius (quads)
	• Assisting muscle:
	  • TFL

Table 4.35 Muscles of Knee Medial/Lateral Rotation

Muscles of Knee Medial Rotation	Muscles of Knee Lateral Rotation
• Popliteus • Semimembranosus • Semitendinosus • Assisting muscles: • Sartorius, gracilis	• Biceps femoris

Table 4.36 Muscles of Foot Dorsiflexion/Plantarflexion

Muscles of Foot Dorsiflexion	Muscles of Foot Plantarflexion
• Tibialis anterior • Extensor digitorum longus • Extensor hallucis longus • Fibularis tertius	• Gastrocnemius • Soleus • Flexor digitorum longus • Flexor hallucis longus • Fibular longus • Tibialis posterior

Table 4.37 Muscles of Foot Inversion/Eversion

Muscles Foot Inversion	Muscles of Foot Eversion
• Tibialis anterior • Tibialis posterior	• Fibularis longus • Fibularis tertius • Fibularis brevis

Table 4.38 Muscles of Toe Flexion/Extension

• Muscles of toe flexion	• Abductor hallucis (1st toe flexion) • Flexor digitorum brevis (2nd–5th PIP joints) • Abductor digiti minimi (5th toe flexion) • Lumbricals (flexes metatarsophalangeal joints) • Flexor hallucis brevis (1st toe metatarsophalangeal joint) • Flexor digit minimi brevis (1st toe metatarsophalangeal joint) • Plantar interossei (toes 3–5 metatarsophalangeal joints) • Dorsal interossei (toes 2–5 metatarsophalangeal joints) • Assisting muscles: • Quadratus plantae (toes 2–5)
• Muscles of toe extension	• Lumbricals (extends IP joints)

Table 4.39 Muscles of Toe Abduction/Adduction

• Muscles of toe abduction	• Abductor hallucis (1st toe abduction) • Abductor digiti minimi (5th toe abduction) • Dorsal interossei (toes 2–5 metatarsophalangeal joints)
• Muscles of toe adduction	• Adductor hallucis (1st toe adduction) • Plantar interossei (toes 3–5 adduction)

terminate topographically.[52] The somatosensory cortex has six layers and has a secondary somatosensory cortex in the parietal lobe to help process the sensory information received by the primary somatosensory cortex.[52]

SOMATOSENSORY REFLEXES

There are several reflexes mediated by the somatosensory system, including the withdrawal reflex, stretch reflex (aka the deep tendon reflex), crossed extensor reflex, Golgi tendon reflex, and flexor reflex.

1. *Withdrawal reflex*: Causes the withdrawal of a body part away from a painful stimulus.
2. *Stretch reflex*: Causes contraction of a muscle and the inhibition of the agonist muscle when a muscle is stretched.
3. *Crossed extensor reflex*: When one limb withdraws from pain, the opposite limb extends to help maintain balance.
4. *Golgi tendon reflex*: Causes a muscle to relax to prevent damage when tension on the muscle is too high.
5. *Flexor reflex*: Causes flexor muscles to contract in response to a painful stimulus.

Certain cervical somatosensory reflexes mirror vestibular reflexes. Similar to vestibular reflexes, these are named after the systems involved: *cervico-ocular reflex* (COR), *cervicocollic reflex* (CCR), and *cervicospinal reflex* (CSR). You will notice that if you were to replace *cervico-* with *vestibulo-*, you would have the vestibular reflexes (VOR, VCR, VSR). You initiate these cervical reflexes by the bending or turning of the head relative to the body.

Muscle spindles and joint receptors in the upper cervical spine provide the proprioceptive information needed for the reflexes.

The vestibular and the corresponding cervical reflexes act to accomplish the same things. While the vestibular reflexes use vestibular afferent information to drive the reflexes, the cervical reflexes use proprioceptive information. A significant difference between these groups of reflexes is that the cervical reflexes are very weak. At best they are useful as a supplement to the vestibular reflexes, with the afferent somatosensory information acting to supplement that of the vestibular system. They may become more important if there is vestibular damage, because then the neck receptors will function as a source of information regarding head motion and position.

Physical damage to the neck may sometimes help explain dizziness. This condition is also known as cervicogenic dizziness. If the patient has a history of neck or head trauma, whiplash injury, or severe degenerative disease of the cervical spine, the clinician must carefully screen the neck to see if symptoms correlate with cervical motions or palpation. Conditions like benign paroxysmal positional vertigo and vascular compression should also be considered.

SENSORY HOMUNCULUS

The sensory homunculus is a representation of which portion of the coronal cut of the postcentral gyrus corresponds with sensations from different parts of the body and can be used to localize lesions based on sensory deficits.[52] There is also a sensory homunculus in the cerebellum that represents points on the cerebellum where cutaneous electrical stimulation produces evoked responses, with evidence suggesting that the cerebellum sharpens the input from its afferent fibers (Figure 4.16).[53]

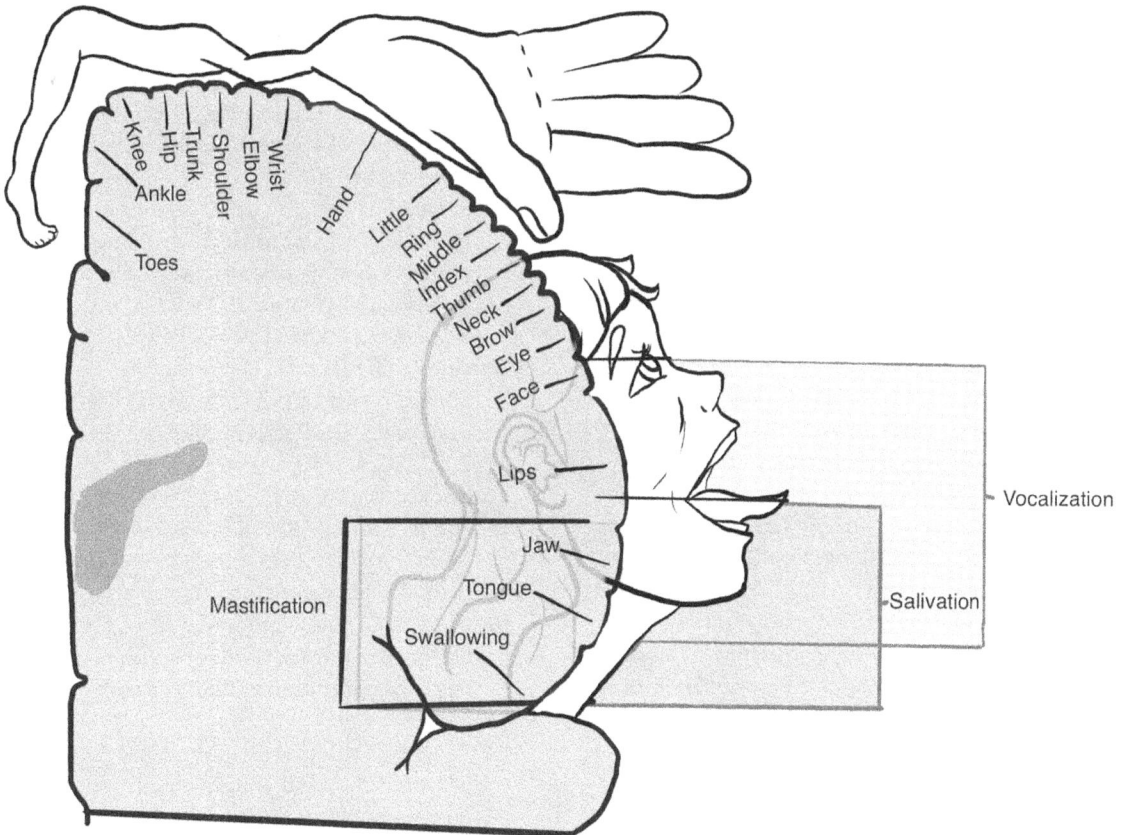

Figure 4.16 Homunculus

REFERENCES

1. Sendic G. Musculoskeletal system. Kenhub. Updated November 3, 2024. https://www.kenhub.com/en/library/anatomy/the-musculoskeletal-system

2. Roussouly P, Gollogly S, Noseda O, Berthonnaud E, Dimnet J. The vertical projection of the sum of the ground reactive forces of a standing patient is not the same as the C7 plumb line: a radiographic study of the sagittal alignment of 153 asymptomatic volunteers. *Spine (Phila Pa 1976)*. May 15 2006;31(11):E320–E325. doi:10.1097/01.brs.0000218263.58642.ff

3. Kim D, Davis DD, Menger RP. Spine sagittal balance. [Updated 2023 Aug 14]. *StatPearls*. Treasure Island (FL): StatPearls Publishing; 2025 Jan. Available from: https://www.ncbi.nlm.nih.gov/books/NBK534858/

4. Gaillard F, Knipe H. Sagittal balance. *Radiopaediaorg*. Radiopaedia.org; 2016. doi:10.53347/rID-49585. Accessed 8/28/2022. https://radiopaedia.org/articles/49585

5. Le Huec JC, Saddiki R, Franke J, Rigal J, Aunoble S. Equilibrium of the human body and the gravity line: the basics. *Eur Spine J*. Sep 2011;20 Suppl 5(Suppl 5):558–563. doi:10.1007/s00586-011-1939-7

6. Anderson BW KM, Black AC, Kharazi KA. Anatomy, Head and Neck, Skull. *StatPearls*. StatPearls Publishing; Updated 2024. Accessed August 11, 2024. https://www.ncbi.nlm.nih.gov/books/NBK499834/

7. Reeves BC, Valcarce-Aspegren M, Robert SM, et al. Isolated unilateral alar ligamentous injury: illustrative cases. *Journal of Neurosurgery: Case Lessons*. 2024;7(14):CASE23664. doi:10.3171/CASE23664

8. Olson K, Joder D. Diagnosis and treatment of cervical spine clinical instability. *Journal of Orthopaedic & Sports Physical Therapy*. 2001;31(4):194–206.

9. Aghoghovwia B. Curvature and movements of the vertebral column. Kenhub. 2024. https://www.kenhub.com/en/library/anatomy/curvature-and-movements-of-the-vertebral-column

10. Ocran E. Joints and ligaments of the vertebral column. Kenhub. 2024. https://www.kenhub.com/en/library/anatomy/joints-and-ligaments-of-the-vertebral-column

11. Physiopedia contributors. Costovertebral Joints. Physiopedia. https://www.physio-pedia.com/index.php?title=Costovertebral_Joints&oldid=353159

12. Wong M, Sinkler MA, Kiel J. Anatomy, Abdomen and Pelvis, Sacroiliac Joint. *StatPearls*. StatPearls Publishing; Updated 2023. Accessed 2024. https://www.ncbi.nlm.nih.gov/books/NBK507801/

13. Elsevier. Interspinous Ligaments (Lumbar Part). Complete Anatomy. Elsevier website. https://www.elsevier.com/resources/anatomy/connective-tissue/joints-of-vertebral-column/interspinous-ligaments-lumbar-part/16994. Accessed August 9, 2025. https://www.elsevier.com/resources/anatomy/connective-tissue/joints-of-vertebral-column/interspinous-ligaments-lumbar-part/16994

14. Safarini OA, Bordoni B. Anatomy, Thorax, Ribs. StatPearls Publishing; Updated 2023. Accessed 2024. https://www.ncbi.nlm.nih.gov/books/NBK538328/

15. Forro SD, Munjal A, JB L. Anatomy, Shoulder and Upper Limb, Arm Structure and Function. *StatPearls*. StatPearls Publishing; Updated 2023. 2024. https://www.ncbi.nlm.nih.gov/books/NBK507841/

16. Arias DG, Black AC, Varacallo M. Anatomy, Shoulder and Upper Limb, Hand Bones. *StatPearls*. StatPearls Publishing; Updated 2023. 2024. https://www.ncbi.nlm.nih.gov/books/NBK547684

17. Joe N. Scapula. Kenhub. Reviewed September 11, 2023. https://www.kenhub.com/en/library/anatomy/scapula

18. Battista C. Scapulothoracic Joint. Ortho Notes. 2024. https://www.orthobullets.com/shoulder-and-elbow/3035/scapulothoracic-joint

19. Wilson Health Ltd. Shoulder Ligaments. Wilson Health Ltd. Accessed 2024, https://www.shoulder-pain-explained.com/shoulder-ligaments.htm

20. Cowan PT, Mudreac A, Varacallo M. Anatomy, Back, Scapula. *StatPearls*. StatPearls Publishing; 2023. Accessed 2024. https://pubmed.ncbi.nlm.nih.gov/30285370/

21. Kadi R MA, Shahabpour M. Shoulder anatomy and normal variants. *J Belgian Soc Radiol*. 2017;101(2):3.

22. Rugg CM, Hettrich CM, Ortiz S, Wolf BR, MOON Shoulder Instability Group, Zhang A. Surgical stabilization for first-time shoulder dislocators: a multicenter analysis. *J Shoulder Elbow Surg*. 2018;27(4):674–685. doi:10.1016/j.jse.2017.10.041

23. Chaudhry SR, Nahian A, Chaudhry K. Anatomy, Abdomen and Pelvis, Pelvis. *StatPearls*. StatPearls Publishing; Updated 2023. Accessed 2024. https://www.ncbi.nlm.nih.gov/books/NBK482258/

24. Contributors CC. Pubic Symphysis. Cleveland Clinic. 2024. https://my.clevelandclinic.org/health/body/23025-pubic-symphysis

25. Chaudhry SR, Imonugo O, Jozsa F, Chaundhry K. Anatomy, Abdomen and Pelvis: Ligaments. *StatPearls*. StatPearls Publishing; Updated 2024. https://www.ncbi.nlm.nih.gov/books/NBK493215/

26. Crumbie L. Ligaments of the Lower Limb. Kenhub. 2024. https://www.kenhub.com/en/library/anatomy/ligaments-of-the-lower-limb

27. O J. The Sciatic Foramena. TeachMeAnatomy. 2024. https://teachmeanatomy.info/pelvis/areas/sciatic-foramen/

28. Sugumar K, Gupta M. Anatomy, Abdomen and Pelvis: Inguinal Ligament (Crural Ligament. Poupart Ligament). *StatPearls*. StatPearls Publishing; Updated 2024. Accessed 2024. https://www.ncbi.nlm.nih.gov/books/NBK542321/

29. Glenister R, S S. Anatomy, Bony Pelvis and Lower Limb, Hip. *StatPearls*. StatPearls Publishing; Updated 2023. 2024. https://www.ncbi.nlm.nih.gov/books/NBK526019/

30. O'Donnell JM, Devitt BM, Arora M. The role of the ligamentum teres in the adult hip: redundant or relevant? A review. *J Hip Preserv Surg*. 2018;5(1):15–22. doi:10.1093/jhps/hnx046

31. Bowman KF, Fox J, Sekiya JK. A clinically relevant review of hip biomechanics. *Arthroscopy*. 2010;26(8):1118–1129. doi:10.1016/j.arthro.2010.01.027

32. Chang A, Breeland G, Black AC, Hubbard JB. Anatomy, Bony Pelvis and Lower Limb: Femur. *StatPearls*. StatPearls Publishing; 2023. Accessed 2024. https://www.ncbi.nlm.nih.gov/books/NBK500017/

33. Gupton M, Imonugo O, Black AC, Launico MV, Terreberry RR. Anatomy, Bony Pelvis and Lower Limb, Knee. *StatPearls*. StatPearls Publishing; Updated 2023. Accessed 2024. https://www.ncbi.nlm.nih.gov/books/NBK500017/

34. Loudon JK. Biomechanics and pathomechanics of the patellofemoral joint. *Int J Sports Phys Thera*. 2016;11(6):820–830.

35. Ficke J, Byerly DW. Anatomy, Bony Pelvis and Lower Limb: Foot. *StatPearls*. StatPearls Publishing; Updated 2023. Accessed 2024. https://www.ncbi.nlm.nih.gov/books/NBK546698/

36. Dave HD, Shook M, Varacallo M. Anatomy, Skeletal Muscle. *StatPearls*. StatPearls Publishing; 2023. Jan., 2024. 2024. https://www.ncbi.nlm.nih.gov/books/NBK537236/

37. Frontera WR, Ochala J. Skeletal muscle: a brief review of structure and function. *Calcified Tissue Int*. 2015;96(3):183–195.

38. Bagher P, Segal SS. Regulation of blood flow in the microcirculation: role of conducted vasodilation. *Acta Physiol*. 2011;202(3):271–284.

39. Dodd LR, Johnson PC. Diameter changes in arteriolar networks of contracting skeletal muscle. *Am J Physiol*. 1991;260(3 Pt 2):H662–H670.

40. Kim S, Jang S. Immediate effects of ankle mobilization on range of motion, balance, and muscle activity in elderly individuals with chronic ankle instability: a pre-post intervention study. *Med Sci Monit*. 2023;29:e941398. doi:0.12659/MSM.941398

41. Rodríguez-Perea Á, Reyes-Ferrada W, Jerez-Mayorga D, et al. Core training and performance: a systematic review with meta-analysis. *Biol Sport*. 2023;40(4):975–992. doi:10.5114/biolsport.2023.123319

42. Chvatal SA, Ting LH. Common muscle synergies for balance and walking. *Front Comput Neurosc.* 2013;7:48. doi:10.3389/fncom.2013.00048

43. Pozzo T, Berthoz A, Lefort L. Head stabilization during various locomotor tasks in humans. *Exp Brain Res.* 1990;82:97–106.

44. Borghese NA, Bianchi L, Lacquaniti F. Kinematic determinants of human locomotion. *Physiology.* 1996;494(3):863–879.

45. Chvatal SA, Ting LH. Voluntary and reactive recruitment of locomotor muscle synergies during perturbed walking. *J Neurosci.* 2012;32:12237–12250. doi:10.1523/JNEUROSCI.6344-11.2012

46. Raizada V, Mittal RK. Pelvic floor anatomy and applied physiology. *Gastroenterol Clin North Am.* 2008;37(3):493–509. doi:10.1016/j.gtc.2008.06.003

47. Madhok SSSN. Hypotonia. *StatPearls.* StatPearls Publishing; Updated 2022. https://www.ncbi.nlm.nih.gov/books/NBK562209/

48. Ganguly JKD, Almotiri M, Jog M. Muscle tone physiology and abnormalities. *Toxins.* 2021;13(4):282. doi:10.3390/toxins13040282

49. Kenneth FSJ. *Muscular Tone and Gait Disturbances.* 6th ed. Elsevier; 2017.

50. Barrett K BS, Boitano S, Brooks H. *Ganong's Review of Medical Physiology.* 25th ed. McGraw-Hill; 2016.

51. Abraira VE, Ginty DD. The sensory neurons of touch. *Neuron.* 2013;79(4):618–639.

52. Raju H, Tadi P. Neuroanatomy, Somatosensory Cortex. *StatPearls.* StatPearls Publishing; Updated 2022. Accessed 2024. https://www.ncbi.nlm.nih.gov/books/NBK555915/

53. Human Neurophysiology Contributors. The cerebellum. humanphysiology.com. 2024. https://humanneurophysiology.com/cerebellum.htm

5

The Cerebrum, Cerebellum, Brainstem, and Cranial Nerves

OVERVIEW

The purpose of the chapter is to provide an overview of the nervous system, and there is an emphasis on structures and clinical signs and symptoms of injury of structures related to the vestibular system.

The nervous system is made up of the central nervous system (CNS) and peripheral nervous system (PNS). The CNS consists of the brain and spinal cord, and the PNS consists of nerves and ganglia (small collections of neurons) located outside of the cranium and vertebral column. The brain is located within the cranium (skull) and controls the majority of our movements, communication/language, memory, emotions, and executive functions (personality, judgment, planning, creativity, etc.). It perceives and interprets the sensations to which we are subjected and makes it possible for us to respond appropriately. It provides a map of our body's position and movement so that we may interact with our world in a meaningful and successful manner. The spinal cord is located within the vertebral column and is the structure that connects the brain and the PNS. The spinal cord is able to mediate simple behaviors such as reflexes and automatic movements.

NEURONS AND GLIAL CELLS

The nervous system contains two principal types of cells: neurons and glial cells.[2] A *neuron* is a highly specialized cell that sends and receives electrochemical signals within the CNS and to/from the PNS. Neurons are comprised of three main parts: a *cell body*, a single *axon*, and multiple (usually) *dendrites* (Figure 5.1). The cell body maintains the neuron's structure and contains the nucleus and specialized organelles that give these cells their special functional properties. The axon is a long and slim process that projects from the cell body and conducts electrical impulses away from the cell body to the axon terminal, where neurons communicate with other neurons, muscle cells, or glands. Some axons are myelinated (covered in a white fatty substance), and others are unmyelinated. Myelin is produced by oligodendrocytes (glial) cells in the CNS and by Schwann cells (which is a type

DOI: 10.1201/9781003524441-5

of glial cell) in the PNS. Myelinated axons have gaps in the myelin (called nodes) that allow the electrical impulses to jump to the next myelin node. This increases the speed of the electrical signal and is the reason that some neurons can communicate with other neurons within milliseconds. Dendrites are unmyelinated processes that emanate from the neuron cell body and look like the branches on a tree. The extent of the branching of dendrites varies between different types of neurons and underlies how they communicate with other neurons.

There are three general classifications of neurons: motor, sensory, and interneurons. Motor neurons project their axons from the CNS to the PNS where their axons are part of cranial and spinal nerves. Sensory neurons have the ability to transduce sensory information into electrical signals in the PNS and carry that information into the CNS. Interneurons are cells that are located entirely within the CNS and act as intermediaries, passing signals to other neurons.

A flow of charged ions across the neuron's membrane shifts the potential electrical energy of the neuron. If a threshold is met, the neuron generates an action potential (a change in the electrical charge) that travels via the axon to other neurons. The point of communication between neurons is the *synapse*. If there is a chemical synapse, the nerve releases chemical messengers called neurotransmitters that bind to receptors on the next neuron and either excite, depress, or modulate their electrical signaling depending upon the receptor. Modulatory neurotransmitters influence the effects (enhance the effects) of other neurotransmitters and also affect a larger number of neurons at the same time. Examples of neurotransmitters include glutamate, epinephrine, norepinephrine, gamma-aminobutyric acid (GABA), glycine, and serotonin.

The mature brain has more than 100 billion neurons,[3,4] and each neuron can connect with between 1,000 and 100,000 other neurons.[4] So the amount and the complexity of signaling and information processing that occurs with the nervous system is incredibly large. It is this electrical signaling between neurons that mediates all human behavior.

Just as there are billions of neurons, there are also billions of glial cells. In fact, about half of the cells of the in the CNS are glia.[5] They have roles in synaptic communication, plasticity, homeostasis, and dynamic monitoring and alterations of CNS structures and function.[5] There are multiple kinds of glial cells, including:[2,5,6]

- Radial glia generate the majority of CNS neurons and glia during embryonic development.
- Oligodendrocytes that produce myelin.
- Astrocytes clear excessive neurotransmitters, stabilize and regulate the blood–brain barrier, and promote synapse formation.
- Ependymal cells secrete cerebrospinal fluid.
- Microglial cells are responsible for phagocytosis that transform into macrophages in response to an injury.

Glial cells in the PNS are primarily Schwann cells.

NEURONS VERSUS NERVES

Neurons are individual cells that are responsible for generating and transmitting impulses for sensation, motor commands to muscles and glands, and interneurons that connect neurons within the CNS. On the other hand, a nerve is a bundle of axons that transmit messages between the CNS to the rest of the body. There are three types of nerves: afferent nerves that carry sensory information from the PNS to the CNS, efferent nerves from the CNS that transmit motor commands as well as autonomic signals to regulate involuntary processes, and mixed nerves that contain both sensory and motor neurons. Nerves are primarily found in the PNS.

THE BRAIN

The brain may be divided into three main parts:

1. Cerebrum
   - Represents ~80% of the brain
   - Divided into two halves (or hemispheres), left and right connected at the corpus collosum
   - Separated into lobes
   - Contains ventricles
   - The surface appears to be wrinkled and has ridges (each called a *gyrus*), valleys (or grooves) each called a *sulcus*, and deep sulci called *fissures*. These wrinkles increase the total cortical area.

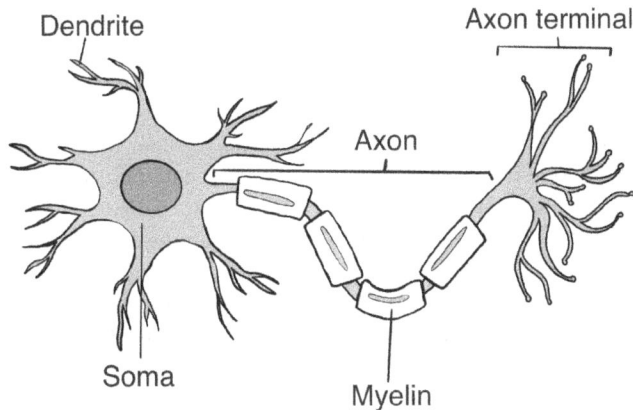

Figure 5.1 Neuronal Anatomy

- The cerebral cortex is formed by the frontal, temporal, parietal, and occipital lobes.
2. Cerebellum
   - Approximately 50% of the brain's neurons.
     - Three zones
       - Lateral zones (there are two)
       - Intermediate zone (between the two lateral zones)
       - The flocculus
     - Three functional areas
       - Cerebrocerebellum (corresponds to the lateral zones)
       - Spinocerebellum (corresponds to the intermediate zone)
       - Vestibulocerebellum (corresponds to the flocculus)
3. Brainstem
   - Connects the brain to the spinal cord.
   - Has three parts
     - Midbrain
     - Pons
     - Medulla oblongata

The brain is composed of gray matter and white matter (named for their appearances). Gray matter has a high concentration of nuclei and neurons with unmyelinated axons, whereas white matter contains neurons and myelinated axons.

MENINGES

There are three layers of membranes and connective tissues called *meninges* that cover the brain and spinal cord that act as a protective covering. The spaces between each of these layers allow for the passage of veins and arteries. These layers are as follows:

1. *Dura mater* is the thick and tough outermost layer that also lines the inner skull. It also extends from the *foramen magnum* to the *filum terminale* and is separated from the walls of the vertebral canal by the epidural space that contains connective tissue. It has two layers: a periosteal layer that is in contact with the skull, and an inner layer.
2. *Arachnoid mater* is a thin and weblike layer of connective tissue that does not contain nerves or blood vessels. There is a subarachnoid space containing cerebral spinal fluid (CSF) between the arachnoid mater and pia mater.
3. *Pia mater* is a thick membrane that surrounds the surface of the brain and has a lot of veins and arteries.

The meninges suspend the CNS and stabilize its shape and position. They are anchored to the skull and spinal column, which constrains movement of the brain with the cranium[2] and spinal cord within the spinal column. There are two potential spaces associated with the dura: the epidural and subdural spaces. The epidural space is the potential space between the cranium and the periosteal layer of the dura.[2] The subdural potential space is between the dura mater (the outermost layer) and the arachnoid mater (middle layer).

BLOOD SUPPLY

The brain is supplied by two arteries: *carotid arteries* (the anterior system) and *vertebral arteries* (the posterior system), each having a left- and right-sided artery. The carotid arteries travel along the front of the neck, while the vertebral arteries travel along the back of the neck. At the base of the brain is a ring-shaped vascular structure where the anterior (internal carotid) and posterior (vertebral) circulations converge to form the *circle of Willis*.[7]

GEEK STUFF

Approximately 60% of people have a complete circle of Willis, while the other 40% have variations that do not form a complete circle.[1]

Strokes along the carotid arteries can cause deficits with speech, vision, motor control, and sensation. Strokes along the vertebral arteries (or after the right and left vertebral artery joins to form the *basilar artery*) can cause changes with level of consciousness, problems with muscle movement, coordination, speech, and vision.

The vertebral and basilar arteries supply the posterior circulation and are the main arteries supplying the brainstem (midbrain, pons, and medulla). While strokes in these arteries are uncommon, they are a disproportionate cause of morbidity and mortality compared to anterior circulation strokes.[8] Often, the main complaints of patients with strokes in these arteries are nausea and vertigo. As these symptoms are often mistaken as non-stroke medical conditions, treatment may be delayed (Table 5.1).[8]

CEREBRUM

The surface of the cerebrum is called the neocortex (2–5 mm thick). The subcortical (below the cortex) area acts as a relay for information between the neocortex and the rest of the body, as well as between different areas of the cortex. Both the neocortex and subcortical nuclei contain cell bodies of neurons and appear as gray (hence the term "gray matter").[4] Subcortical white matter, on the other hand, is deeper in the brain and acts as a communication network to different parts of the gray matter. The spinal cord, on the other hand, has white matter on the outside with gray matter inside.

The cerebrum has been described as having between four and six lobes, depending upon the author, and is the largest part of the brain. All agree that there are at least four lobes: frontal, parietal, temporal, and occipital (Figure 5.2 and Table 5.2). Some authors consider the limbic system to be part of the temporal lobe. Other authors consider the insular cortex to be a lobe on its own, and it is in the lateral sulcus separating the temporal lobe from the parietal and frontal lobes.

FRONTAL LOBE

Concerned with emotions, reasoning, movement planning, creativity, judgement, problem solving, and parts of speech, the frontal lobe is divided into three main areas: *prefrontal cortex*, *primary motor cortex*, and *supplementary motor cortex*. Some authors describe a fourth area: *motor speech* (Broca's area).[2]

The premotor cortex is anterior (rostral) to the primary motor cortex with 30% of axons in the corticospinal tract originating there. The neurons in the lateral frontal lobe seem to be involved in the selection of movements based on environmental events, while those in the medial premotor cortex assist in movement selection as well as movements that are initiated internally rather than externally.[10] Its main job is to prepare for movement.[11] The primary motor cortex plans, controls, and executes voluntary movements, and is anterior to the central sulcus. The primary motor cortex is somatotopically organized and is represented by the motor homunculus depicting movement production in different body regions.[11]

The supplementary motor cortex is located on the medial surface of the premotor cortex and is thought to be involved in coordination and postural stabilization.[11]

Table 5.1 Arteries Supplying the Brain, and Deficits from a Stroke

Arteries of the Brain	Deficits from a Cerebrovascular Accident (CVA) by Artery[9]	Lobe(s)/Regions of the Brain Supplied
Anterior cerebral (ACA)	• Leg weakness • Difficulty thinking and making decisions	• Superior parts of the frontal lobe • Anterior parts of the parietal lobe • Parts of the primary sensory cortex
Middle cerebral (MCA)	• Hemiplegia • Blindness • Language	• Portions of the frontal, temporal, and parietal lobes
Posterior cerebral (PCA)	• Vision • Hemiparesis of extremities and face • Vertical gaze palsy	• Occipital lobe • Inferior temporal lobe • Posterior parietal lobe • Midbrain
Vertebral basilar	• Dizziness/vertigo • Ipsilateral facial paralysis with contralateral limb weakness • Difficulty speaking • Vomiting/nausea • Loss of proprioception and vibration sense • Ataxia • Loss of facial pain and temperature • Intention tremor • Pupillary palsy • Hypersomnolence • Amnesia • Visual hallucinations	Brainstem • Midbrain • Pons • Medulla Cerebellum
Anterior inferior cerebellar artery (AICA) (from basilar artery)	• Vertigo • Truncal ataxia • Horizontal nystagmus • Dysmetria • Loss of hearing • Dysarthria • Vomiting	Cerebellum

Symptoms of injuries to the frontal lobe include the loss of fine motor control, and the inability to plan a sequence of complex movements or to do multiple-step tasks. Nonmotor symptoms include the loss of spontaneity, loss of flexible thinking, persistence of a single thought, the inability to attend to a task, emotional lability and mood changes, and the inability to understand humor.

The blood supply for the frontal lobe is the anterior cerebral artery (ACA), which arises from the termination of the internal carotid artery.

PARIETAL LOBE

The parietal lobe[12,13] is divided into two functional regions—sensation/perception, and integration of sensory input (primarily with the visual system)—and occupies about a quarter of each hemisphere. It integrates sensory information to form a single perception, and allows us to understand spatial relationships and do math computations. It is involved in the perception of touch, temperature, pain, proprioception, and advanced perception of

Lateral View

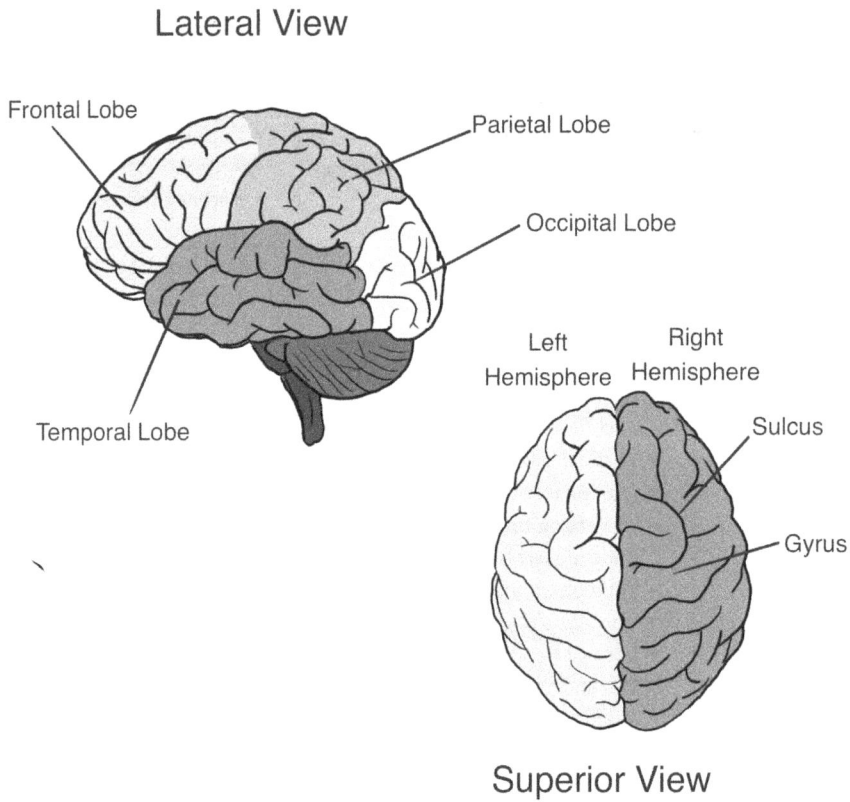

Frontal Lobe

Parietal Lobe

Occipital Lobe

Temporal Lobe

Left Hemisphere

Right Hemisphere

Sulcus

Gyrus

Superior View

Figure 5.2 The Cerebrum

Table 5.2 Lobes of the Brain

Number of Lobes	Lobes	Author
4	Frontal, parietal, temporal, occipital	Regina Bailey
5	Frontal, parietal, temporal, occipital, insula	Janice Evans
6	Frontal, parietal, temporal, occipital, insula, limbic	Sophie Stewart

visual and auditory information. It helps us learn complex and precise movements, such as writing. Calculation and language are controlled by the parietal lobe on the dominant side, while sensory visuospatial processing occurs on the nondominant side. The parietal lobe creates an internal schema of our bodies, knowing where body parts are located and their position in space without needing to see them.

Important areas of the parietal lobe include:

- *Primary somatosensory area*
  - The primary somatosensory area receives information regarding temperature, pain, vibration, proprioception, and fine touch.
- *Parietal association cortex*
  - The superior parietal lobule assists in planned movements, spatial reasoning, and spatial attention. The lateral intraparietal sulcus is responsible for eye movements in response to an external stimulus. The medial area helps to calculate distances of objects from our nose used during reaching movements. The ventral area receives information from auditory, visual, somatosensory, and vestibular systems. The anterior area interprets the size, shape, and position of objects.

- *Optic radiations*
  - There are two loops of fibers (optic radiations) carrying information from the lateral geniculate nucleus of the thalamus to the visual area (V1 of the occipital lobe). The lower division carries information from the superior part of the visual field (inferior retinal field) through the temporal lobe to the occipital lobe, while the dorsal loop runs through the parietal lobe and carries information from the inferior part of the visual field.[12]

The blood supply for the parietal lobe is as explained in Table 5.3.

Signs/symptoms of parietal damage include the inability to read and write (agraphia), difficulty distinguishing left from right, the inability to do math, and the inability to feel temperature, pressure, vibration, or pain. You may also have the inability to recognize objects by touch. There are vision deficits that arise from parietal damage, including the loss of control while shifting your gaze (ocular motor apraxia), missing objects you are reaching for while looking at them (optic ataxia), or the lack of being able to see how an object fits into a setting (e.g., seeing a tree but not the forest) (Table 5.4).

TEMPORAL LOBE

The temporal lobe[14] is the second largest of the brain's lobes and makes up about 20% of the cerebral cortex.[15] Involved in hearing and auditory processing and speech perception, the temporal lobe is the key to being able to understand meaningful speech and to make sense of different sounds and pitches; episodic memory; phonological, social, and visual cognitive functions; and facial recognition. It is also involved in speech production.

It is located anterior to the occipital lobe and posterior to the frontal lobe and is inferior to the lateral fissure (aka lateral sulcus). It may be subdivided into the superior temporal lobe, middle temporal lobe, and the inferior temporal lobe. The hippocampus and the amygdala are both located in the temporal lobe. It may be classified into four systems: lateral temporal system, polar temporal system, inferior temporal system, and inferior temporal system.

Table 5.3 Parietal Lobe Blood Supply

Parietal Lobe Location	Blood Supply
Lateral surface	• Middle cerebral artery (branch of the Internal carotid artery)
Medial surface	• Anterior cerebral artery (branch of the Internal carotid artery) • Posterior cerebral artery
Posterior surface	• Posterior cerebral artery

Table 5.4 Signs of Parietal Damage

Parietal Side of Damage	Symptoms
Left side (Gerstmann syndrome)	• Right-left confusion • Agraphia • Difficulty with math • Aphasia • Agnosia (inability to recognize and identify objects) • Right-side neglect/inattention (rare)
Right side	• Left-side neglect/inattention • Difficulty making things (constructional apraxia) • Denial of deficits • Impaired drawing ability
Bilateral (Balint syndrome)	• Ocular apraxia • Inability to integrate visual scenes • Optic ataxia

Lateral Temporal System

Functions of the lateral temporal system include motion, speech, and facial processing; language comprehension (*Wernicke's area*—typically in the left hemisphere and involves part of the parietal lobe); audiovisual integration; and perceptual and conceptual acoustic sound processing, "processing visual information, including working memory for short-term visual maintenance of information."[16,17] It also is responsible for the conscious retrieval of conceptual knowledge and automatic retrieval of semantic information (meaning and veracity of information).[16]

Polar Temporal System

Functions of the polar temporal system include processing language, social cues, emotions, auditory and visual aspects of facial recognition, and emotional processing of auditory, olfactory, and visual stimuli.[16]

Inferior Temporal System

Functions of the inferior temporal system include contribution to declarative memories (memories that can be thought of and verbalized) and semantic knowledge, and incorporating item information with spatio-temporal information. Some studies suggest it is relevant for working memory maintenance, reading, object recognition, and facial recognition.[16]

Medial Temporal System

Functions include involvement in spatial information processing, memory consolidation and rapid encoding of new associations, episodic memory (the ability to remember a specific occasion in the past and its time and place),[18] facial recognition, and visuospatial processing.[16] It is crucial for semantic memory (the ability to recall general facts about the world).[18]

Hippocampus

The hippocampus is responsible for creating declarative memories.[18]

Amygdala

The amygdala is found in the medial temporal lobe and is associated with fear, anxiety, reward processing, reward learning and motivation, aggression, maternal instinct, sexual behavior, and eating and drinking behaviors. It is also involved in the regulation of perception, attention, and explicit memory. It is implicated in the psychiatric illness of addiction and autism.[19-22]

Signs and Symptoms of Temporal Damage

Common symptoms include memory problems, difficulty understanding language or writing (*alexia*), acalculia (like alexia, but for numbers and math), seizures, severe or frequent feelings of anxiety or pain, confusion, and changes in vision.[15]

OCCIPITAL LOBE

The occipital lobe is the smallest lobe of the cerebrum and accounts for about 18% of total neocortical volume. It is posterior to the parietal and temporal lobes of each hemisphere. It functions to process vision and works with other parts of the brain to help us understand what we see.

The Visual Cortex

The visual cortex, which resides in the occipital lobe of the brain, receives, processes, and integrates visual information from the retinas. This is the part of the brain that allows you to "see." It is divided into five regions (V1–V5) based on their structure (cell type) and function.

Table 5.5 lists the regions of the visual cortex.[23,24]

Damage to the visual cortex can cause *cortical blindness*, which is typically the result of a stroke in the posterior cerebral artery.[25] Other causes of cortical blindness include infection, eclampsia, traumatic brain injury, encephalitis, meningitis, medications, and hyperammonemia.[23]

Damage to bilateral visual cortices can cause complete cortical blindness, which is sometimes accompanied by Anton–Babinski syndrome, which is when a patient is blind but denies having any visual impairment (Table 5.6).[23]

Table 5.5 Regions of the Visual Cortex

Visual Cortex Region	Function
V1	V1 is the largest and most important layer of the visual cortex. V1 is divided into six layers, each having a different function. It receives projections from the LGN (thalamus) and responds to specific types of visual cues such as the orientation of edges and lines. It allows you to see but not recognize what you see. V1 receives input from both the magnocellular as well as parvocellular pathways. The output of V1 projects to V2, V3, V4, V5.
V2	V2 is called the "secondary visual cortex." It receives information from V1 and responds to differences in color, spatial frequency, moderately complex patterns, object orientation, and recognition. Information leaving V2 splits into magnocellular and parvocellular pathways. It has feedback connections to V1 and feedforward connections to V3–V5.
V3	Along with V4 and V5, this layer is concerned with the recall of visual memory relating to objects (object recognition).
V4	Object orientation, spatial frequency, and color. Along with V3 and V5, V4 is concerned with the recall of visual memory relating to objects (object recognition). The output of V4 is mainly to the inferior temporal cortex.
V5	V5 is called the "middle temporal visual area" and determines the speed and direction of moving objects. Along with V3 and V4, V5 is also concerned with the recall of visual memory relating to objects (object recognition).

Table 5.6 Blood Supply to the Occipital Lobe

Occipital Lobe Part		Blood Supply
• Posterolateral surface • Cuneate gyrus • Lingual gyrus	Posterior cerebral artery	• Occipital branch (divides into medial and lateral occipital arteries)
• Cuneus		• Parietooccipital artery
• Visual cortex • Inferior cuneus • Lingual gyrus		• Calcarine artery

INSULA

The insular cortex[26] is in the lateral sulcus of the brain and can be divided into anywhere between 2 and 13 subdivisions. It is involved in central auditory processing, taste, olfaction, vestibular processing, emotions, the detection of novel stimuli, and assists in speech production. It serves a wide variety of functions, including sensory, affective processing (how the brain processes emotions), and high-level cognition. It is a primary visceral–somatic region contributing to visceral sensory and motor responses and somatic sensory responses, especially in the face, tongue, and upper limbs, as well as processing somatosensory information from all over the body. By stimulating the insular cortex with electricity, the following sensations were elicited: tingling, electric, warm, cold, shiver, constriction sensations, and auditory distortions. The blood supply to the insula is listed in Table 5.7.[26]

Table 5.7 Blood Supply to the Insula

Insula Part	Blood Supply
• Anterior • Middle • Posterior short gyri	M2 segment of middle cerebral artery (MCA) (superior trunk)
• Posterior long gyri	Inferior trunk of the MCA

LIMBIC

The limbic area of the brain[27] sits below the cerebrum, lateral to the thalamus, and above the brainstem. It processes emotion, memory, and motivational processes that connect to other parts of the brain. It contains components of the visual, auditory, and somatosensory systems. It contains the hypothalamus, anterior thalamic nuclei, habenular commissure,[28] the olfactory bulbs, hippocampus, parahippocampal gyrus, fornix, mammillary body, septum pellucidum, amygdala, cingulate gyrus, and entorhinal cortex.[29]

Functionally, it assists in processes related to spatial memory, learning, motivation, emotional processing, and social processing. According to Crumbie, a quick way to remember the functions of the limbic system is to think of the five F's:[30]

- Feeding (satiety and hunger)
- Forgetting (memory)
- Fighting (emotional response)
- Family (sexual reproduction and maternal instincts)
- Fornicating (sexual arousal)

Hypothalamus

The hypothalamus maintains the body's homeostasis by controlling endocrine, autonomic, and somatic behavior. It regulates feeding, escape and fear from predators,[27] and the acute-phase immune response.[31]

Olfactory Bulbs

"The olfactory bulbs are involved in the sense of smell."[27]

Hippocampus

The hippocampus is important for short-term memory, longer-term memory, and spatial memory.[32]

Parahippocampal Gyrus

The parahippocampal gyrus is located in the cortical region surrounding the hippocampus, it has a role in scene recognition as well as memory encoding and retrieval.[33]

Fornix

Functionally, the fornix is associated with cognition, memory, emotions, and sexual responses. The word *fornix* comes from Latin and means "arch." It is shaped like the letter *C* and is comprised of white matter nerve bundles and fibers. It is located below the corpus callosum and is the largest single pathway of the hippocampus connecting to various subcortical structures. There is a posterior pillar (*crura*) for each hemisphere that end at the mammillary bodies.[27] It begins in the hippocampus and "stretches longitudinally to the diencephalon and basal forebrain forming an arch of the thalamus."[34]

Damage to bilateral components of the limbic system is rare, however, asymmetry and volume loss are common for schizophrenia.

Amygdala

Located in the medial temporal lobe and part of the limbic system, the amygdala is involved in processing the emotional responses of fear, anxiety, and aggression, as well as processing memory and decision-making.[35]

Cingulate Gyrus

Located immediately above the corpus callosum, the cingulate gyrus is involved in emotion formation, learning, memory, and links behavior and motivational outcomes.[27,36,37]

Mammillary Bodies

The mammillary bodies are a pair of rounded structures inferior to the third ventricle, posterior to the pituitary gland and the floor of the hypothalamus, and anterior to the interpeduncular fossa. The mammillary bodies are associated with recollective memory. Damage to either mammillary body, typically from prolonged thiamine shortages, may result in amnesia.[38]

Septum Pellucidum

Comprised of two layers of both white and gray matter, the septum pellucidum is a thin triangular membrane positioned between the two cerebral hemispheres and separates the anterior horns of the lateral ventricles and is connected to the lower part of the corpus callosum.[39]

Habenular Nuclei

The two habenular nuclei are located above the pineal gland and recess.[40] The habenula is divided into the medial habenula and lateral habenula. The medial habenular is a mass of cholinergic neurons, while the lateral habenula contains dopaminergic and serotonergic neurons.

Functionally, the habenular nuclei receive afferent fibers from the basal ganglia and limbic system, and act to integrate olfactory, visceral, and somatic afferent pathways. The medial habenula regulates mood and fear memory, while the lateral habenula is involved in behavioral expression, emotional expression, and sleep mechanism control.

VENTRICLES

There are four ventricles, which are interconnected cavities in the cerebrum, that are filled with cerebrospinal fluid produced in the ventricles and cushions the brain.

Two Lateral Ventricles

There is one lateral ventricle in each hemisphere. They are C-shaped and separated from each other by the septum pellucidum, and communicate with the third ventricle through the interventricular foramen. The lateral ventricle is comprised of the central body of the ventricle and three horns (anterior, posterior, and inferior).[41]

- *Central body*: It is located within the parietal lobe and extends from the interventricular foramen anteriorly to the corpus collosum posteriorly. The medial wall is mostly formed by the septum pellucidum and the body of the fornix (the C-shaped nerve fibers of the hippocampus) in the lower part. The floor is formed by the following (in order from lateral to medial): the body of the caudate nucleus, stria terminalis (a band of fibers running the ventricular surface of the thalamus and separates the thalamus and caudate nucleus) and thalamostriate vein, lateral part of the superior

surface of the thalamus, and the choroid plexus.[41]
- *Anterior horn*: Also referred to as the frontal horn, this ventricle lies in the frontal lobe.
- *Posterior horn*: Also called the occipital horn, lies in the occipital lobe.
- *Inferior horn*: The longest of the horns, it forms a curve around the posterior thalamus and descends posterolaterally and then anteriorly into the temporal lobe.

Third Ventricle

This ventricle is slit-like and lies between the two thalami and part of the hypothalamus.

Fourth Ventricle

Found in the hindbrain, this ventricle is tent-like and broad, and is bounded by the pons and cranial half of the medulla anteriorly and the cerebellum posteriorly. It is continuous superiorly with the cerebral aqueduct and inferiorly with the central canal of the spinal cord.[41]

Disturbances of the CSF flow may lead to hydrocephalus (excessive fluid accumulation in the brain).

BASAL GANGLIA

The basal ganglia (BG) consist of a cluster of nuclei found in the neocortex deep within the white matter that is primarily involved in motor control (Figure 5.3). The BG forms part of the extrapyramidal

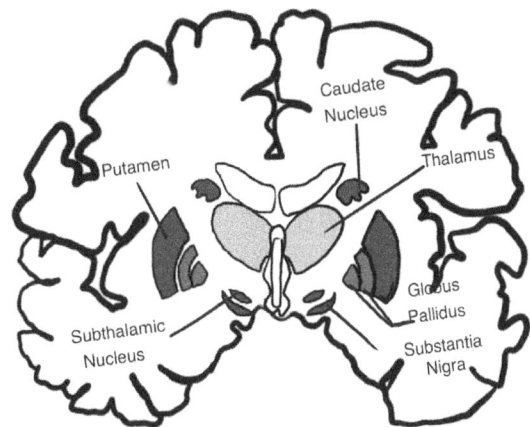

Figure 5.3 Basal Ganglia

motor system (tracts that do not pass through the pyramids carrying involuntary motor signals to the spinal cord) but works in tandem with the pyramidal (carrying voluntary motor signals to the spinal cord) and limbic systems.[42] It chooses which actions to allow and which to inhibit during motor movements[43] and uses two pathways—the direct and indirect pathway—to fine-tune our voluntary movements. Along with other higher cortical functions, the BG plans and modulates skeletal muscle movement, including eye movements, blinking, walking, and facial expressions, as well as being involved with working memory, reward processing, and motivation.[42] There are a number of disorders linked to BG deficits, including Huntington disease,

Parkinson disease, restless leg syndrome, Tourette syndrome, Meige syndrome, Wilson disease, attention deficit hyperactivity disorder (ADHD), autism, schizophrenia, obsessive-compulsive disorder, mood disorders, insomnia, anxiety, addiction, and basal ganglia stroke.

The BG consists of five pairs of nuclei that include the caudate nucleus and putamen (together referred to as the *striatum*), globus pallidus (consisting of the globus pallidus interna and externa), subthalamic nucleus, and substantia nigra.

As mentioned, there are two major pathways in the BG: the direct pathway (DP) that promotes movement and the indirect pathway (IP) that inhibits movement (Figures 5.4 and 5.5). Both

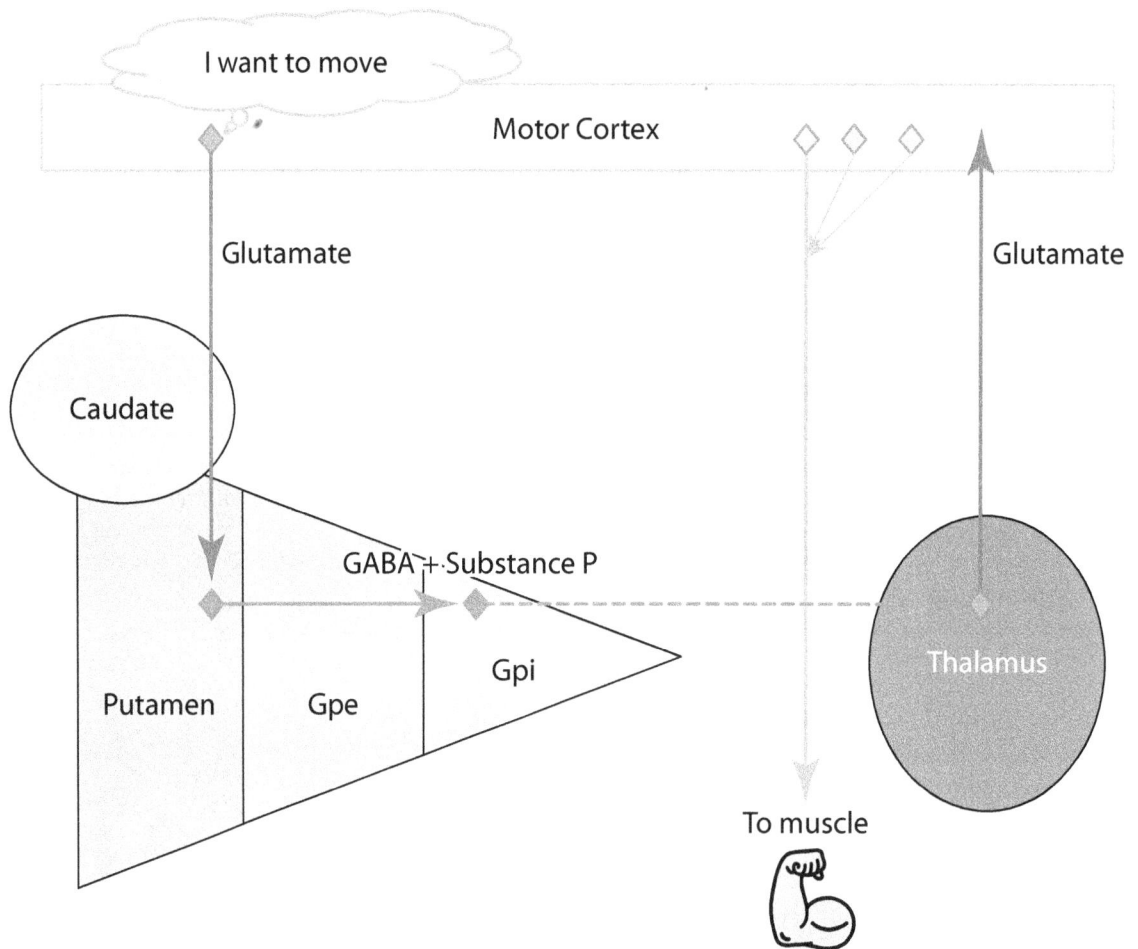

Figure 5.4 Basal Ganglia Direct Pathway

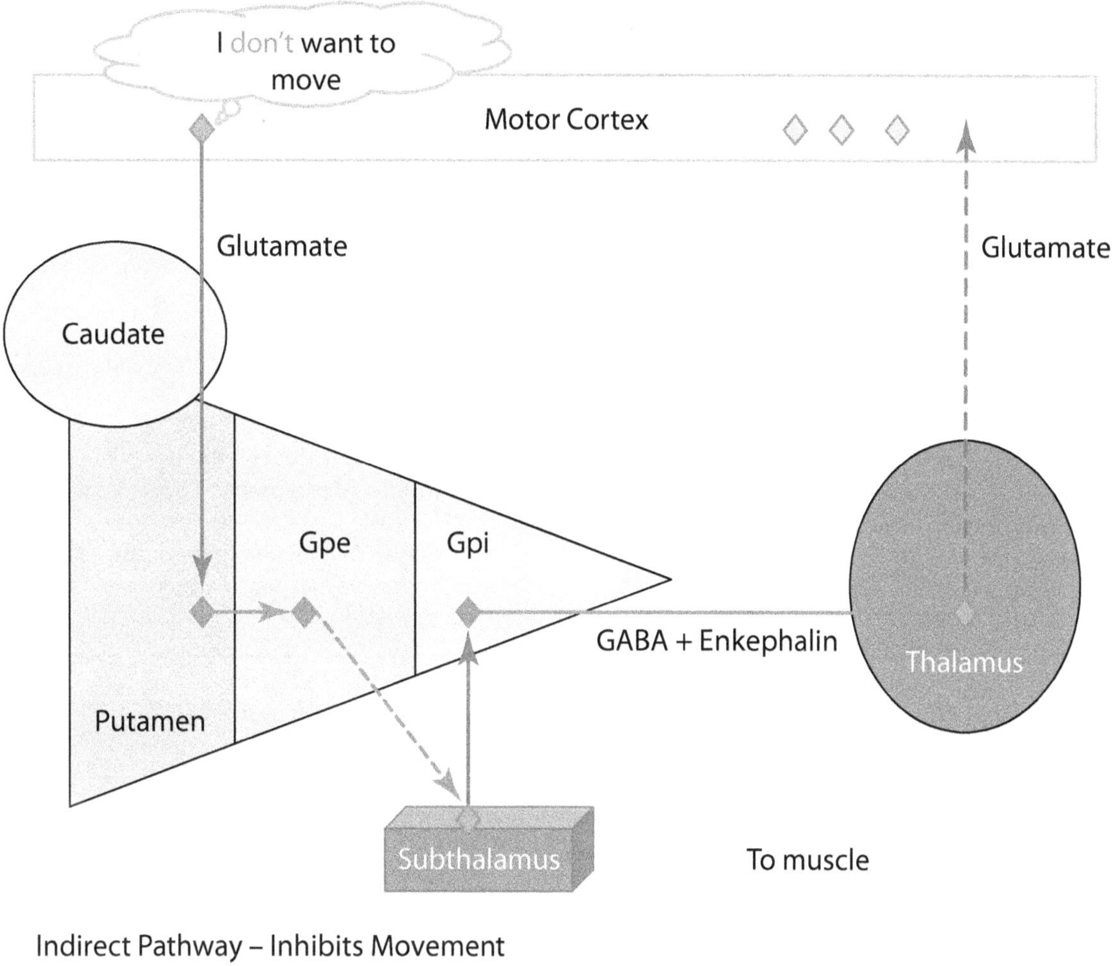

Indirect Pathway – Inhibits Movement

Figure 5.5 Basal Ganglia Indirect Pathway

pathways begin with an "action" signal from the motor cortex using the neurotransmitter glutamate. In the DP, the signal is first sent to the caudate/putamen, where it synapses with and activates inhibitory neurons. The now activated inhibitory neurons send GABA and substance P to the globus pallidus interna (GPi), where it synapses with and inhibits the firing of other neurons that send information to the thalamus. Since the thalamus is not inhibited, it sends action signals back to the motor cortex, that sends action signals to the skeletal muscles, turning them on (see Figure 5.4).

GEEK STUFF

Here is a mnemonic to remember the basal ganglia nuclei:

Put a Carrot and Glazed Pancakes under the Thalamus Sunday Night.

- **put**amen, **ca**udate (nucleus), **gl**obus **pal**lidus, under the thalamus = **su**bthalamic nucleus, **su**bstantia **ni**gra

The IP has to find a way to inhibit the thalamic action signal, so it takes an indirect path to send an inhibitory message to it. The IP begins with an action signal from the motor cortex to the caudate and putamen that synapses with and activates in inhibitory neurons. The inhibitory neurons in the caudate/putamen send an inhibitory signal to the globus pallidus externa (GPe) where it synapses and inhibits the firing of other inhibitory neurons to the subthalamus. Since the subthalamus is not inhibited, it sends an action signal to the GPe where it synapses with and activates inhibitory neurons. The now activated inhibitory neurons in the GPi send inhibitory signals using GABA and enkephalin to the thalamus, where it inhibits the firing of an action signal back to the motor cortex. Since there is no longer an action signal sent back to the motor cortex, no neurons there are activated, and no messages are sent to the skeletal muscles and no movement occurs.

Obviously, we modulate our movements that allow us to either tap someone on the shoulder or give a punch. We do this using dopamine from the substantia nigra pars compacta, which sends dopamine to the caudate/putamen to synapse on D1 and D2 receptors. Dopamine will enhance or dampen the inhibitory signals sent from the caudate/putamen and enhance movements. Think of the volume button on your radio. The radio plays music, but the volume control determines how loud the sound is, just as dopamine modulates the force/speed of movement. When we flex our arms and make our biceps bulge, we need to reduce the activation of the triceps muscle to allow elbow flexion. Dopamine plays a role in fine-tuning these muscle activities. Acetylcholine (Ach), on the other hand, acts in the opposite manner to dopamine. Where dopamine excites, Ach will inhibit. Where dopamine inhibits, Ach will excite.

After the fine-tuned information is sent back to the cortex, the orders (impulses) are sent to the skeletal muscles through the tracts of the pyramidal motor system.[42]

Neurotransmitters used in the BG include acetylcholine, dopamine, GABA, glutamate, and serotonin. These neurotransmitters exert control on D1–D5 receptors to modulate output.

GEEK STUFF

Direct pathway

- Facilitates cortically initiated movements.
- Enhanced conduction through the direct pathway leads to hyperkinesia.
- Inhibited conduction through the direct pathway leads to hypokinesia.

Indirect pathway

- Suppresses potentially conflicting or unwanted motor activity.
- Enhanced conduction through the indirect pathway leads to hypokinesia or akinesia.
- Inhibited conduction through the indirect pathway leads to hyperkinesia or dyskinesia.

DIENCEPHALON

The diencephalon is superior and anterior to the brainstem or midline at the base of the cerebrum and includes the thalamus, hypothalamus, epithalamus, and subthalamus.

Thalamus

The thalamus is a relay station with almost all pathways (sensory and motor) going to the cerebral cortex carrying specific information going through it.[2] Motor systems that connect from the cerebral cortex to the cerebellum, projections between the basal nuclei and cerebral cortex, and limbic projections to the cerebral cortex typically also involve the thalamus.[2] Blood supply for the thalamus is provided by the posterior cerebral artery.[44]

Hypothalamus

Forming the floor and also located in the medial wall of the third ventricle, the hypothalamus is the autonomic control center of the brain regulating visceral responses, temperature, the wake–sleep cycle, and some limbic system functions.[2,44]

Epithalamus

Located in the posterior part of the roof and the adjoining part of the lateral wall of the third ventricle, it contains among other structures the pineal gland. This endocrine gland secretes melatonin in response to darkness, and other hormones that have a regulatory influence on many endocrine organs.[44]

Subthalamus

Lying below the posterior part of the thalamus and lateral to the hypothalamus and continuous with the upper ends of the red nucleus and subtantia nigra,[2,44] the subthalamic nucleus is involved with motor control in coordination with the basal ganglia. Containing glutaminergic neurons projecting to the GPi, stimulation of the GPi ultimately will inhibit movement. Damage to the subthalamus will result in hemiballismus.[45]

CEREBELLUM

The word *cerebellum* is Latin for "little brain," as it protrudes from under the posterior inferior cerebral cortex in the back of the brain and is located in the posterior cranial fossa behind the fourth ventricle and is behind the pons and medulla oblongata.[46] It represents only 10% of the total weight of the brain but contains roughly 50% of the brain's neurons.[2] The cerebellum is important for being able to perform everyday voluntary activities and is essential to upright posture and the ability to balance, but does not initiate these motions. When assessing patients with balance deficits or complaints of dizziness, the cerebellum and brainstem must be a consideration as when there are deficiencies in cerebellar function due to trauma or disease, a person may have difficulty with balance, walking, speaking, coordinating fine motor movements, may display ataxic movements, tremors, dizziness, or nystagmus. Unlike the motor cortex where one cerebral hemisphere controls the contralateral skeletal muscles, the cerebellum influences the ipsilateral side of the body.[2] It receives information from the spinal cord, cerebral cortex, and vestibular nuclei, and sends information through the brainstem. Major jobs of the cerebellum include:

- Adjusting motor responses by comparing planned movements to sensory data regarding actual movements.
- Modulates force and range of motion of movements.
- Involved in motor learning

CEREBELLAR ANATOMY

The cerebellum is comprised of two hemispheres with each of its three lobes being separated by two transverse fissures. The primary fissure is shaped like a V and separates the anterior and posterior lobes, while the posterolateral fissure separates the posterior lobe from the flocculonodular lobe.[46]

The cerebellum has:

- Three lobes
- Three zones
- Three functional areas
- Three pairs of peduncles
- Three pairs of cerebellar nuclei

The cerebellum is folded in half (think of an omelet or taco) with the anterior lobe being superior and anterior, and the posterior lobe making up the rest of the fold, and the flocculonodular lobe making up the inside of the omelet. The cortex of the cerebellum is covered by gray matter but has a white core and is folded like an accordion that is fused at the midline.[46] See Figure 5.6.

If you take the cerebellum and lay it flat, it is easier to describe the zones and functional areas. See Figure 5.7.

The three cerebellar zones correspond to the functional zones:

1. Lateral zone (cerebrocerebellum functional zones)
2. Intermediate zone (spinocerebellum functional zone)
3. Flocculonodular zone (vestibulocerebellum function zone)

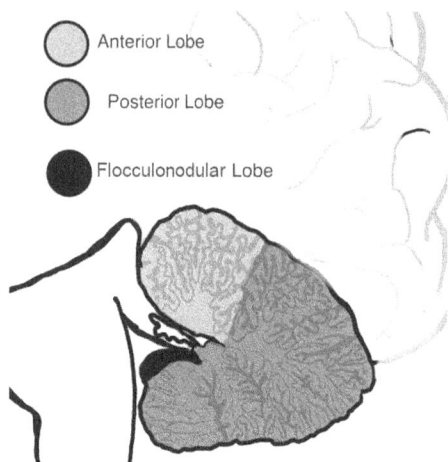

Figure 5.6 Lobes of the Cerebellum

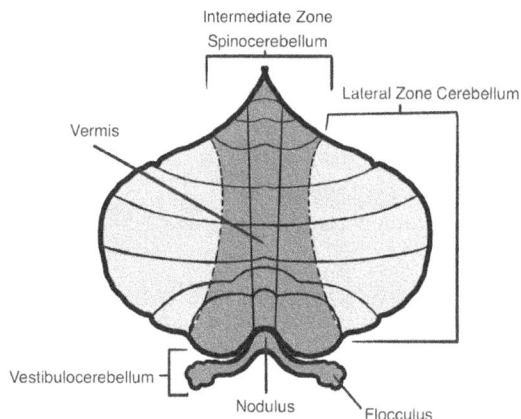

Figure 5.7 Cerebellar Zones

Functional Areas

CEREBROCEREBELLUM

The cerebrocerebellum is comprised of the lateral hemispheres of the cerebellum.[47] It plans movements, coordinates muscle activation, is important for visually guided movements, and is involved in motor learning. It receives input from the cerebral cortex (parietal lobe) via the pons. Output from the cerebrocerebellum goes to the thalamus and then the premotor cortex, the primary motor area, and the red nucleus.

Lesions of the cerebrocerebellum (lateral cerebellar zones) result in errors in the direction, force, speed, and amplitude of movements. Deficits you may see include dysmetria (past-pointing), dysdiadochokinesia (impaired rapid-alternating movements), rebound phenomena (lack of force control), and intention tremors.

SPINOCEREBELLUM

The spinocerebellum is comprised of the intermediate zone and near the midline of the cerebellum.[47] It regulates body movements and aids in error correction and receives input from the dorsal column of the spinal cord, the trigeminal nerve (CN V), visual system, auditory system, and the spinocerebellar tract. The vermis, which is part of this zone and runs along the middle, is involved in posture, limb movements, and trunk and eye movements. The spinocerebellum receives information regarding limb sensations of touch, proprioception, and pressure sensation from the spinal cord. Adjacent to the vermis, the spinocerebellum (intermediate zone) controls distal extremities, while the rest of the cerebrocerebellum (lateral zones) plans sequential movements of the entire body.[46] The spinocerebellum (including the vermis) contains two maps of the body that represent sensory input. Output from the spinocerebellum goes to the deep cerebellar nuclei, and then to the cerebral cortex and brainstem. Lesions of this zone result in deficits of whole-body posture, locomotion, and eye motions. The cerebellum also has a homunculus, which is a representation of the parts of the cerebellum that correspond to contralateral motor and sensory functions (Figure 5.8).

VESTIBULOCEREBELLUM

The vestibulocerebellum is comprised of the flocculonodular lobe as well as the lingula (the anterior tip of the spinocerebellum).[47] It controls balance, posture, and ocular reflexes, especially visual fixation. It is focused on spatial awareness and balance. It receives information from the vestibular system, and auditory and visual systems. Along with the vermis of the spinocerebellum, it is involved with all classes of eye movements. When there are deficits to this zone you may see nystagmus and/or vestibular function loss, and disturbed balance and gait.

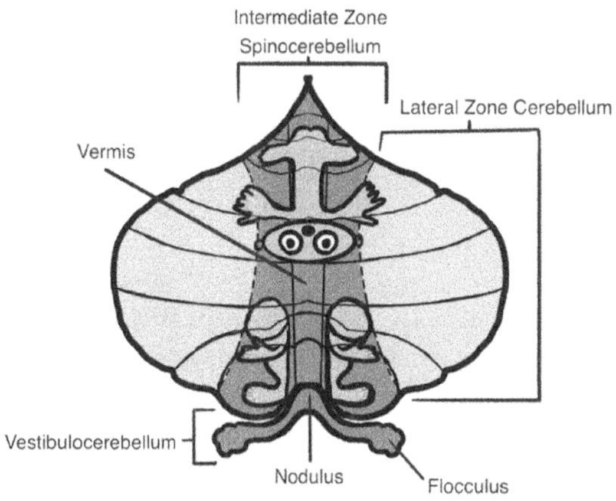

Figure 5.8 Cerebellar Homunculus

Cerebellar Nuclei

There are three paired cerebellar nuclei (one in each cerebellar hemisphere). They are the fastigial nucleus, interposed nucleus (comprise of the globose and emboliform nuclei), and the dentate nucleus. These nuclei can be separated into a rostrolateral group and a caudomedial group, with the rostrolateral group being made up of the emboliform and dentate nuclei and the caudomedial group comprised of the fastigial and globose nuclei.

GEEK STUFF

A mnemonic to remember the cerebellar nuclei is:

Denise Embraces Global Fasting.

- dentate, emboliform, globose, fastigial

DENTATE NUCLEI

Named for its dentate (serrated) edge, these nuclei are the largest of the cerebellar neurons. They are involved in the modulation with conscious thought and visuospatial function,[48] modulating movements of skeletal muscles of the extremities and oculomotor muscles.[49] Deficits of the dentate nucleus usually result in cerebellar ataxia.[48]

Afferent connections to the dentate nuclei include proprioception information via the spinocerebellar tract (through the inferior cerebellar peduncle).

Efferent connections send signals through the superior cerebral peduncle and decussate to the contralateral thalamus that then connects to the premotor cortex, prefrontal gyri, posterior parietal areas, and basal ganglia.[48,50,51]

GLOBOSE AND EMBOLIFORM NUCLEI

These nuclei are lateral to the fastigial nucleus, with the globose nuclei being closer to the fastigial nucleus and the emboliform nucleus being closer to the dentate nucleus. Together they are called the "interposed nucleus" as they are located 'between' the dentate and fastigial neuclei.[52] Efferent proprioceptive information is sent to the lateral thalamus and then relayed to the precentral gyrus that sends regulatory signals down the lateral corticospinal tract to distal muscles. Proprioceptive information is also sent to the red nucleus then down the rubrospinal tract to manage distal flexor muscles.[52]

FASTIGIAL NUCLEI

Fastigial nuclei are closest to the midline in the anterior segment of the superior vermis and play a role in motor control by sending signals to the brainstem and cranial nerves that deal with eye movement, as well as assist with feeding, cardiovascular, respiratory, and immune functions, as well as regulating defecation and micturition function.[53] Afferent connections to the fastigial nuclei include signals from the inferior olive, medullary/pontine reticular formation, and hypothalamus. In monkeys, it has been found that afferent connections from the flocculus to the fastigial nucleus play a role in mediating visual–vestibular interactions.[54] Efferent pathways include connections to the primary motor cortex,[55,56] vestibular nuclei, and medullary/pontine reticular formations;[53,57,58] and to the brainstem (to regulate head, face, and eye movements),[59] the hypothalamus, and limbic system.[60,61]

Afferent Connections

The following areas send afferent connections to the cerebellum: the skin, muscles, tendons, and joints, olivary nucleus, vestibular nuclei, cortex, and trigeminal nucleus.

Efferent Connections

Information is sent from the cerebellum to the extensor muscles via the cerebellovestibular tract, the brainstem via the cerebelloreticular tract, the thalamus via the cerebellothalamic tract, and to the motor systems of the brainstem via the cerebellorubral tract.[47]

Peduncles

The word *peduncle* is Latin for "little foot." There are three pairs of peduncles—the superior, middle, and inferior—connecting the cerebellum to the rest of the brain and CNS. In general, most of the afferent nerve fibers enter the cerebellum via the middle (from the pons) and inferior peduncles (from the medulla oblongata), with the bulk of the efferent fibers exiting through the superior peduncle to the midbrain. The superior cerebellar peduncle is mostly an efferent pathway transmitting information from the cerebellar nuclei to the upper motor neurons in the red nucleus as well as the superior colliculi, with information then relayed to the thalamus, primary motor cortex and premotor cortex.[62] The middle cerebellar peduncle is an afferent pathway from the pons, with information relayed from the cerebral cortex and superior colliculus.[62] The inferior cerebellar peduncle (also called the restiform body) contains both efferent to the vestibular nuclei and reticular formation, while afferent fibers arrive from the vestibular nuclei, spinal cord, and several regions of the brainstem gray matter.[62]

Blood Supply

The cerebellum is supplied by a posterior blood supply system (vertebrobasilar artery system) of three paired arteries (Table 5.8).[46]

Cerebellar Damage

Cerebellar damage, no matter the cause, results in errors in movement on the same side as the damage.[62] Somatic and visual inputs are represented in a topographic fashion in the cerebellum, and damage to one part of the cerebellum may cause movement difficulties for one part of the body, but other parts will not be affected.[62] Depending on the location of the damage, deficits may include a wide-based and unsteady gait, hypotonia, dysdiadochokinesia, intentional tremors, staccato speech, trunk ataxia, limb ataxia, dysmetria, rebound phenomena, nystagmus, and imbalance. Oculomotor abnormalities following cerebellar damage include vertical skew deviations, esotropia (usually greater with distance viewing), dysconjugate saccades, and dysconjugate vestibular responses.

An easy way to remember some cerebellar signs is using the word DANISH:[63]

- D: dysdiadochokinesia and dysmetria
- A: ataxia
- N: nystagmus
- I: intention tremor
- S: speech (slurred or scanning)
- H: hypotonia

Table 5.9 lists the types of cerebellar dysfunctions and their causes.[63]

Some of the principal cerebellar complications are described next.

Table 5.8 Blood Supply to the Cerebellum

Cerebellar Location	Blood Supply
• Most of the cerebellar cortex • Cerebellar nuclei • Superior cerebellar peduncles	Superior cerebellar artery (SCA) (a branch of the basilar artery)
• *Anterior* portion of the inferior cerebellum • Middle cerebellar peduncle	Anterior inferior cerebellar artery (AICA) (a branch of the basilar artery)
• *Posterior* inferior portion of the cerebellum • Inferior cerebellar peduncle	Posterior inferior cerebellar artery (PICA) (the largest branch of the vertebral artery)

Table 5.9 Causes of Cerebellar Dysfunction

Cerebellar Dysfunction	Most Important Causes

Unilateral	• Unilateral posterior circulation ischemic/hemorrhagic stroke
	  • Part of lateral medullary syndrome (LMS)
	  • Hemiparesis with ataxia following lacunar stroke
	• Multiple sclerosis
	• Space-occupying lesions (SOL) in the posterior cranial fossa (abscess from tuberculosis, staph), tumors
	• Unilateral cerebellar–pontine angle lesions or SOL (e.g., neurofibromatosis, schwannoma)
	• Multiple system atrophy

Bilateral	• Multiple sclerosis • Posterior circulation stroke • Bilateral cerebellar–pontine angle lesions or tumors • Paraneoplastic syndromes • Multiple system atrophy (MSA) • Toxins and drugs: Alcohol, phenytoin, lithium, carbamazepine • Metabolic: Hypothyroidism, B12 deficiency, Wilson disease, celiac disease • Infections: Enteroviruses, HIV, neurosyphilis, toxoplasmosis, borreliosis, Creutzfeldt–Jakob disease • Inflammation: Miller Fischer variant of Guillain–Barré syndrome • Hereditary: Friedreich ataxia, Von Hippel–Lindau syndrome, spinocerebellar ataxias, ataxia telangiectasia
Spastic paresis with cerebellar signs	• Multiple sclerosis • Friedreich ataxia • Spinocerebellar ataxia • Arnold–Chiari malformation • Syringomyelia, syringobulbia

Dandy Walker Syndrome

This is a congenital malformation where there is a partial or absent vermis. Symptoms include slow motor development, convulsions, vomiting, and a large fourth ventricle (and increased intracranial pressure).[47]

Arnold–Chiari Malformation

Arnold–Chiari malformations describe a group of deformities that include the cerebellum, pons, and medulla oblongata.[64] These malformations are classified based on anatomical defect and morphology and are listed[64] in Table 5.10.

Presentation of Chiari I includes headaches and/or neck pain (80%), exacerbated with a Valsalva maneuver. Other common symptoms include ocular disturbances, dizziness, hearing loss, vertigo, gait ataxia, and general fatigue. Other signs and symptoms that may be observed or reported with Chiari malformation include myelopathy (with loss of pain and temperature sensations but preserved fine touch and proprioception) and motor weakness.[66,67] Cerebellar signs include ataxia, dysmetria, and nystagmus. Cranial nerve deficits from CN IX, X, XI, and XII may be present. Sleep apnea may occur. Also, it is not uncommon for no clinical manifestations to occur.[64]

In terms of the cerebellum, this is a congenital malformation in which the cerebellar tonsils fall below the foramen magnum obstructing blood flow inside the skull, as well as obstructing cerebrospinal

Table 5.10 Chiari Malformation Classifications

Malformation Classification	Characterizations
Chiari I	Least severe, characterized pointed cerebellar tonsils projecting 5 mm below the foramen magnum
Chiari II	Brainstem herniation and towering cerebellum Herniated cerebellar tonsils and vermis
Chiari III	Herniation of the cerebellum with or without the brainstem into low occipital or high cervical meningoencephalocele (an abnormal sac of flue, brain tissue, and meninges extending through a defect in the skull)
Chiari IV	No longer used
Chiari V	Most severe, characterized by cerebellar agenesis (the brain develops without a cerebellum) with occipital lone descent and herniation through the foramen magnum[65]

fluid flow. Symptoms include headaches, neck pain, tingling of hands/feet, vomiting, and fatigue.[47]

Alcoholism

Alcoholism may cause thiamine (B1) deficiency that leads to cerebellar degeneration. Symptoms include balance problems, vertigo, hypotonia, diplopia, nystagmus, ataxia, tremors, unsteady and uncoordinated gait, wide-based gait, and motor skills deficits.[68]

According to Kheradmand and Zee, there are three principle cerebellar syndromes: floccular–parafloccular syndrome, ventral uvula–nodular syndrome, and oculomotor vermis–caudal fastigial nuclei syndromes.[69]

Floccular–Parafloccular Syndrome

This syndrome affects eye motion. The flocculus and paraflocculus are responsible for haze holding, smooth pursuit, vestibular ocular reflex cancellation (VOR-C), controlling amplitude and direction of rotational VOR, and preventing post-saccadic drift. Keeping this in mind, the cardinal signs of this syndrome include:

1. *Pursuit deficits*: Smooth tracking is impaired when the head is still, and VOR-C is impaired when the head is moving.
2. Impaired gaze holding with the eyes drifting centripetally (toward the center).
3. Downbeat nystagmus.

Ventral Uvula–Nodular Syndrome

The nodulus and adjacent ventral uvula are the most caudal aspects of the vermis and act upon low-frequency components of the VOR via projects to the velocity–storage mechanism of the vestibular nuclei. The velocity storage mechanism slows the decay of nystagmus during constant-velocity head rotations and extends the duration of the VOR response. It also improves the VOR at lower head rotation frequencies.

Lesions of the nodulus result in:

- An increase in duration of the VOR response to constant velocity input.
- Loss of habituation to repetitive stimulation.
- Tilt suppression of post-rotary nystagmus no longer occurs.
- VOR no longer reorients to the axis of rotation that normally occurs with an imposed linear acceleration.
- Periodic alternating nystagmus (PAN) are horizontal jerk-type nystagmus that change direction every few minutes.

Lesions to both the nodulus and uvula result in:

- Abnormally directed slow phases of nystagmus during low-frequency head rotation around an earth-vertical axis.
- Sustained optokinetic stimulation with the head upright and after horizontal head shaking.

- Alterations to smooth pursuit and optokinetic nystagmus.

Oculomotor Vermis–Caudal Fastigial Nuclei Syndromes

- *Dorsal vermis lobules V–VII and posterior fastigial nucleus lesions*: Changes in saccade accuracy, latency, adaptation, and dynamic properties; changes in smooth pursuit and pursuit adaptation.
- *Fastigial oculomotor region lesions*: Hypermetria and hypometria in both horizontal directions, contralateral pursuit impairment.

Wallenberg Syndrome

Occlusion of the posterior inferior cerebellar artery (PICA) will cause Wallenberg syndrome and includes the following signs/symptoms: dysphagia and dysarthria resulting from paralysis of the ipsilateral palatal and laryngeal muscles; analgesia of the ipsilateral side of the face; vertigo, nausea, vomiting, and nystagmus; ipsilateral Horner syndrome; ipsilateral limb ataxia and contralateral loss of sensations of pain and temperature.[46,70]

BRAINSTEM

The brainstem is located toward the base of the brain and consists of the *midbrain, pons,* and *medulla oblongata.* It connects the cerebrum to the spinal cord and cerebellum, and deals with alertness, arousal, breathing, heart rate, and blood pressure. Ten of the twelve cranial nerves (CNs) arise from nuclei in the brainstem (Figure 5.9).

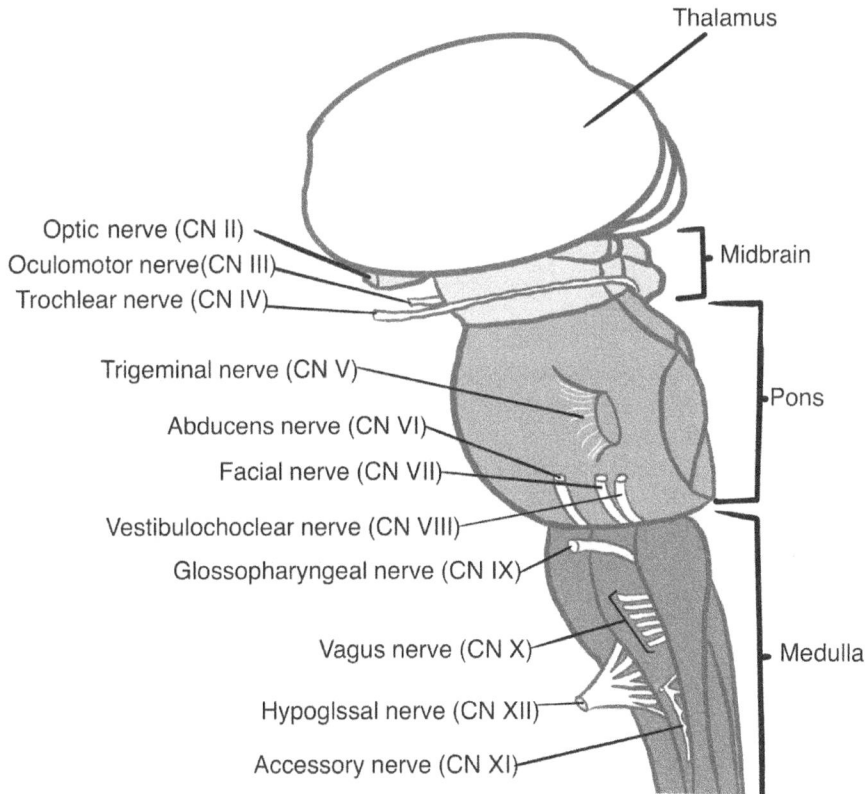

Figure 5.9 Brainstem

MIDBRAIN

Connecting the pons and diencephalon, the midbrain (also called the mesencephalon) contains the cerebral aqueduct, which connects the third ventricle superiorly with the fourth ventricle inferiorly. The midbrain may be separated into three sections: tectum, tegmentum, and cerebral peduncles.

The midbrain has several parts that have specialized functions:

- CN III (oculomotor nerve)
- CN IV (trochlear nerve)
- Edinger–Westphal nucleus (parasympathetic eye innervation)
- Red nucleus (contralateral coordinating motor control, locomotion)
- Substantia nigra (dopamine production, reward system)
- The reticular formation passes through (motor function)
- The superior and inferior colliculi (vision and hearing)
- The thalamus (integrates and sends sensory information)
- The hippocampus passes through (which regulates short-term memory)
- The hypothalamus (controls the nervous system)
- The pineal body (controls melatonin to regulate sleep)

Tectum

The tectum is posterior to the cerebral aqueduct, which is a narrow conduit for cerebrospinal fluid between the third and fourth ventricles, and contains the bilateral superior and inferior colliculi, which are shaped like hills (the name *colliculi* is derived from a Latin word meaning "hill"). The superior colliculi are involved with visual reflexes, and the inferior colliculi are involved in processing auditory information.

Tegmentum

Located between the cerebral aqueduct and the pars compacta substantia nigra contains two areas

named for colors: red nucleus (involved in coordination of movements) and periaqueductal gray matter (involved in pain processing).[71] The tegmentum is also involved in alertness.

Cerebral Peduncle

The two cerebral peduncles are comprised of white matter, are cylindrical shaped, and are separated by a space called the interpeduncular fossa. Do not confuse these with the three pairs of cerebellar peduncles. The ventral and dorsal sides of each peduncle are separated by the *substantia nigra* (black substance), which produces the neurotransmitter dopamine, which is needed for motor control, cognitive executive function, and limbic (emotion) activity, and acts as part of the basal ganglia. The substantia nigra has two parts, the dorsal pars compacta containing the neurons that produce dopamine, and the pars reticulata that contains neurons that produce the inhibitory neurotransmitter GABA.

Ascending and Descending Pathways

See Table 5.11.

Midbrain Injury

Injury or damage to the midbrain may cause difficulty with coordinated movement, posture, disequilibrium, speaking, swallowing, vision, hearing, loss of sensation, and memory. CN III damage can cause a palsy where the eye presents down and out, dilated pupil, blurred vision, diplopia, and head tilt toward the unaffected side to compensate for the oculomotor palsy.

PONS

Connecting the medulla oblongata inferiorly to the midbrain superiorly and cerebellum posteriorly via the middle cerebellar peduncles, the pons contains cranial nerves VI (abducens nerve), VII (facial nerve), and VIII (vestibulocochlear nerve).[73] The anterior portion of the pons is convex. Functionally, it influences the sleep cycle and level of alertness, relays and regulates pain signals from

Table 5.11 Ascending/Descending Pathways of the Midbrain

Ascending Pathways of the Midbrain[72]	Descending Pathways of the Midbrain[72]
• *Superior cerebellar peduncles* contain the cerebellothalamic and cerebellorubral tracts. • *Medial longitudinal fasciculus* connects the oculomotor, trochlear, abducens, Edinger–Westphal, vestibular, reticular, and spinal accessory nuclei. • *Medial lemniscus* continues on the dorsal column of the spinal cord and carries information regarding vibration, light touch, skin stretch, proprioception, temperature, texture, pressure, and discrimination to the thalamus. • *Lateral lemniscus* conveys auditory information from the cochlear nucleus to the contralateral inferior colliculus. • *Trigeminal lemniscus* carries information regarding tactile, pain, and temperature sensations from the face to the thalamus. • *Spinal lemniscus* conveys pain, temperature sensation, non-discriminative touch, and pressure to the thalamus.	The *crus cerebri* is the most ventral area of a cerebral peduncle and is composed of three descending pathways to the pons (collectively called the longitudinal pontine fibers when they are in the pons): • Corticospinal • Corticonuclear • Corticopontine pathways

Table 5.12 Ascending/Descending Neural Tracts of the Pons

Pons Ascending Tracts	Pons Descending Tracts
• Medial lemniscus • Lateral lemniscus • Spinal lemniscus (spinothalamic tract) • Trigeminal lemniscus (trigeminothalamic tract) • Superior cerebellar peduncle	• Corticospinal • Corticobulbar (corticonuclear) • Corticopontine

the body, eye movement, manages breathing, and assists in balance and movement.

Ascending and Descending Neural Tracts of the Pons

See Table 5.12.[74]

Vestibular Nuclei

The vestibular nuclei are located at the junction of the pons and medulla, and project to the contralateral vestibular nuclei, spinal cord, cerebellum, thalamus, and motor nuclei of the extraocular muscles. It has the job of maintaining balance, posture, head position, and clear vision during head movement.[75] The four main vestibular nuclei are the lateral, medial, superior, and inferior (descending) (Table 5.13).[75,76]

Connections to the Peripheral Vestibular System

Afferent vestibular information travels along CN VIII (vestibulocochlear nerve) from the peripheral vestibular system of the inner ear, through the internal auditory canal, through the cerebellar–pontine angle to arrive at the vestibular nuclei. Most of the input from the crista ampullaris of the anterior and lateral semicircular canals arrives at the superior and medial vestibular nuclei, while the inferior and lateral nuclei receive information from the inferior semicircular canals, utricle, and saccule.[76]

Table 5.13 Vestibular Nuclei

Vestibular Nucleus	Function
Lateral vestibular nucleus	Aids in the vestibulospinal reflex (VSR) and sends axons via the lateral vestibulospinal tract to maintain balance.
Medial vestibular nucleus	Mediates the vestibular–ocular reflex (VOR).
Superior vestibular nucleus	Aids in coordination and postural adjustments and related eye movements, and communicates with the flocculonodular lobe of the cerebellum. It plays a role in the conscious perception of gravity and movement.
Inferior (descending) vestibular nucleus	Receives information regarding head tilt and gravity.

Connections with the Cortex

The superior and lateral vestibular nuclei project to the thalamus, which relays signals to the primary vestibular cortex of the parietal lobe (adjacent to the primary motor cortex). Other identified connections include one to the primary somatosensory cortex, and another between the somatosensory and motor cortices.[76]

Connections with the Cerebellum

Projections from the vestibular nuclei to the inferior olivary nucleus are relayed to the inferior cerebellar peduncle and then to the ipsilateral cerebellar vermis, flocculus, and nodulus.[76] Some first-order neurons of the vestibular Scarpa's ganglion, after passing through the inferior cerebellar peduncle, synapse directly with the ipsilateral vestibulocerebellum, vermis, and fastigial nucleus.[76]

Pons Injury

Pons infarct presentations vary from the common "crossed syndrome" with ipsilateral cranial nerve palsy and contralateral motor and/or sensory impairment to the less common pure motor hemiparesis or hemiplegia, and pure sensory impairment.[77] Clinical presentations of the anatomical/arterial territories are classified as follows.[77]

VENTRO-CAUDAL PONTINE INFARCT

This is caused by decreased blood flow in the paramedian perforating arteries from the basilar artery and causes the following symptoms:

contralateral motor hemiparesis or hemiplegia (corticospinal tract), ipsilateral facial nerve palsy, ipsilateral abducens palsy, contralateral decreased pain, and temperature sensation (lateral spinothalamic tract).

MID-PONTINE BASE INFARCT

Caused by decreased blood flow in the paramedian arteries from the basilar artery. Symptoms depend on the area of pons affected:

- *Pontine nucleus*: Ipsilateral ataxia
- *Trigeminal nerve fibers*: Ipsilateral face sensorimotor weakness
- *Corticospinal tract*: Hemiparesis

TEGMENTAL PONTINE SYNDROME

This syndrome can affect many structures, including cranial nerves (V, VI, VII, VIII), medial lemniscus, medial longitudinal fasciculus, respiratory centers, and the pontine reticular formation.

Rostral Pontine Syndrome

Blood flow obstruction in the anterior inferior or superior cerebellar arteries cause:

- *Trigeminal nuclei*: Ipsilateral facial sensory disturbances and masticator paralysis
- *Tectospinal tract*: Impaired blinking
- *Lateral spinothalamic tract and medial lemniscus*: Contralateral hemisensory loss
- *Superior cerebellar peduncle*: Ipsilateral hemiataxia

Caudal Pontine Syndrome

Blood flow loss in the circumferential or anterior inferior cerebellar artery presents as:

- *Medial longitudinal fasciculus*: Ipsilateral conjugate gaze palsy and nystagmus
- *Abducens nucleus*: Ipsilateral impaired eye abduction
- *Middle cerebellar peduncle*: Ipsilateral hemiataxia
- *Lateral spinothalamic tract and medial lemniscus*: Contralateral hemisensory loss

MULTIPLE PONTINE INFRACTS

Infarcts primarily affecting the territory of the perforating arteries results in:
- *Corticobulbar fibers*: Pseudobulbar palsy (dysarthria, dysphagia, face and tongue weakness, emotional lability). Some individuals present with pathological crying or laughing.

BILATERAL PONTINE INFARCTS

Caused by impaired blood flow in the basilar artery. Presents with:

- Tetraplegia
- Impaired consciousness
- Locked-in syndrome (tetraplegia, bilateral facial paralysis, pharyngeal, and horizontal gaze palsy with retained consciousness and cognition)

ANATOMICAL LOCATIONS OF PONTINE INFARCTS

See Table 5.14.[77]

MEDULLA OBLONGATA

Connecting the brainstem to the spinal cord, the medulla oblongata (or simply medulla), contains cranial nerves IX (glossopharyngeal nerve), X (vagus nerve), XI (accessory nerve), and XII (hypoglossal nerve).

It is comprised of the cardiovascular-regulation system, descending motor tracts, ascending sensory tracts, and the aforementioned cranial nerves. About 85% to 90% of motor neurons decussate at the lower medulla to form the lateral corticospinal tract.[78,79]

Pyramids

The medullary pyramids are paired white matter pyramid or ridge-shaped structures that contain the axons of the corticospinal and corticonuclear (sometimes called the corticobulbar) tracts (motor fibers) whose cell bodies are in the motor cortex (upper motor neurons). Together these tracts are also called pyramidal tracts.

The lateral corticospinal tract descends in the lateral funiculus and synapses with lower motor neurons at each level of the spine, controlling gross and fine motor movements. Non-decussating fibers descend in the anterior corticospinal tract and control proximal muscles and trunk muscles.[79]

Table 5.14 Signs/Symptoms of Pons Infarct by Location

Location of Pons Infarct	Signs/Symptoms
Medial	• Contralateral hemiparesis • Internuclear ophthalmoplegia (affects one or all extraocular muscles; may cause blurred vision and/or diplopia, loss of ocular range of motion, dysconjugate eye movements, or ptosis) • Conjugate horizontal gaze paresis
Lateral	• Contralateral hemisensory loss • Ataxia
Caudal	• Ipsilateral lower motor neuron palsy of the facial nerve • Abducens palsy • Sensorineural hearing loss • Vertigo

The corticonuclear tract travels from the primary motor cortex through the corona radiata, the internal capsule, then the brainstem. It innervates voluntary muscles of the eyes and eyelids. The corticobulbar tract connects the motor cortex and brainstem, and innervates muscles of the face, tongue, and throat.

Extrapyramidal System

Main functions of the extrapyramidal system include maintaining posture and regulating involuntary motor functions.[80] It adjusts muscle tone and controls movements that are originally voluntary but then become automatic through exercise and learning, performs movements that make voluntary movements more natural, and inhibits involuntary movements.[80] To accomplish this it involves parts of the cerebral cortex, cerebellum, thalamus, reticular substance, and basal ganglia.[80]

Olivary Body

The olives are oval or ridge-shaped on the anterior medulla, lateral to the pyramids near the border of the medulla and the pons. There are two parts to the olivary nuclei: inferior and superior. The inferior olivary nucleus acts as a relay between the spine and cerebellum integrating motor and sensory information for cerebellar motor learning and function, while the superior olivary nucleus assists in the perception of sound localization and analysis and acts as a relay between the inferior colliculi and the cochlear nuclei.[81] The cerebellum receives modulatory inputs from the inferior olive that receives motor, sensory, and proprioceptive input from the spine, the motor cortex, motor information from the red nucleus, and eye movement information from the superior colliculus. Next, the information is relayed via the contralateral inferior cerebellar peduncle to the cerebellar nuclei.[81] The signals from the inferior olive are thought to be used to fine-tune movement and process error signals regarding the external environment.

Medullary Injury

There are significant syndromes that occur when there is damage to the medulla.[78]

LATERAL MEDULLARY SYNDROME (WALLENBERG SYNDROME)

This is the most common syndrome due to medullary stroke due to vertebral artery thrombosis or dissection. Signs/symptoms include vertigo, Horner syndrome (sweating, decreased pupil size, and ptosis), headache, dysphonia, pain, impaired facial sensation, vertical nystagmus, dysphagia, and ipsilateral ataxia. Contralaterally, there is impaired pain and temperature sensations of the upper and lower extremities.

MEDIAL MEDULLARY SYNDROME (DEJERINE SYNDROME)

This is contralateral arm and leg paralysis caused by a lack of blood flow to the pyramidal decussation. In about 50% of cases, the contralateral face is also affected. If the medial longitudinal fasciculus is damaged, there may be nystagmus or ipsilateral tongue paralysis.

There are uncommon syndromes as well, which include bilateral medial medullary syndrome, hemimedullary syndrome, and Babinski–Nageotte and Cestan–Chenais syndromes.

CRANIAL NERVES

The twelve pairs of cranial nerves are so named because they originate within the skull and begin in the nuclei of the brain. They are labeled with Roman numerals I through XII based on their location, with CN I (the olfactory nerve) being the closest to the anterior part of the skull. CN I and CN II are different than the other cranial nerves in that they are the only two that begin in the cerebrum. Cranial nerves III, IV, and VI are grouped together because they innervate the six extraocular eye muscles (Table 5.15).

Table 5.15 Cranial Nerve Origins and Exits

CN	Origin	Exits the Skull Via
I	Roof of nasal cavity (olfactory mucosa)	Olfactory foramina of the cribriform plate of the ethmoid bone to the olfactory bulb below the frontal lobe
II	The retina	Optic canal to the optic chiasm
III	Midbrain (at the level of the superior colliculus)	Superior orbital fissure (inside of annulus of Zinn)
IV	Midbrain (at the level of the inferior colliculus)	Superior orbital fissure (outside of annulus of Zinn)
V	Pons (primarily) (also, midbrain, medulla, and spinal cord)	1. V1 branch: Superior orbital fissure (outside of annulus of Zinn) 2. V2 branch: Foramen rotundum 3. V3 branch: Foramen ovale
VI	Pons (inferior part) at pontomedullary junction	Superior orbital fissure (inside of annulus of Zinn)
VII	Pons (primarily)	1. Internal acoustic meatus (internal auditory canal) 2. Stylomastoid foramen
VIII	Pontomedullary junction (some nuclei are in the pons while others are in the medulla)	Internal acoustic meatus (internal auditory canal)
IX	Medulla (primarily)	Jugular foramen
X	Medulla	Jugular foramen
XI	Medulla (cranial part) (primarily) Cervical spinal cord (C1–C5) (spinal part)	1. Jugular foramen (the cranial component and some spinal component) 2. Foramen magnum (spinal component)
XII	Medulla (primarily)	Hypoglossal canal of the occipital condyles

GEEK STUFF

To recall the CNs that control eye movement, remember the following as if it were a chemical formula: LR6 SO4 ATR3.

- *LR6*: The 6th CN supplies the lateral rectus muscle.
- *SO4*: The 4th CN supplies the superior oblique muscle.
- *ATR3*: All the rest of the eye muscles are supplied by the 3rd CN.

The cranial nerves and their functions are in Table 5.16.[82,83]

CRANIAL NERVE LOCATIONS

You can remember the location of the CNs by using the Rule of 4s, where the first four CNs exit the brain (CN 1 and 2) and midbrain (CN 3 and 4), the next four (CN 5–8) exit the pons, and the last four (CN 9–12) exit the medulla.

CRANIAL NERVE DAMAGE

There are many possible causes of cranial nerve damage, including strokes, traumatic brain injuries, infections, increased intracranial pressure, nerve palsies, hypertension, cancer, diseases (such as multiple sclerosis, Lyme, Guillain–Barre, herpes zoster, lupus, Wernicke encephalopathy, Parkinson disease, and cavernous sinus disease), inflammation, tumors, and congenital conditions.

Table 5.16 Cranial Nerves and Their Functions

CN	Nerve	Sensory or Motor	Function
I	Olfactory	Sensory	• Relays information regarding smell
II	Optic	Sensory	• Relays vision information
III	Oculomotor	Motor	• Responsible for motor innervation to four of the six extraocular eye muscles (superior and inferior recti, inferior oblique, and medial rectus) • Controls pupil size and accommodation for near vision
IV	Trochlear	Motor	• Innervates the superior oblique muscle
V	Trigeminal	Sensory and motor	The largest CN has three divisions: 1. *V1 branch*: Ophthalmic (sensory information from the scalp, forehead, conjunctiva, and upper eyelids) 2. *V2 branch*: Maxillary (sensory information from the checks, upper lip, skin of the nose, nasal cavity) 3. *V3 branch*: Mandibular (sensory information from the ears, lower lip, and chin), innervates muscles of the mastication and ears (tensor tympani, tensor veli palatini)
VI	Abducens	Motor	• Innervates the lateral rectus muscle
VII	Facial	Sensory and motor	• Relays information regarding taste form most of the tongue (anterior two-thirds of tongue) • Relays information from the outer part of the ear (touch, pain, temperature) • Innervates muscles of facial expression, closing the eyelid, the stapedius (middle ear), and some of the jaw muscles (mastication) • Innervates glands for salivation, nasal glands, palatine glands, and tear production (lacrimal glands)
VIII	Vestibulocochlear	Sensory	• Cochlear portion: Relays information regarding sound • Vestibular portion: Relays information regarding balance, head motion, and position
IX	Glossopharyngeal	Sensory and motor	• Relays information regarding taste from the back part of the tongue • Relays touch, pain, temperature, and taste from the posterior one-third of the tongue • Relays sensory information from the sinuses, tonsils, pharynx, soft palate, part of the ear, and part of the nasopharynx • Relays information from the baroreceptors and chemoreceptors of the carotid sinus • Innervates the stylopharyngeus muscle of the throat for voluntary pharynx elevation during swallowing and speaking • Innervates the parotid gland

(Continued)

Table 5.16 (Continued)

CN	Nerve	Sensory or Motor	Function
X	Vagus	Sensory and motor	• It is the main parasympathetic nerve (~90% of parasympathetic outflow) • Relays sensations from the ear canal and parts of the throat • Relays sensations from chest and trunk organs (e.g., heart, lungs, liver, spleen, stomach, gallbladder, pancreas, kidneys, and intestines) • Relays information from the aortic arch including baroreceptors, and the partial pressures of O_2 and CO_2 • Relays taste information from the root of the tongue and epiglottis • Innervates throat muscles for swallowing, speech and coughing • Innervates muscles of organs in the chest and trunk, including digestive tract, and sweating
XI	Accessory	Motor	• Innervates muscles of the neck (rotation, flexion, extension) and elevates and retracts the scapulae
XII	Hypoglossal	Motor	Innervates most of the tongue muscle: • Intrinsic muscles: curls tongue • Extrinsic muscles: elevated, depresses, protracts tongue

GEEK STUFF

Mnemonics to remember the cranial nerves:

• Oh, Oh, Oh, To Touch And Feel Very Good Velvet, such A Heaven.

Another mnemonic is:

• On Occasion Our Trusty Truck Acts Funny, Very Good Vehicle Any How.

A mnemonic to remember which are sensory (words beginning with S), which are motor (words beginning with M), or both (words beginning with B) in order of cranial number:

• Some Say Money Matters, But My Brother Says Big Brains Matter More.

A way to remember what each CN is responsible for is to draw a person using the CN number (you can look at the list of CNs to figure this one out).

Damage to various cranial nerves can cause:

• CN I: Affects the ability to smell.
• CN II: Blindness.
• CN III: Produces the inability to move eyes correctly causing diplopia, difficulty opening eyes, and impairs pupil constriction.
• CN IV: Inability to abduct and intort the eye causing vertical and torsional diplopia. The patient typically tilts their head to the contralateral side to compensate for lack of intorsion.
• CN V: May cause neuralgia, difficulty chewing food or speaking, and facial numbness.
• CN VI: Inability to abduct the eye causing horizontal diplopia. The patient presents with one eye adducted.
• CN VII: (Bell palsy 70%, trauma 10–23%, neoplasm 2.2–5%).[84] May cause weakness or paralysis of facial muscles, as well as impaired corneal reflex, orbicularis oculi reflex, and orbicularis oris reflex. Damage in the cerebellopontine angle may additionally decrease saliva and tear secretion, cause a loss of taste in the anterior two-thirds of the tongue, and

cause hyperacusis.[85] Patients may be unable to close their eyes.

- CN VIII: May cause nystagmus, vertigo, nausea, and hearing loss.
- CN IX: "Glossopharyngeal nerve lesions produce difficulty swallowing; impairment of taste over the posterior one-third of the tongue and palate; impaired sensation over the posterior one-third of the tongue, palate, and pharynx; an absent gag reflex; and dysfunction of the parotid gland."[86]
- CN X: "Vagus nerve lesions produce palatal and pharyngeal paralysis; laryngeal paralysis; and abnormalities of esophageal motility, gastric acid secretion, gallbladder emptying, and heart rate; and other autonomic dysfunction."[86]
- CN XI: Produces decreased shoulder motion and pain that radiates to the upper back, neck, and ipsilateral arm.
- CN XII: Supranuclear lesions cause an uncoordinated tongue with slow and spastic movements and are typically caused by strokes or pseudobulbar palsies. Infranuclear lesions lead to tongue weakness and atrophy. Bilateral lesions produce profound difficulty swallowing and speaking.[87]

SPINAL CORD

OVERVIEW

Extending from the foramen magnum of the skull, the spinal cord extends to the first or second lumbar vertebrae, where it terminates as the *conus medullaris* (medullary cone). The *cauda equina* (horse's tail) is a collection of spinal nerve roots that emerge from the spinal cord below the L1 vertebra. The *filum terminale* is a thin fibrous cord extending from the end of the conus medullaris to the 1st coccygeal vertebra (Co1) and anchors the distal end of the spinal cord. In the center is a central canal that contains cerebrospinal fluid traveling to the ventricles in the brain.[88] The spinal cord travels through and is protected by the vertebral canal of the vertebral column with further protection provided by the meninges that surround the spinal cord. It is divided into four main regions (cervical, thoracic, lumbar, and sacral) and one coccygeal region. Altogether, there are 31 pairs of spinal nerves with each nerve exiting the vertebral column through the intervertebral foramina to innervate a portion of the body (Table 5.17). The spinal nerves have two roots: an anterior (ventral) root that is responsible for efference motor signals to skeletal muscles of the trunk and limbs as well as preganglionic autonomic fibers to blood vessels and internal organs; and a posterior (dorsal) root that is responsible for afferent sensory information from peripheral receptors from skin, bones, joints, muscles, and internal organs.[89]

Each spinal nerve is formed by the merging of an anterior root that transmits motor information and exits the spine through the anterolateral sulcus, and a posterior root that has a sensory ganglion and transmits sensory information. The posterior roots originate from the posterior horns of the gray matter and exit through the posterolateral sulcus of the spinal cord.[90] The roots merge just before the intervertebral foramen and form the spinal nerve

Table 5.17 Spinal Cord Regions and Spinal Levels

Number of Nerve Pairs	Region	Spinal Level(s)	Explanation
8	Cervical nerves	C1–C7	The nerves of C1 through C7 exit above the corresponding spinal segment, with C8 nerve exiting below C7. (Note: There are eight cervical spinal nerves but only seven cervical spinal segments.)
12	Thoracic nerves	T1–T12	All of the rest of the spinal nerves exit below the spinal segment.
5	Lumbar nerves	L1–L5	
5	Sacral nerves	S1–S5	
1	Coccygeal nerve	Co1	

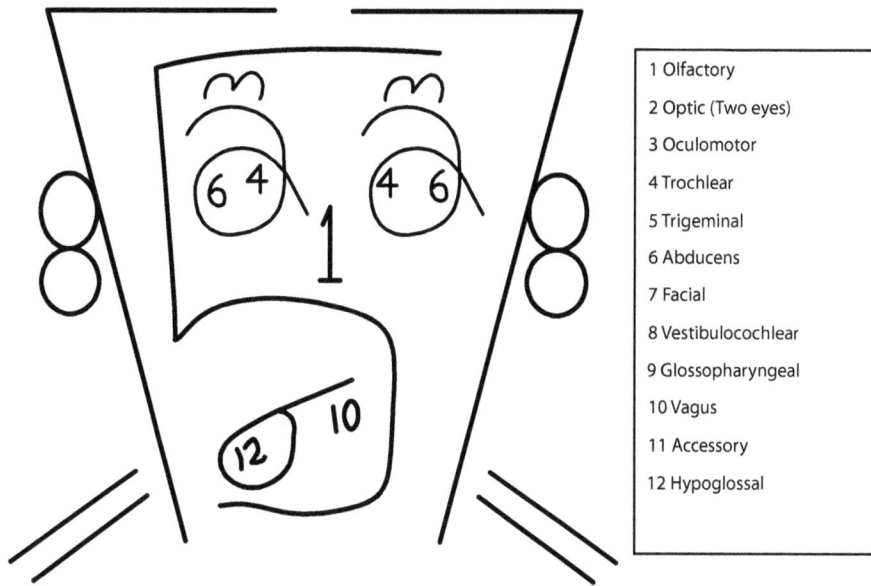

Figure 5.10 Cranial Nerve Face

1 Olfactory
2 Optic (Two eyes)
3 Oculomotor
4 Trochlear
5 Trigeminal
6 Abducens
7 Facial
8 Vestibulocochlear
9 Glossopharyngeal
10 Vagus
11 Accessory
12 Hypoglossal

trunk, which divides into four branches: anterior ramus, posterior ramus, communicating ramus, and meningeal ramus (Figure 5.11).

GEEK STUFF

A mnemonic to remember where the spinal cord terminates is SCULL.

• **S**pinal **C**ord **U**ntil **L**2 (LL)

Upper versus Lower Motor Neurons

Upper motor neurons are nerve fibers that are responsible for communication between the brain to the spinal cord. Lower motor neurons are nerve fibers responsible for communication between the spinal cord to muscles.[91]

ASCENDING AND DESCENDING NEURAL TRACTS

Neural highways, called *pathways*, are found in the white matter of the spinal cord. You will recall that the white matter is on the outside of the spinal cord, while gray matter is on the inside. On each side of the spinal cord, the white matter is divided into an anterior, lateral, and posterior funiculus (or bundle of axons). You may also hear these funiculi referred to as the anterior, lateral, or posterior columns. Ascending tracks take information to the brain, whereas descending tracts carry information from the brain (Figure 5.12 and Table 5.18).

Ascending Tracts

ANTERIOR FUNICULUS

(Anterior/lateral) spinothalamic tract (STT): This pathway is comprised of an anterior and lateral pathway that run together and can be considered one pathway.[92] Keep in mind that the anterior STT is considered to be in the anterior funiculus, while the lateral STT is in the lateral funiculus. This tract decussates two levels above the entry level and then ascends in the ventrolateral aspect of the spinal cord white matter. This is a sensory tract that carries information regarding pain and temperature via the lateral STT, while the anterior STT carries crude touch and pressure information from the skin from the anterior part of the pathway to the somatosensory area of the thalamus.

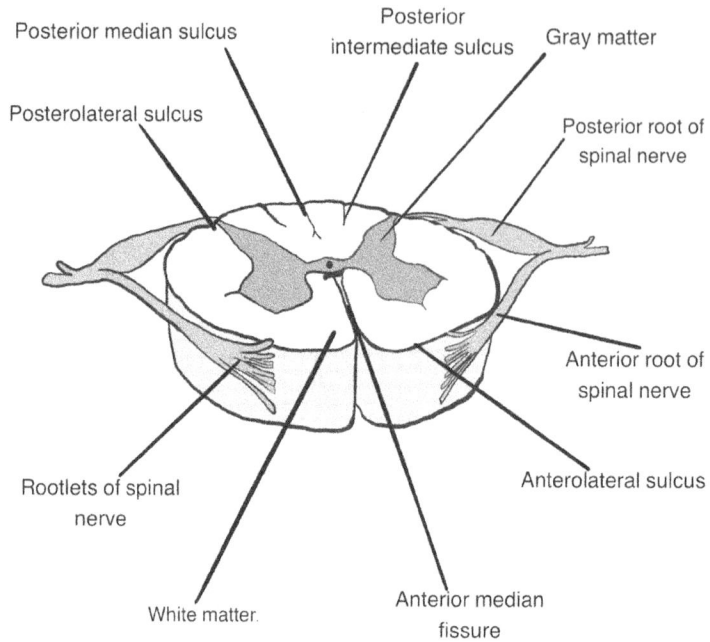

Figure 5.11 Spinal Cord Cross Section

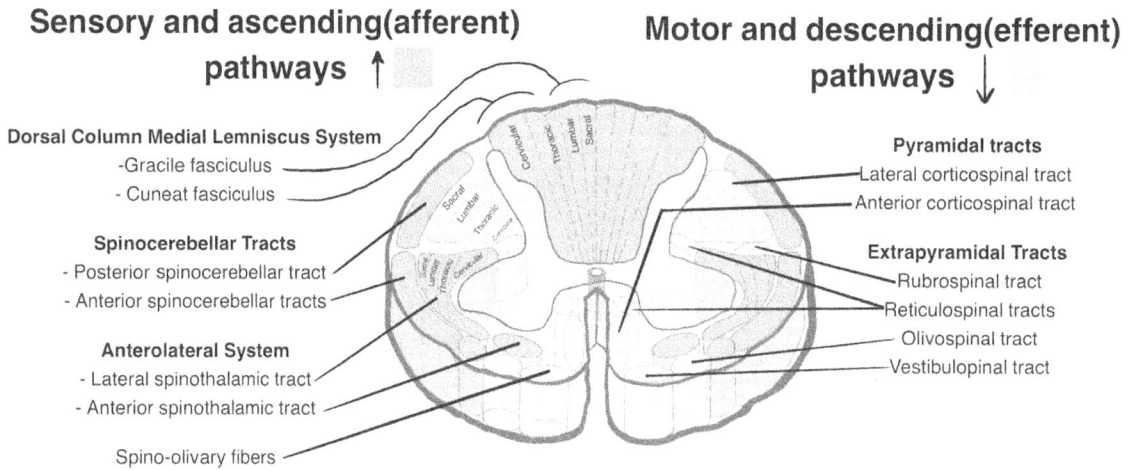

Figure 5.12 Spinal Cord Ascending/Descending Tracts

Table 5.18 Ascending/Descending Spinal Cord Neural Tracts by Funiculus

Funiculus	Important Ascending Sensory Tracts
Anterior funiculus	• Anterior spinothalamic tract
Lateral funiculus	• Dorsal (posterior) spinocerebellar tract • Ventral (anterior) spinocerebellar tract • Spinotectal tract • Lateral spinothalamic tract
Posterior funiculus	• Fasciculus gracilis • Fasciculus cuneatus
Funiculus	**Important Descending Motor Tracts**
Anterior funiculus (medial motor systems)	• Anterior corticospinal tract (pyramidal tract) • Tectospinal tract (extrapyramidal tract) • Vestibulospinal tract (extrapyramidal tract) • Reticulospinal tract (extrapyramidal tract)
Lateral funiculus (lateral motor systems)	• Lateral corticospinal tract (pyramidal tract) • Rubrospinal tract (extrapyramidal tract)
Posterior funiculus	• None

Lesions on one side of the body will cause pain and temperature deficit for contralateral levels below. Conditions that may affect the STT include Brown–Séquard syndrome, syringomyelia, anterior spinal artery syndrome, and lesions to the thalamus.[92]

LATERAL FUNICULUS

- *Lateral spinothalamic tract*: Discussed earlier along with the anterior STT.
- *Dorsal (posterior) spinocerebellar tract (DSCT)*: A somatosensory tract carrying unconscious proprioceptive information from muscle spindles and Golgi tendon organs of the lower limbs and trunk to the cerebellum. Information is transmitted to Clarke's nucleus in the posterior gray horn and ascends on the ipsilateral side, entering the cerebellum through the inferior peduncle and ending in the vermis and paravermis in the anterior lobe of the cerebellum.[93] Damage to the DSCT results in ataxia (loss of coordination).[94]

  Clinical scenarios that may cause DSCT dysfunction include: Friedreich ataxia, vitamin E deficiency, tabes dorsalis, Brown–Séquard syndrome, and vitamin B12 deficiency.[93]
- *Ventral (anterior) spinocerebellar tract (VSCT)*: Running parallel to the DSCT, the VSCT carries motor information. While the DSCT remains ipsilateral, the VSCT decussates twice, first at the level of Clarke's nucleus where it ascends contralaterally to the side of input and enters the cerebellum through the contralateral superior cerebellar peduncle where it decussates back to the ipsilateral side of input within the cerebellum.[93]
- *Spinotectal tract*: The function of this tract is believed to be the transmission of nociceptive (pain) information, as well as facilitating the reflexive head movements toward noxious stimuli.[95] The fibers of this tract cross and ascend in the anterolateral white column of the spinal cord, and project medially at the level of the midbrain to the superior colliculus and periaqueductal gray matter, and terminate in the contralateral superior colliculus.[95]

POSTERIOR FASCICULUS

- *Fasciculus gracilis*: The fasciculus gracilis carries sensory information from level T6 and below, and includes mechanoreceptors from the lower extremities regarding fine touch and two-point discrimination, conscious proprioception, and vibration. The nerves enter the spinal cord through the medial dorsal root entry zone. Once in the spinal cord, the central axon gives off collateral branches that terminate in the spinal gray matter to facilitate spinal reflexes.[96] Ultimately, the fasciculus gracilis, which travels the length of the spinal cord, terminates and synapses at the nucleus gracilis in the caudal medulla on the floor of the fourth ventricle.

The gracilis nucleus forms part of the dorsal column medial lemniscus pathway (an ascending bundle of myelinated axons) in a three-order system that includes first-order neurons that bring information from the ipsilateral side of the body, then second-order neurons from the gracile and cuneate nucleus decussate and combine to form the medial lemniscus and travel to the thalamus. From the thalamus, third-order neurons relay information to the primary somatosensory cortex of the cerebrum.[97]

- *Fasciculus cuneatus*: This bundle of nerves begins in the mid-thoracic level and runs lateral to the fasciculus gracilis with nerve fibers coming from the upper thoracic and cervical dorsal roots of the spinal cord, carrying tactile, vibration, and proprioception from the upper body and extremities.[95] After decussating in the medulla, fibers form the internal arcuate tract and medial lemniscus, and terminate with third-order neurons in the thalamus that ultimately go to the sensorimotor cortex.[95]

Descending Tracts

The descending tracts carrying motor information are structurally arranged into lateral and medial tracts but are also divided into pyramidal tracts that originate in the motor cortex carrying voluntary motor signals to the brainstem and spinal cord, and extrapyramidal tracts that originate in the brainstem that do not pass through the pyramids carrying involuntary motor signals used for muscle tone, balance, posture, and modulation of motor plans.[98] Each tract is comprised of two interconnecting neurons: a first-order upper motor neuron in the cerebral cortex or brainstem and traveling in the anterior gray horn of the spinal cord, and a second-order lower motor neuron that travels from the spinal cord to the skeletal muscles.

ANTERIOR FUNICULUS (MEDIAL MOTOR SYSTEMS)

- *Corticospinal tract (pyramidal tract)*: Controlling voluntary movements of the trunk and limbs, this motor pathway runs from the motor cortex and descend through the coronal radiata, internal capsule, cerebral peduncle, pons, and then into the medulla where the majority of fibers decussate (and form the lateral corticospinal tract), while some remain ipsilateral (forming the anterior corticospinal tract). Here they go into the *anterior* and *lateral* corticospinal tracts that descend the spinal cord and synapse with lower motor neurons in the anterior gray horn.[98] The anterior corticospinal tract descends in the anterior funiculus, while the lateral corticospinal tract descends in the lateral funiculus.

  Controlling trunk muscles, the anterior corticospinal tract is formed from the undecussated fibers or the corticospinal tract at the level of the bulbo-medullary junction and descends in the anterior funiculus of the spinal cord where they decussate at the spinal level, then innervate to synapse with a lower motor neuron in the anterior gray horn of the spinal cord.[98]

- *Tectospinal tract*: This extrapyramidal tract is involved in orienting the eyes and head toward sound and originates in the contralateral superior colliculus, which primarily is involved with visual reflexes, but also receives auditory information, and projects caudally and crosses at the dorsal tegmental decussation and ultimately joins the medial longitudinal fasciculus.[99] It is not associated with a particular muscle group but is involved in a startle auditory reflex and turns the neck and head toward a sudden sound.[99]

- *Vestibulospinal tract*: Located at the junction of the pons and medulla, there are four main vestibular nuclei that receive information from CN VIII. One of the projections leaving the nuclei is the vestibulospinal tract that originates from the lateral and inferior vestibular nuclei and travels through the ventral white matter for the entire spinal cord.[100] Collateral nerves from the lateral vestibulospinal tract synapse with medial motoneurons that innervate proximal muscles of the limbs in the ventral gray horn and facilitate the contraction of the forelimb and hindlimb muscles to maintain balance and posture.[100]

- *Reticulospinal tract*: Carrying orders from the reticular formation, this tract descends via the medial (pontine) reticulospinal tract or the lateral (medullary) reticulospinal tract. The medial reticulospinal tract originates in the pontine reticular formation and descends the ventromedial spinal cord in the ipsilateral anterior funiculus.[80] The medial reticulospinal tract is also stimulated by the ascending spinothalamic tract. It synapses with the interneurons, then gamma motor neurons, and inhibits the limb flexors and stimulates limb extensors to maintain balance and make postural adjustments.[101]

The lateral reticulospinal tract originates in the medullary reticular formation and descends the ipsilateral anterolateral funiculus[80] and synapses with interneurons in the intermediate gray matter of the spinal cord, and then gamma motor neurons to flex the limbs and inhibit limb extensors to maintain balance and make postural adjustments.[101]

LATERAL FUNICULUS (LATERAL MOTOR SYSTEMS)

- *Lateral corticospinal tract (pyramidal tract)*: The main job of the lateral corticospinal tract is to carry orders from the upper motor neurons of the primary motor cortex in the precentral gyrus to activate the contralateral limb muscles for voluntary movement.[91] It travels from the primary motor cortex through the corona radiata ipsilaterally, the posterior limb of the internal capsule, the cerebral peduncle, and ventral pons, decussating in the medulla, and descending contralaterally in the spinal cord to synapse with a lower motor neuron to the muscle.[91,102]

- *Rubrospinal tract*: Originating in the red nucleus of the midbrain, this tract decussates in the caudal midbrain and forms a contralateral tract in the lateral funiculus. It transmits signals into the red nucleus from the motor cortex and cerebellum to the spinal cord and ventral horn lamina to synapse with alpha and gamma motor neurons to stimulate the flexor muscles, and along with the corticospinal tract, controls hand and finger movements.[80]

DERMATOMES AND MYOTOMES

Dermatomes are areas of skin innervated by sensory fibers from a single spinal nerve. These areas were first mapped in 1933 and have since undergone revision and create a pattern. Some landmarks are used to identify dermatomal levels (see Table 5.19).

A full dermatome map is presented in Figure 5.13.

Myotomes are a group of muscles innervated by a single spinal nerve. The myotome map is not precise due to variations in muscle innervation. Myotomes C1–T12 are typically tested with the patient seated (Table 5.20 and Figure 5.14).

Myotomes L1–S3 are tested with the patient lying supine (Table 5.21).

Table 5.19 Dermatome Landmarks

Dermatome Spinal Level	Landmark
C6	Thumb
C7	Middle finger
C8	Little finger
T1	Anteromedial forearm and arm
T2	Medial forearm and arm to axilla
T4	Nipple
T6	Xyphoid process
T10	Umbilicus
L3	Medial knee
L4	Anterior knee and medial malleolus
L5	Doral surface of the foot and the first three toes
S1	Lateral malleolus

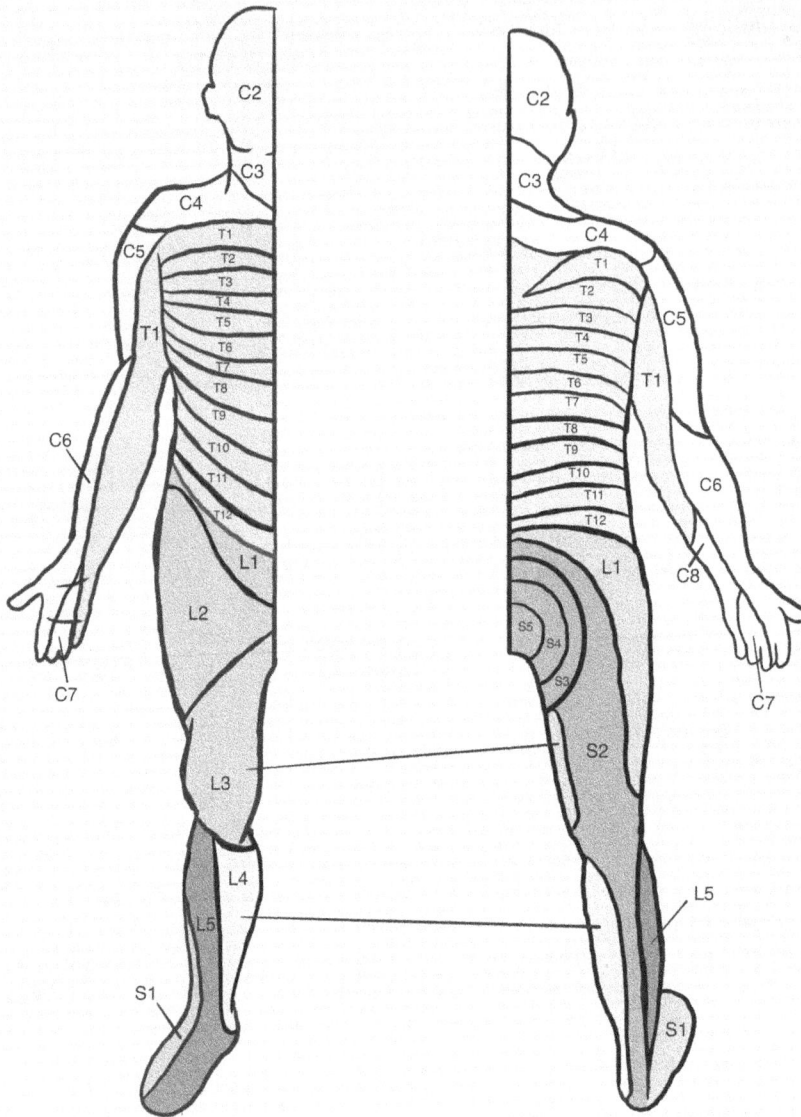

Figure 5.13 Dermatome Map

CENTRAL PATTERN GENERATORS (CPG)

CPG are defined as networks of neurons capable of enabling the production of rhythmic motor behaviors.[104] According to Steuer and Guertin, "Several CPGs localized in brainstem and spinal cord areas have been shown to underlie the expression of complex behaviors such as deglutition, mastication, respiration, defecation, micturition, ejaculation, and locomotion."[104] CPG for locomotion are mostly located in the lumbar region of the spinal cord and are local interneurons.[88] There is behavioral evidence suggesting CPG neurons undergo adaptations and plasticity changes following cervical or thoracic spinal cord injury, but at the cellular level there is only indirect evidence.[88]

Table 5.20 Cervical and Thoracic Myotome Actions

Myotome Spinal Level	Muscle Action(s) of Cervical and Thoracic Myotomes[103]
C1–C2	• Flexion of the neck
C3 and CN XI	• Lateral flexion of the neck
C4 and CN XI	• Elevation of the shoulder
C5	• **Shoulder abduction**, lateral rotation, and flexion
C5–C6	• Flexion of the arm at the shoulder joint
C6	• Supination at the shoulder joint • **Elbow flexion** • Extending the wrist
C6–**C7**	• **Elbow extension**
C6–C8	• Medial rotation, adduction, and extension of the arm at the shoulder
C7–C8	• Pronation at the shoulder joint • Flexion and extension of the digits of the hand at the metacarpophalangeal and interphalangeal joints
C8	• Extension of the thumb at the metacarpophalangeal joint • Ulnar flexion at the wrist joint • **Wrist flexion**
T1	• Abduction of finger III metacarpophalangeal joints • Adduction of finger II, III, IV at the metacarpophalangeal joints
T2-T12	• These nerves innervate the thoracic and abdominal wall muscles

Note: Bolded myotome levels and muscle actions are often tested during a neural examination.

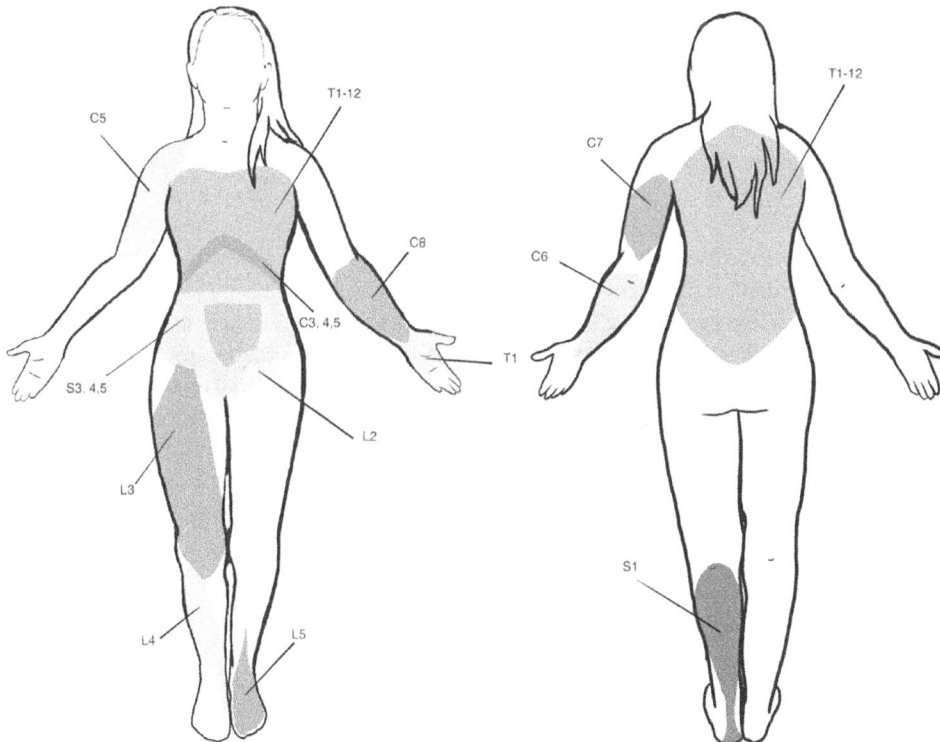

Figure 5.14 Myotome Map

Table 5.21 Lumbar and Sacral Myotome Actions

Myotome Spinal Level	Muscle Action(s) of Lumbar and Sacral Myotomes[103]
L1–**L2**–L3	• **Hip flexion** and • Hip medial (internal) rotation
L1–L4	• Hip adduction
L1, L5	• Hip lateral (external) rotation
L3–**L4**	• **Knee extension**
L4–L5	• Hip extension • Inversion of the foot at the intertarsal joints
L4–S1	• Dorsiflexion of the foot at the ankle joint
L5–S1	• Hip abduction • Eversion of the foot
L5–S2	• Flexion of the leg at the knee joint
L5	• **Ankle dorsiflexion** • Toe extension
S1–S2	• **Ankle plantarflexion**
S2–S3	• Toe adduction
S3–S4	• Anal reflexive contraction of the external anal sphincter
S3–S5	• Rectal and/or bladder dysfunction

Note: Bolded myotome levels and muscle actions are often tested during a neural examination.

REFLEX ARCS

Simple reflexes, such as a withdrawal reflex when you step on something sharp, are mediated locally within one or two spinal segments by a simple neural spinal cord pathway. These are either one or two (or more) synapses.[88] These simple reflexes may be autonomic and related to organs, eyes, and blood vessels, or somatic and related to skeletal muscle responses.[88] Monosynaptic reflex arcs (1a) are the simplest and fastest, mediate inputs from muscle spindles activated by muscle stretch (e.g., tendon reflexes), and play a role in postural adjustments.[88] The 1b reflex arc (known as the inverse myotatic reflex) is associated with input from Golgi tendon organs. This is a two-synapse reflex and mediates a wide range of muscle activity.[88]

The "flexion reflex (withdrawal reflex)" is associated with pain receptors in the skin and is takes three or more synapses to activate ipsilateral flexor muscles, and two interneurons for ipsilateral extensor inhibition. If the stimulus is strong or intense, it may activate contralateral pathways to activate extension of the contralateral limb.[88]

SPINAL CORD INJURIES (SCI)

Most SCI are the result of violence and motor vehicle accidents, with sports-related SCI occurring most often in males between the ages of 16 and 30 years of age.[105] As a result of injury to the spinal cord, SCI may be classified in different ways. First, they may be classified by the type of injury, either primary or secondary. Next, they may be named for the amount of injury, such as complete or incomplete. The most common cause of SCI is the result of motor vehicle accidents. Other causes besides trauma include malignancies, chronic tuberculosis,[105] strokes, cancer, stenosis, and inflammation.

Primary injuries are most commonly the result of direct mechanical spinal cord trauma, but may also be due to cord compression from vertebral fractures, malignancies, hematomas, abscesses, distraction injuries, and lacerations.[105] Secondary injuries are the result of changes, such as inflammation, from the primary injury, begin within minutes of the primary injury, and may last for months.[105]

SCI are graded using the American Spinal Injury Association (ASIA) Impairment Scale.[105,106]

Table 5.22 Spinal Cord Syndromes

Syndrome	Structures Involved	Losses below the Level of Injury That May Be Caused	Preserved
Central cord	CST, SST	• More pronounced weakness to Upper extremities vs. lower extremities (CST) • Pain and temperature sensation (SST) • Bladder dysfunction	• Sacral • Bowel control is usually spared
Anterior cord	SST, CST	• Bilateral pain and temperature sensation (SST) • Motor paralysis (CST) • Occasional autonomic dysfunction	• Proprioception • Vibration sense • Fine touch • 2-point discrimination
Posterior cord	DC	• Decreased tactile, vibration, and proprioception sensations	• Pain and temperature • Motor function
Brown–Séquard	DC, STT, CST	• Ipsilateral loss of motor control (CST) • Ipsilateral Loss of proprioception, tactile, and vibration sensations (DC) • Contralateral pain and temperature deficits (STT)	• Clinical presentation depends on severity and location of injury
Cauda equina and conus medullaris syndromes	Cauda equina (L1–L5) Conus medullaris (L3–L5)	• Loss of Achilles tendon reflex • Weakness to one or both lower extremities • Loss of bowel/bladder and sexual function control (men) • Saddle anesthesia and sensory deficits to lower extremities	• Clinical presentation depends on severity and of injury
Neurogenic shock	Cervical ganglia	• Loss of sympathetic tone • Hypotension • Bradycardia	

- *ASIA A*: Complete injury with loss of motor and sensory function.
- *ASIA B*: Incomplete injury with preserved sensory function but complete loss of motor function.
- *ASIA C*: Incomplete injury with preserved motor function below the injury level. Less than half of these muscles have Medical Research Council (MRC) grade 3 strength.
- *ASIA D*: Incomplete injury with preserved motor function below the injury level. At least half of these muscles have MRC grade 3 strength.
- *ASIA E*: Normal motor and sensory examination

Complete versus Incomplete

Complete SCI (CSCI) occurs when there is a complete transection of the spinal cord that prevents the transmission motor, sensation, and autonomic nerve signals across the injury. Patients with CSCI will have loss of sensation and motor control below the level of the injury. CSCI presentations include:

- *Lumbosacral injuries*: Loss of motor control and sensation to lower extremities; loss of control of bowel, bladder, and sexual function.
- *Thoracic injuries*: Includes the signs and symptoms of lumbosacral injuries, as well as the loss

of torso motor control and sensation resulting in postural deficits.

- *Cervical injuries*: Includes signs and symptoms of thoracic injuries, as well as the loss of motor control and sensation of upper extremities resulting in quadriplegia.
- *Cervical injuries above C5*: Includes signs and symptoms of cervical injuries as well as the loss of diaphragm innervation, compromising respiration.

Spinal Cord Syndromes

Incomplete SCI (ISCI) may be classified as central cord syndrome, anterior cord syndrome, posterior cord syndrome, Brown–Séquard syndrome, conus medullaris syndrome, or neurogenic shock.[105] Spinal cord tracts that are affected may include the corticospinal tract (CST), spinothalamic tract (STT), and dorsal columns (DC).

Central cord syndrome most often is the result of a hyperextension injury of the cervical spine causing spinal cord impingement and is the most common form of ISCI.[107] Clinical presentations are variable and depend on the extent of the injury to the nerve root and are the result of compression of the spinothalamic and corticospinal tracts.[107] Presentation includes upper and lower extremity weaknesses (worse in the upper extremities), a varying degree of sensory loss, and difficulty with fine motor control and ambulation. As the tracts that correspond to the upper extremities are medial, they are affected more than those of the lower extremities, which are more lateral, with sacral tracts being most lateral (and therefore unaffected). Prognosis is variable, with most patients having substantial neurologic recovery with hand function returning last.[107]

Anterior cord syndrome (also called ventral cord syndrome) results from any condition that causes infarction of the ventral two-thirds of the spinal cord, such as from car accidents, falls, spinal cord tumors, herniated discs, or other etiologies. Occasionally, autonomic dysfunction results from the occlusion of the anterior spinal artery that supplies the anterior two-thirds of the spinal cord.[108] Presentation includes motor, pain, and temperature loss below the level of injury. Prognosis is poor due to the lack of acute treatment options,[108] but better

than for those with cerebral infarction.[109] For more in-depth information, see "Anterior Spinal Artery Syndrome" by Sandoval and De Jesus.[108]

Posterior cord syndrome occurs frequently from infectious, toxic, or metabolic causes, more so than from traumatic causes.[105] It is the rarest form of ISCI. The presentation includes impairments in proprioception, vibration sense, and kinesthesia. Common location of injury is to the posterior columns and dorsal horns of the spinal cord (dorsal column medial lemniscal pathway). Prognosis is generally favorable compared to complete SCI.[110]

Brown–Séquard syndrome (BSS) occurs from a hemisection of the spinal cord. Presentation includes weakness or paralysis, proprioceptive deficits ipsilaterally, and loss of pain and temperature contralaterally.[111] Most common causes include trauma (most common) from gunshot wounds, stab injuries, motor vehicle accidents, blunt trauma, and falls causing vertebra fractures, with lesser common non-traumatic causes such as vertebral disc herniation, cysts, cervical spondylosis, tumors, multiple sclerosis, radiation, and decompression sickness.[111] Prognosis varies depending on the cause of the injury and the extent of damage. BSS has better long-term prognosis than either anterior or central cord syndromes.[111]

"Cauda equina and conus medullaris syndromes have overlap in anatomy and clinical presentation."[112] Cauda equina syndrome results from compression of the spinal cord or nerve roots from L1–L5 (more often L3–L5). These syndromes are rare and are more common in young men. Presentation includes back pain/sciatica, lower extremity (LE) weakness and changes in LE sensation, saddle anesthesia, absent or decreased rectal tone, bladder dysfunction, decreased or absent bulbocavernosus reflex, and impotence in men.[112] Prognosis is linked to the timing of intervention (surgical decompression).

Neurogenic shock results from the disruption of normal sympathetic control over vascular tone causing hypoperfusion of organ tissues and often arises from spinal cord injuries (especially those above the level of T6).[113] Presentation includes hypotension accompanied by bradycardia, with warm and pink skin. This condition needs to be differentiated from hypovolemic shoch, cardiogenic shock, and septic shock. Prognosis is influenced by the severity of spinal cord injury, response to treatment strategies, and the existence and severity of neurological deficits at initial assessment.[113]

REFERENCES

1. Lazorthes G, Gouazé A, Santini J.-J, Salamon G. The arterial circle of the brain (circulus arteriosus cerebri). *Anatomica Clinica.* 1979;1(3):241–257.
2. Vanderah TW, Gould DJ. *Nolte's the Human Brain: An Introduction to its Functional Anatomy.* Elselvier; 2021.
3. Stiles J, Jernigan T. The basics of brain development. *Neuropsychol Rev.* 2010;20(4):327–348.
4. Pakkenberg B, Gundersen H. Neocortical neuron number in humans: effect of sex and age. *J Compar Neurol.* 1997;384(2):312–320.
5. Allen NJ, Lyons DA. Glia as architects of central nervous system formation and function. *Science.* Oct 12 2018;362(6411):181–185.
6. Wei DC, Morrison EH. Histology, Astrocytes. StatPearls Publishing; 2023. https://www.ncbi.nlm.nih.gov/books/NBK545142/
7. Enyedi M, Scheau C, Baz RO, Didilescu AC. Circle of Willis: anatomical variations of configuration. A magnetic resonance angiography study. *Folia Morphol (Warsz).* 2023;82(1):24–29. doi:10.5603/FM.a2021.0134
8. Alwood BT, RH D. Vertebrobasilar Stroke. StatPearls Publishing; 2023, 2025. https://www.ncbi.nlm.nih.gov/books/NBK556084/
9. Carolina UoN. Blood vessels of the brain. Accessed 10/07/2023, 2023. https://www.med.unc.edu/neurology/wp-content/uploads/sites/716/2018/05/blood-vessels-of-the-brain-1.pdf
10. Purves D, Augustine G, Fitzpatrich D, et al. *Neuroscience.* 2 ed. The Premotor Cortex. Sinauer Associates; 2001.
11. Mytilinaios D. Motor Cortex. Updated 2022. Accessed 10/07/2023, 2023. https://www.kenhub.com/en/library/anatomy/motor-cortex
12. Shahid s. Parietal Lobe. Ken Hub. Updated 07/20/2023. Accessed 10/07/2023, 2023. https://www.kenhub.com/en/library/anatomy/parietal-lobe
13. Clinic C. Parietal Lobe. Cleveland Clinic. Updated 01/08/2023. Accessed 10/07/2023, 2023. https://my.clevelandclinic.org/health/body/24628-parietal-lobe
14. Patel A, Nicole GM, Biso R, Fowler. JB. Neuroanatomy, Temporal Lobe. StatPearls Publishing; 2023. Accessed 24/7/2023.
15. Temporal Lobe. The Cleveland Clinic. Accessed 10/08/2023, 2023. https://my.clevelandclinic.org/health/body/16799-temporal-lobe
16. Baker C, Briggs R, Milton C, et al. A connectomic atlas of the human cerebrum-chapter 6: the temporal lobe. *Oper Neurosurg.* 2018;(Dec)(Suppl 1):S245–S294.
17. Baylis G, Rolls E, Leonard C. Functional subdivisions of the temporal neocortex. *J Neuroscience.* 1987;February(2):330–342.
18. Knierim J. The hippocampus. *Curr Biol.* 2015;25(23):R1116–R1121.
19. Janak P, Tye K. From circuits to behaviour in the amygdala. *Nature.* 2015;517(7534):284–292.
20. LeDoux J. The amygdala. *Curr Biol.* 2007;17(20):R868–R874.
21. Yang Y, Wang J. From structure to behavior in basolateral amygdala-hippocampus circuits. front neural circuits. *Front Neural Circuits.* 2017;11:86.
22. McDonald A, Mott D. Functional neuroanatomy of amygdalohippocampal interconnections and their role in learning and memory. *J Neurosci Res.* 2017;95(3):797–820.
23. Huff T, Mahabadi N, Tadi P. Neuroanatomy, Visual Cortex. StatPearls Publishing; 2022.
24. Bron A, Tripathi R, Triapthi B. The Retina. *Wolff's Anatomy of the Eye and Orbit.* 8th ed. Taylor & Francis; 1998:chap 14.
25. Sceleanu A. Arteries of visual cortex. *Oftalmologia.* 2002;54(3):87–90. Arterele cortexului vizual occipital.
26. Uddin L, Nomi J, Hebert-Seropian B, Ghaziri J, Boucher O. Structure and function of the human insula. *J Clin Neurophysiol.* 2017;34(4):300–306.

27. Torrico T, Abdijadid S. Neuroanatomy, Limbic System. StatPearls Publishing; 2023. January, 2023. https://www.ncbi.nlm.nih.gov/books/NBK538491/

28. Hariri A, Bookheimer S, Mazziotta J. Modulating emotional responses: effects of a neocortical network on the limbic system. *Neuroreport.* 2000;11(1):43–48.

29. Catani M, Dell'acqua F, Schotten MTd. A revised limbic system model for memory, emotion and behaviour. *Neurosci Biobehav Rev.* 2013;37(8):1724–1737.

30. Crumbie L. Limbic System. Kenhub. Updated 8/8/2023. Accessed 10/01/2023, 2023.

31. Bear M, Reddy V, Bollu P. Neuroanatomy, Hypothalamus. StatPearlsPublishing; 2022. October, 2022. https://www.ncbi.nlm.nih.gov/books/NBK525993/

32. Squire L. Memory and the hippocampus: a synthesis from findings with rats, monkeys, and humans. *Psychol Rev.* 1992;99(2):195–231.

33. Epstein R, Kanwisher N. A cortical representation of the local visual environment. *Nature.* 1998;392(6676):598–601.

34. Sendic G. Fornix of the brain. Kenhub. Updated 8/8/2023. Accessed 10/14/2023, 2023. https://www.kenhub.com/en/library/anatomy/fornix-of-the-brain

35. Amunts K, Kedo O, Kindler M, et al. Cytoarchitectonic mapping of the human amygdala, hippocampal region and entorhinal cortex: intersubject variability and probability maps. *Anat Embryol (Berl).* 2005;210(5–6):343–352.

36. Hadland K, Rushworth M, Gaffan D, Passingham R. The effect of cingulate lesions on social behaviour and emotion. *Neuropsychologia.* 2003;41(8):919–931.

37. Cingulate binds learning. *Trends Cogn Sci.* 1997;97(1):2

38. Mammillary Body. Healthline. Accessed 10/14/2023, 2023. https://www.healthline.com/human-body-maps/mammillary-body#1

39. Chiswo R. Septum Pellucidum. Kenhub. Accessed 10/14/2023, 2023. https://www.kenhub.com/en/library/anatomy/septum-pellucidum

40. Loukopoulou C. Habenula. Kenhub. Accessed 10/14/2023, 2023. https://www.kenhub.com/en/library/anatomy/the-habenular-nuclei

41. Shenoy SS, Lui F. Neuroanatomy, Ventricular System. StatPearls Publishing; 2023. https://www.ncbi.nlm.nih.gov/books/NBK532932/

42. Andruşca A. Basal Ganglia. Kehhub. Updated 10/30/2023. Accessed 11/11/2023, https://www.kenhub.com/en/library/anatomy/basal-ganglia

43. Young CB, Reddy V, Sonne J. Neuroanatomy, Basal Ganglia. StatPearls Publishing; 2023. Accessed 11/11/2023.

44. Crumbie L. Thalamus. Kenhub. Accessed 2/10/2024, https://www.kenhub.com/en/library/anatomy/thalamus

45. Basinger H, Joseph J. Neuroanatomy, Subthalamic Nucleus. StatPearls Publishing; 2022. https://www.ncbi.nlm.nih.gov/books/NBK559002/

46. Jimsheleishvili S, Dididze M. Neuroanatomy, Cerebellum. StatPearls Publishing; 2023. Accessed 2/16/2024, https://www.ncbi.nlm.nih.gov/books/NBK538167/

47. Shahid S. Afferent and Efferent Pathways of the Cerebellum. KEN HUB. Accessed 10/01/2023, 2023. https://www.kenhub.com/en/library/anatomy/afferent-and-efferent-pathways-of-the-cerebellum

48. Leon ASd, Das JM. Neuroanatomy, Dentate Nucleus. StatPearls Publishing; 2023. Accessed 2/17/2024. https://www.ncbi.nlm.nih.gov/books/NBK554381/

49. Soteropoulos DS, Baker SN. Bilateral representation in the deep cerebellar nuclei. *J Physiol.* 2008;586(4):1117–1136.

50. Bostan AC SP. The basal ganglia and the cerebellum: nodes in an integrated network. *Nat Rev Neurosci.* 2018;19(6):338–350.

51. Dum RP, Strick PL. An unfolded map of the cerebellar dentate nucleus and its projections to the cerebral cortex. *J Neurophysiol.* 2003;89(1):634–639.

52. Crumbie L. Cerebellar Nuclei and Tracts. KenHub. Accessed 2/17/2024, https://www.kenhub.com/en/library/anatomy/cerebellum-nuclei-tracts

53. Yu M, Wang S-M. Neuroantomy, Nucleus Fastigial. StatPearls Publishing; 2023. Accessed 2/17/2024. https://www.ncbi.nlm.nih.gov/books/NBK547738/

54. Fuchs AF, Robinson FR, Straube A. Participation of the caudal fastigial nucleus in smooth-pursuit eye movements. I. Neuronal activity. *J Neurophysiol*. 1994;72(6):2714–2728.

55. Kelly RM, Strick PL. Cerebellar loops with motor cortex and prefrontal cortex of a nonhuman primate. *J Neuroscience*. 2003;23(23):8432–8444.

56. Allen GI, Tsukahara N. Cerebrocerebellar communication systems. *Physiol Rev*. 1974;54(4):957–1006.

57. Ito M. Cerebellar circuitry as a neuronal machine. *Prog Neurobiol*. 2006;78(3–5):272–303.

58. Ito M. The modifiable neuronal network of the cerebellum. *Jpn J Physiol*. 1984;34(5):781–792.

59. Zhang XY, Wang JJ, Zhu JN. Cerebellar fastigial nucleus: from anatomic construction to physiological functions. *Cerebellum Ataxias*. 2016;3:9.

60. Harper JW, Heath RG. Anatomic connections of the fastigial nucleus to the rostral forebrain in the cat. *Exp Neruol*. 1973;39(2):285–292.

61. Heath RG, Harper JW. Ascending projections of the cerebellar fastigial nucleus to the hippocampus, amygdala, and other temporal lobe sites: evoked potential and histological studies in monkeys and cats. *Exp Neruol*. 1974;45(2):268–287.

62. Purves D, Augustine GJ, Fitzpatrick D, Katz LC, LaMantia A-S. *Neuroscience*. Sinauer Associates; 2001.

63. Ataullah A, Naqvi I. Cerebellar Dysfunction. StatPearlsPublishing; 2023. Updated 1/2023. Accessed 10/15/2023. https://www.ncbi.nlm.nih.gov/books/NBK562317/

64. Hidalgo JA, Tork CA, Varacallo M. Arnold-Chiari Malformation. StatPearls Publishing; 2023. https://www.ncbi.nlm.nih.gov/books/NBK431076/

65. Tubbs R, Muhleman M, Loukas M, Oakes W. A new form of herniation: the Chiari V malformation. *Childs Nerv Syst*. 2012;28(2):305–307.

66. Rogers J, Savage G, Stoodley M. A systematic review of cognition in Chiari I malformation. *Neuropsychol Rev*. 2018;28(2):176–187.

67. Jayamanne C, Fernando L, Mettananda S. Chiari malformation type 1 presenting as unilateral progressive foot drop: a case report and review of literature. *BMC Pediatr*. 2018;18(1):34.

68. Cerebellar Degeneration. Cleveland Clinic. Accessed 10/15/2023, 2023.

69. Kheradmand A, Zee D. Cerebellum and oculomotor control. *Front Neurol*. 2011;2:53. https://www.ncbi.nlm.nih.gov/pmc/articles/PMC3164106/

70. Javalkar V, Khan M, Davis D. Clinical manifestations of cerebellar disease. *Neruol Clin*. 2014;32(4):871–879.

71. Grujičić R. Tectum and Tegmentum. Kenhub. Updated August 8, 2023. Accessed 10/20/2023, 2023. https://www.kenhub.com/en/library/anatomy/midbrain-pons-nuclei-tracts

72. Vasković J. Midbrain (Mesencephalon). Kenhub. Accessed 10/20/2023, 2023. https://www.kenhub.com/en/library/anatomy/midbrain-pons-gross-anatomy

73. Basinger H, Hogg JP. Neuroanatomy, Brainstem. StatsPearls; 2023. https://www.ncbi.nlm.nih.gov/books/NBK544297/

74. Ocran E. Pons. Kenhub. Accessed 10/20/2023, 2023. https://www.kenhub.com/en/library/anatomy/pons-en

75. Hernandez E, Das. JM. Neuroanatomy, Nucleus Vestibular. StatPealrs Publishing; 2022. October 17, 2022. Accessed 1/07/2024. https://www.ncbi.nlm.nih.gov/books/NBK562261/

76. Vasković J. Vestibular System. KenHub. Accessed 1/07/2024. https://www.kenhub.com/en/library/anatomy/the-vestibular-system

77. Malla G, Jillella DV. Pontine Infarction. StatPearls Publishing; 2023. Accessed 10/20/2023. https://www.ncbi.nlm.nih.gov/books/NBK554418/

78. Iordanova R, Reddivar AKR. Neuroanatomy, Medulla Oblongata. StatPearls Publishing; 2023. Accessed 10/20/2023. https://www.ncbi.nlm.nih.gov/books/NBK551589/

79. AbuHasan Q, Munakomi S. Neuroanatomy, Pyramidal Tract. StatPearls Publishing; 2023. Accessed 11/05/2023. https://www.ncbi.nlm.nih.gov/books/NBK545314/

80. Lee J, Muzio MR. Neuroanatomy, Extrapyramidal System. StatPearls Publishing; 2022. Updated 1/2023. Accessed 1/06/2024, 2024. https://www.ncbi.nlm.nih.gov/books/NBK554542/

81. Paul MS, Das JM. Neuroanatomy, Superior and Inferior Olivary Nucleus (Superior and Inferior Olivary Complex). StatPearls Publishing; 2023. https://www.ncbi.nlm.nih.gov/books/NBK542242/

82. Seladi-Shulman J, Hobbs H. The 12 Cranial Nerves. Healthline. Updated 02/07/2023. Accessed 10/28/2023, 2023. https://www.healthline.com/health/12-cranial-nerves

83. Vasković J. 12 Cranial Nerves. Kenhub. Accessed 10/28/2023.

84. Walker N, Mistry R, Mazzoni T. Facial Nerve Palsy. StatPearls Publishing; 2023. Accessed 10/28/2023. https://www.ncbi.nlm.nih.gov/books/NBK549815/

85. Dulak D, Naqvi I. Neuroanatomy, Cranial Nerve 7 (Facial). StatPearls Publishing; 2023. Accessed 10/28/2023. https://www.ncbi.nlm.nih.gov/books/NBK526119/

86. Walker H. Hall W, Hurst J, eds. *Clinical Methods: The History, Physical, and Laboratory Examinations*. 3rd ed. Butterworths; 1990. https://www.ncbi.nlm.nih.gov/books/NBK386/

87. Kim S, Naqvi I. Neuroanatomy, Cranial Nerve 12 (Hypoglossal). StatPearls Publishing; 2022. Accessed 11/03/2023. https://www.ncbi.nlm.nih.gov/books/NBK532869/

88. Guertin PA. Central pattern generator for locomotion: anatomical, physiological, and pathophysiological considerations. *Front Neurol*. 2013;3:183.

89. Kahn Y, Lui F. Neuroanatomy, Spinal Cord. StatPearls Publishing; 2023. January, 2023. Accessed 01/01/2024. https://www.ncbi.nlm.nih.gov/books/NBK559056/

90. Vasković J. Spinal Cord. Kenhub. Updated 11/03/2023. Accessed 11/05/2023. https://www.kenhub.com/en/library/anatomy/the-spinal-cord

91. Javed K, Reddy V, Lui F. Neuroanatomy, Lateral Corticospinal Tract. StatPearlsPublishing; 2023. July 24, 2023. 1/06/2024, 2024. https://www.ncbi.nlm.nih.gov/books/NBK534818/

92. Al-Chalabi M, Reddy V, Gupta S. Neuroanatomy, Spinothalamic Tract. StatPearls Publishing; 2023. Accessed 12/14/2023. https://www.ncbi.nlm.nih.gov/books/NBK507824/

93. Koh M, Markovich B. Neuroanatomy, Spinocerebellar Dorsal Tract. StatPearls Publishing; 2023. August 8, 2023. Accessed January, 2023. https://www.ncbi.nlm.nih.gov/books/NBK556013/

94. Marzvanyan A, Alhawaj A. Physiology, Sensory Receptors. StatPearls Publishing; 2013. January, 2023. https://pubmed.ncbi.nlm.nih.gov/30969683/

95. Baxter R. Ascending Tracts of the Spinal Cord. Kenhub. Accessed 12/14/2023, https://www.kenhub.com/en/library/anatomy/ascending-tracts-of-the-spinal-cord

96. Al-Chalabi M, Reddy V, Alsalman. I. Neuroanatomy, Posterior Column (Dorsal Column). StatPearls Publishing; 2023. January, 2023. Accessed 12/14/2023. https://www.ncbi.nlm.nih.gov/books/NBK507888/

97. Chopra S, Tadi P. Neuroanatomy, Nucleus Gracilis. StatPearl Publishing; 2023. January, 2023. Accessed 01/01/2024. https://www.ncbi.nlm.nih.gov/books/NBK546640/

98. Andruşca A. Descending tracts of the spinal cord. KenHub. Accessed 01/01/2024. https://www.kenhub.com/en/library/anatomy/descending-tracts-of-the-spinal-cord

99. Reynolds N, Khalili YA. Neuroanatomy, Tectospinal Tract. StatPearls Publishing; 2023. January, 2023. https://www.ncbi.nlm.nih.gov/books/NBK549916/

100. Yoo H, Mihalia D. Neuroanatomy, Vestibular Pathways. StatPearls Publishing; 2022. January, 2023. 1/06/2024, 2024. https://www.ncbi.nlm.nih.gov/books/NBK557380/

101. Vasković J. Reticulospinal tract. KenHub. Updated November 03, 2023. Accessed 1/06/2024, 2024. https://www.kenhub.com/en/library/anatomy/reticulospinal-tract

102. Kraskov A, Baker S, Soteropoulos D, Kirkwood P, Lemon R. The Corticospinal Discrepancy: Where are all the Slow Pyramidal Tract Neurons? *Cereb Cortex.* August 14, 2019 2019;29(9):3977–3981.

103. Osika A. Myotomes. Kenhub. Accessed 11/05/2023, https://www.kenhub.com/en/library/anatomy/myotomes

104. Steuer I, Guertin PA. Central pattern generators in the brainstem and spinal cord: an overview of basic principles, similarities and differences. *Rev Neurosci.* 2019;30(2):107–1064.

105. Bennett J, Das JM, Emmady PD. Spinal Cord Injuries. StatPearls Publishing; Updated 2024. https://www.ncbi.nlm.nih.gov/books/NBK560721/

106. Roberts TT, Garrett RL, Cepela DJ. Classifications In Brief: American Spinal Injury Association (ASIA) Impairment Scale. *Clin Orthopaed Relat Res.* 2017;475(5):1499–1504. doi:10.1007/s11999-016-5133-4

107. Ameer MA, Tessler J, Munakomi S, Gillis CC. Central Cord Syndrome. StatPearls Publishing; Updated 2023. https://www.ncbi.nlm.nih.gov/books/NBK441932/

108. Sandoval JI, De Jesus O. Anterior Spinal Artery Syndrome. StatPearls Publishing; Updated 2024. https://www.ncbi.nlm.nih.gov/sites/books/NBK560731/

109. Santana JA, Dalal K. Ventral Cord Syndrome. StatPearls Publishing; Updated 2023. https://www.ncbi.nlm.nih.gov/books/NBK541011/

110. Physiopedia contributors. Posterior Cord Syndrome. Physiopedia. 2025. https://www.physio-pedia.com/index.php?title=Posterior_Cord_Syndrome&oldid=365801

111. Shams S, Davidson CL, Arain A. Brown-Séquard Syndrome. StatPearls Publishing; Updated 2024. https://www.ncbi.nlm.nih.gov/books/NBK538135/

112. Rider LS, Marra EM. Cauda Equina and Conus Medullaris Syndromes. StatPearls Publishing; Updated 2023. https://www.ncbi.nlm.nih.gov/books/NBK537200/

113. Dave S, Dahlstrom JJ, Weisbrod LJ. Neurogenic Shock. StatPearls Publishing; Updated 2023. https://www.ncbi.nlm.nih.gov/books/NBK459361/

6

Cognition and Spatial Memory

Chapter Goals

1. Define cognition
2. Identify the effects of cognitive deficits on balance
3. Explain how we use spatial memory
4. Describe the effect of gait speed on falls

It has been established that memory and cognition play a role in a person's ability to maintain balance. Many studies have found that people with vestibular dysfunction have impaired spatial navigation. Recall, balance is divided into static and dynamic balance, and we need to use both to navigate our worlds in an efficient way. Just as there are different types of balance, we have different types of memory. *Executive function* has been defined as the "ability to process feedback, interpret life's good and bad moments, and react in an appropriate way to events."[1] *Episodic memory* is a form of long-term memory that includes details of past events that we have already experienced. *Cognition* is "the process by which knowledge and understanding is developed in the mind."[2] Cognition has six neuropsychological domains: executive function, visuospatial skills, memory, attention/concentration, abstract reasoning, and language.[3]

Conditions that may impact cognition include brain injury, mental illness, neurological disorders, genetic syndromes and abnormalities, prenatal drug exposure, malnutrition, heavy metal poisoning, neonatal jaundice, hypoglycemia, hypothyroidism, prematurity, hypoxia, child abuse, cancer therapy, autism, systemic lupus, stroke, dementia, delirium, depression, schizophrenia, chronic alcohol abuse, substance abuse, brain tumors, vitamin deficiencies, hormone imbalance, drugs, some chronic diseases (e.g., Parkinson's, Alzheimer's, Huntington's, HIV), meningitis, and other infections.[3]

COGNITION

Cognition allows us to assess our environment and consciously decide on actions that may affect our balance, such as deciding which path to take or whether to use an assistive device. "Cognition helps to have an effective adaptation to changing environments."[4] However, it has been found in one small study that elderly adults with mild cognitive impairment had poorer static balance than those with normal cognition.[5] Another study concluded that balance and executive functions are related to each other, with physical activity and depression being associated with balance gait speed.[6] This study of 84 individuals also stated that cognitive and physical training can be performed to prevent balance and executive function declines.[6]

In a systematic review and meta-analysis, investigators found a significant association between executive function and dynamic balance when comparing 18 studies.[7] In the same review, when comparing four studies examining the relationship between episodic memory and static balance, they

DOI: 10.1201/9781003524441-6

found that faster (mental) processing speeds were associated with better static and dynamic balance.[7]

Divandari et al. found that "the strength of association between cognition and balance appears to be domain-specific and task-specific." They further discovered that executive function showed the strongest correlation with balance, processing speed and global cognition had moderate correlations, and episodic memory showed a small association with dynamic balance.[7] Other researchers have also found that postural balance depends on task difficulty.[8,9]

A study by Popp et al. of 16 subjects with unilateral vestibular loss, 18 with bilateral vestibulopathy, and 17 healthy controls found that those with bilateral vestibular loss performed worse than controls on tests of visuospatial abilities, rapid processing, and memory and executive function, while subjects with unilateral damage performed worse on visuospatial abilities.[10,11]

A meta-analysis by Iso-Markku et al. suggests physical activity might postpone cognitive decline, but only to a very small extent.[12]

The best cognitive assessment methods for vestibular scientists and clinicians to use are yet to be determined, and multiple domains and subdomains of cognition, including attention, executive function, memory, and visual–spatial ability, are associated with vestibular disorders.[13]

SPATIAL MEMORY AND NAVIGATION

"Spatial memory refers to one's stored spatial representations of environments, which are subsequently used to help them navigate within those environments."[14-16] It is integral to our everyday lives and encompasses "everything from remembering how to get home to finding your favorite cereal in the grocery store."[17] "The hippocampus has been found to be one of the core regions of the brain for special navigation, using multiple sensory modalities (e.g., vision and vestibular) to gather information regarding location-specific information to form a global "cognitive map."[18-20] The availability of multisensory input improves memory-guided spatial navigation.[18] One can

deduce that when sensory input is impaired that memory-guided spatial navigation may become impaired. The vestibular system facilitates numerous functions from basic reflexes (vestibulo-ocular reflex, vestibulospinal reflex, vestibulocollic reflex) that assist postural control to higher cognitive processes such as spatial navigation, spatial memory, and bodily self-consciousness.[21] In fact, Dieterich and Brandt found that bilateral peripheral vestibulopathy impaired spatial memory, navigation, mental rotation, sensory response inhibition, and auditory and visual working memory, as well as cognitive-motor interference in dual tasking.[22]

According to Liu et al., there are two common strategies used during navigation: a landmark-based navigation relying on visual landmarks and a vector-based navigation that uses vestibular signals for continuously updating one's heading and position.[21,23-25]

The vestibular system has direct connections to the prefrontal cortex, insula, and hippocampus, which are key areas responsible for higher cognitive functions.[11] Vestibular signals are transmitted through the vestibular nuclei and thalamus to cortical areas and the hippocampal system for spatial perception.[21] Vestibular semicircular canal input is sent to head direction cells of the hippocampus and is thought to directly contribute to the ability to recognize which direction someone is facing.[26] The cerebral cortex (cognitive functions) has several areas containing vestibular-related signals when studied in humans using functional magnetic resonance imaging (fMRI), magnetoencephalography, or positron emission tomography (PET), indicating that the signals are broadly distributed in the cortices and form a vestibular network.[21,27-31] Liu et al. point out the regions of the cortex exhibiting vestibular signals also process visual and somatosensory information, and state there is probably not a pure (cortex) vestibular region of the brain, but instead discuss "multisensory integration/interaction."[21]

Spatial exploration behavior and spatial memory differences between young adults and those in midlife can be seen. This suggests that both behaviors are sensitive to age effects.[14]

Using magnetic resonance imaging, hippocampal volume atrophy was found in subjects with bilateral vestibulopathy.[32] The same subjects showed marked deficits in spatial memory and navigation.[32] The hippocampus builds our internal map of the world and our place/position in it, and relies on the vestibular system (as well as vision and somatosensory systems) to provide information about our body positions and motion. The vestibular system and the hippocampus are relevant to spatial navigation.[11] It is uncertain whether damage to the maculae (utricle/saccule) or the vestibulo-ocular reflex is more relevant to spatial navigation.[11]

There are a few tests that are low-tech and may be performed in a clinic to test visual/vestibular perception. One is the Subjective Visual Vertical (SVV) test, in which a patient is asked to judge a line with respect to the perceived direction of gravity (e.g., tell me when the line is straight up and down).[13] There are many ways to administer the test, from the bucket test, in which a patient looks into a bucket held in front of their eyes, to virtual reality versions. SVV is a valid and reliable perceptual test; however, abnormal percepts of verticality are not only due to vestibular dysfunction, and therefore the test lacks specificity.[13,33–39] Less than 2 degrees of error is considered a normal value.[13,40–42]

Other tests look at spatial navigation ability and include the Triangle Completion Test (TCT) and Gait Disorientation Test (GDT).[13] The TCT involves blindfolding a patient and leading them along two segments of a triangle, and then asking them to independently rotate and complete the triangle by returning to the starting point.[43] In a study by McLaren et al., the TCT showed poor test–retest reliability both in the real world and in virtual reality.[43] In the GDT, the patient's times are compared when walking 6.096 meters (20 feet) with the eyes open versus closed. According to the authors of the study, the GDT had good reliability for vestibular-impaired participants, 75% sensitivity, and excellent inter-rater reliability.[44] Scores $\geq$4.5 seconds differentiate vestibular-impaired from healthy adults.[13]

DOES VESTIBULAR THERAPY IMPROVE SPATIAL NAVIGATION?

In a study by Cohen and Kimball, 53 subjects with chronic vestibulopathies completed 4 weeks of vestibular exercises, after which gait velocity increased and angle of veering decreased over time, leading the authors to conclude that performing exercises that create visual–vestibular interaction leads to reduced spatial disorientation.[13,45] One study suggests that the most effective approach to enhancing the visual–spatial working memory of individuals with mild cognitive impairments involves exercising at least 3 times per week at moderate intensity for over 60 minutes each for more than 3 months.[46]

FUNCTIONAL ASSESSMENT TOOLS LINKED TO COGNITIVE IMPAIRMENT

TIMED UP AND GO (TUG) TEST

- Cognitive change was predicted by the TUG in individuals with subjective cognitive decline.[47]
- In one study, slower baseline TUG scores were associated with faster cognitive decline.[47]
- A test time greater than 8.1 seconds is an indicator of cognitive frailty.[48]

Grip Strength

- Low grip strength is associated with more risk of onset of cognitive decline and dementia.[49]

Five Times Sit to Stand

- Cutoff score of >12.47 helps to identify cognitive frailty.[48]

GAIT SPEED AND COGNITION

An included sign of some cognitive conditions includes slow gait speed. According to Tsang et al., "Self-perceived balance confidence and gait speed influence falls."[50] Studies have shown a higher fall risk with gait speeds that are slower than 0.6 to 1.0 m/s in community-dwelling adults, and several studies suggested faster gait speeds decrease fall risk.[50] One study of 2,705 subjects (average age 78.5 years) compared falls in the elderly with and without mild cognitive impairment and found no evidence that the association between gait speed and fall risk varied by mild cognitive impairment status.[51] It would seem that the slow gait speed is placing patients at risk of falls, whether it is associated with cognitive deficits or not. However, gait abnormalities without dementia is a significant predictor of the risk of developing dementia,[52] and slow gait speeds predict transition to cognitive impairment.[53]

Some cognitive deficits that place patients at a higher risk of falls include dementia, motoric cognitive risk syndrome, and cognitive frailty.

MEMORY AND COGNITION TESTING

There are many bedside tests of memory and cognition. This chapter will review a couple of common free tests of memory and cognition.

MONTREAL COGNITIVE ASSESSMENT (MoCA)

The MoCA is a highly sensitive valid assessment to detect mild cognitive impairment (MCI). It assesses short-term memory, visuospatial abilities, executive functions, attention/concentration, working memory, language, and orientation to time and place. It is a free assessment tool that may be downloaded at mocacognition.com.

CLOCK-DRAW TEST

It is expected that the patient will be able to draw the numbers of the clock in the correct positions, as well as the clock hands. It has good inter-rater and test–retest reliability, high sensitivity and specificity, concurrent validity, and predictive validity.[54] Patients are scored as follows:

- One point for drawing a closed circle.
- One point for putting all 12 numbers on the clock.
- One point for having numbers in the correct place.
- One point for having the hands pointing in the correct direction.

This test is a screen for cognitive decline in older adults and discriminates healthy individuals from those with dementia and Alzheimer's.[18]

CLOCK-DRAW TEST INSTRUCTIONS

1. Instruct the patient to "Draw a clock, putting in all of the numbers, and set the hands for 10 after 11."
2. The patient should have a copy of the correctly drawn clock on the upper part of the paper and are allowed to copy it.

INTERPRETATION OF THE CLOCK-DRAW TEST

- There have been many different scoring systems since the test was first used.
- Any score <4 should be cause for concern.

Mini-Cog

The Mini-Cog© is a test that consists of a delayed three-item recall and a clock-drawing test and takes less than 10 minutes to administer. Detailed instructions and printable tests are available on the Mini-Cog website (https://mini-cog.com).

MINI-COG INSTRUCTIONS

Delayed recall:

1. The instructor says, "I am going to say three words that I want you to remember now and later. The words are banana, sunrise, chair (or the word set you have chosen). Please say them now."
2. The patient has three tries to repeat the words, and you may repeat the words for each try.
3. If they are unable to repeat the words back to you after three tries, go to the clock drawing test.

Clock drawing: Say the following phrases in order:

1. "Please draw a clock in the circle." It is acceptable to provide a sheet of paper with the circle already drawn for the person.
2. "Put all the numbers in the circle."
3. When step 2 is completed, say, "Now set the hands to show ten past eleven."
4. Ask the person to recall the three words, saying "What were the three words I asked you to remember?" Administer this part of the test even if the person did not accurately repeat the three words earlier.

Key things to remember:

- Unlike the clock-draw test, the clock drawing portion of the Mini-Cog provides the circle of the clock already drawn.

Scoring:

- Recall score: One point for each correctly recalled word without prompt.
- Clock drawing: Two points for a normal clock that includes all the numbers in correct order with two hands present, one pointing to 11 and one pointing to 2 (hand length is not scored). Zero points for an abnormal clock drawing.

MINI-COG INTERPRETATION

- Clinically important cognitive impairment: Scores of 0, 1, or 2
- Lower likelihood of dementia: Scores of 3, 4, or 5

REFERENCES

1. Contributors M-W. Executive Function. Merriam-Webster, Incorporated. 2024. https://www.merriam-webster.com/dictionary/executive%20function
2. Oxford Leaners Dictionary Contributors. Cognition. 2024. https://www.oxfordlearnersdictionaries.com/definition/english/cognition?q=Cognition
3. Gonzalez Kelso I, P T. Cognitive Assessment. StatPearls Publishing; 2022. Accessed 2024. https://www.ncbi.nlm.nih.gov/books/NBK556049/
4. Liu Y, Ma W, Li M, et al. Relationship between physical performance and mild cognitive impairment in Chinese community-dwelling older adults. Clin Interv Aging. 2021;16:119–127. doi:10.2147/CIA.S288164
5. Qi L, Zhou M, Mao M, Yang J. The static balance ability on soft and hard support surfaces in older adults with mild cognitive impairment. PLoS One. 2023;18(12):e0295569. doi:10.1371/journal.pone.0295569
6. Ödemişlioğlu-Aydın EA, Aksoy S. Evaluation of balance and executive function relationships in older individuals. Aging Clin Exp Res. Nov 2023;35(11):2555–2562. doi:10.1007/s40520-023-02534-4
7. Divandari N, Bird M, Vakili M, Jaberzadeh S. The association between cognitive domains and postural balance among healthy older adults: a systematic review of literature and meta-analysis. Curr Neurol Neursci Rep. 2023;23(11):681–693. doi:10.1007/s11910-023-01305-y
8. Ghai S, Ghai I, Efenberg AO. Effects of dual tasks and dual- task training on postural stability: a systematic review and meta-analysis. Clin Interv Aging. 2017;12:557–577.
9. Stuhr C, Hughes CML, Stöckel T. Task-specific and variability-driven activation of cognitive control processes during motor performance. Sci Rep. 2018;8(1):10811. doi:10.1038/s41598-018-29007-3
10. Popp P, Wulff M, Finke K, Rühl M, Brandt T, Dieterich M. Cognitive deficits in patients with a chronic vestibular failure. J Neurol. 2017;264:554–563. doi:10.1007/s00415-016-8386-7
11. Aedo-Sanchez C, Riquelme-Contreras P, Henríquez F, Aguilar-Vidal E. Vestibular dysfunction and its association with cognitive impairment and dementia. Font Neurosci. 2024;18:1304810. doi:10.3389/fnins.2024.1304810
12. Iso-Markku P, Aaltonen S, Kujala UM, et al. Physical activity and cognitive decline among older adults: a systematic review and meta-analysis. J Am Med Asso. 2024;7(2):e2354285. doi:10.1001/jamanetworkopen.2023.54285
13. Grove CR, Klatt BN, Wagner AR, Anson ER. Vestibular perceptual testing from lab to clinic: a review. Font Neurol. 2023;14:1265889. doi:10.3389/fneur.2023.1265889
14. Puthusseryppady V, Cossio D, Yu S, et al. Less spatial exploration is associated with poorer spatial memory in midlife adults. Front Aging Neurosci. 2024;16:1382801.
15. Wolbers T, Hegarty M. What determines our navigational abilities? Trend Cognitive Sci. 2010;14:138–146. doi:10.1016/j.tics.2010.01.001
16. Johnson A, Varberg Z, Benhardus J, Maahs A, Schrater P. The hippocampus and exploration: Dynamically evolving behavior and neural representations. Font Human Neurosci. 2012;6:216. doi:10.3389/fnhum.2012.00216

17. Puthusseryppady V, Cossio D, Chrastil ER. Spatial memory and hippocampal remapping: Who will age well? *Proc Natl Acad Sci U S A*. 2024;16(3):e2319952121. doi:10.1073/pnas.2319952121

18. Iggena D, Jeung S, Maier PM, Ploner CJ, Gramann K, Finke C. Multisensory input modulates memory-guided spatial navigation in humans. *Commun Biol*. 2023;6(1):1167. doi:10.1038/s42003-023-05522-6

19. Nyberg N, Duvelle É, Barry C, Spiers HJ. Spatial goal coding in the hippocampal formation. *Neuron*. 2022;110:394–422. doi:10.1016/j.neuron.2021.12.012

20. O'Keefe J, Burgess N, Donnett JG, Jeffery KJ, Maguire EA. Place cells, navigational accuracy, and the human hippocampus. *Biol Sci*. 1998;353:1333–1340. doi:10.1098/rstb.1998.0287

21. Liu B, Shan J, Gu Y. Temporal and spatial properties of vestibular signals for perception of self-motion. *Front Neurol*. 2023;14:1266513. doi:10.3389/fneur.2023.1266513

22. Dieterich M, Brandt T. Central vestibular networking for sensorimotor control, cognition, and emotion. *Curr Opin Neurol*. 2024;37(1):74–82. doi:10.1097/WCO.0000000000001233

23. Etienne AS, Jeffery KJ. Path integration in mammals. *Hippocampus*. 2004;14:180–192. doi:10.1002/hipo.10173

24. Gallistel CR. *The Organization of Learning*. The MIT Press; 1990.

25. Valerio S, Taube JS. Path integration: how the head direction signal maintains and corrects spatial orientation. *Nat Neurosci*. 2012;15:1445–1453. doi:10.1038/nn.2315

26. Grove CR, Klatt BN, Wagner AR, Anson ER. Vestibular perceptual testing from lab to clinic: a review. *Front Neurol*. 2023;14:1265889. doi:10.3389/fneur.2023.1265889

27. Deutschländer A, Bense S, Stephan T, Schwaiger M, Brandt T, Dieterich M. Sensory system interactions during simultaneous vestibular and visual stimulation in P E T. *Human Brain Mapping*. 2002;16:92–103. doi:10.1002/hbm.10030

28. Lopez C, Blanke O, Mast FW. The human vestibular cortex revealed by coordinate-based activation likelihood estimation meta-analysis. *Neuroscience*. 2012;212:159–179. doi:10.1016/j.neuroscience.2012.03.028

29. Smith AT, Wall MB, Thilo KV. Vestibular inputs to human motion-sensitive visual cortex. *Cerebral Cortex*. 2012;22:1068–1077. doi:10.1093/cercor/bhr179

30. Fredrickson JM, Schwarz D, Kornhuber HH. Convergence and interaction of vestibular and deep somatic afferents upon neurons in the vestibular nuclei of the cat. *Acta Oto-Laryngologica*. 1966;61:168–188. doi:10.3109/00016486609127054

31. Ödkvist LM, Schwarz DWF, Fredrickson JM, Hassler R. Projection of the vestibular nerve to the area 3a arm field in the squirrel monkey (Saimiri sciureus). *Brain Res*. 1974;21:97–105. doi:10.1007/BF00234260

32. Brandt T, Schautzer F, Hamilton DA, et al. Vestibular loss causes hippocampal atrophy and impaired spatial memory in humans. *Brain*. 2005;128:2732–2741. doi:10.1093/brain/awh617

33. Ashish G, Augustine AM, Tyagi AK, Lepcha A, Balraj A. Subjective visual vertical and horizontal in vestibular migraine. *J Int Adv Otol*. 2017;13:254–258. doi:10.5152/iao.2017.4056

34. Min KK, Ha JS, Kim MJ, Cho CH, Cha HE, Lee JH. Clinical use of subjective visual horizontal and vertical in patients of unilateral vestibular neuritis. *Otol Neurotol*. 2007;28:520–525. doi:10.1097/01.mao.0000271674.41307.f2

35. Wang C, Winnick A, Ko Y, Wang Z, Chang T. Test-retest reliability of subjective visual vertical measurements with lateral head tilt in virtual reality goggles. *Tzu Chi Med J*. 2021;33:294–300. doi:10.4103/tcmj.tcmj_207_20

36. Michelson PL, McCaslin DL, Jacobson GP, Petrak M, English L, Hatton K. Assessment of subjective visual vertical (SVV) using

the bucket test and the virtual SVV system. *Am J Audiol.* 2018;27:249–259. doi:10.1044/2018_AJA-17-0019

37. Dai T, Kurien G, Lin V. Mobile phone app vs bucket test as a subjective visual vertical test: a validation study. *J Otolaryngol.* 2000;49:1–3. doi:10.1186/s40463-020-0402

38. Dieterich M, Brandt T. Perception of verticality and vestibular disorders of balance and falls. *Front Neurol.* 2019;10:172. doi:10.3389/fneur.2019.00172

39. Brandt T, Dieterich M, Danek A. Vestibular cortex lesions affect the perception of verticality. *Annals Neurol.* 1994;35:403–412. doi:10.1002/ana.410350406

40. Akin FW, Murnane OD, Pearson A, Byrd S, Kelly JK. Normative data for the subjective visual vertical test during centrifugation. *J Am Acad Audiol.* 2011;22:460–468. doi:10.3766/jaaa.22.7.6

41. Friedmann G. The influence of unilateral labyrinthectomy on orientation in space. *Acta Oto-Laryngological (Stockh).* 1971;(71):289–298.

42. Zakaria MN, Salim R, Tahir A, Zainun Z, Mohd Sakeri NS. The influences of age, gender and geometric pattern of visual image on the verticality perception: a subjective visual vertical (SVV) study among Malaysian adults. *Clin Otolaryngol.* 2019;44:166–171. doi:10.1111/coa.13255

43. McLaren R, Chaudhary S, Rashid U, Ravindran S, Taylor D. Reliability of the triangle completion test in the real-world and in virtual reality. *Front Human Neurosci.* 2022;16:945953. doi:10.3389/fnhum.2022.945953

44. Grove CR, Heiderscheit BC, Pyle GM, Loyd BJ, Whitney SL. The gait disorientation test: a new method for screening adults with dizziness and imbalance. *Arch Phys Med Rehabil.* 2021;102(4):582–590. doi:10.1016/j.apmr.2020.11.010

45. Cohen HS, Kimball KY. Improvements in path integration after vestibular rehabilitation. *J Vestibular Res* 2002;12:47–51. doi:10.3233/VES-2002-12105

46. Deng J, Wang H, Fu T, et al. Physical activity improves the visual-spatial working memory of individuals with mild cognitive impairment or Alzheimer's disease: a systematic review and network meta-analysis. *Front Public Health.* 2024;12:1365589. doi:10.3389/fpubh.2024.1365589

47. Borda MG, Ferreira D, Selnes P, et al. Timed up and go in people with subjective cognitive decline is associated with faster cognitive deterioration and cortical thickness. *Dementia Geriatric Cognitive Disorders.* 2022;51(1):63–72. doi:10.1159/000522094

48. Kim GM, Kim BK, Kim Dr, Liao Y, Park JW, Park H. An association between lower extremity function and cognitive frailty: A sample population study from the KFACS Study. *Int J Environ Res Public Health.* 2021;18(3):1007. doi:10.3390/ijerph18031007

49. Cui M, Zhang S, Liu Y, Gang X, Wang G. Grip strength and the risk of cognitive decline and dementia: a systematic review and meta-analysis of longitudinal cohort studies. *Front Aging Neurosci.* 2021;13:625551. doi:10.3389/fnagi.2021.625551

50. Tsang CSL, Lam FMH, Leung JCS, TCY K. Balance confidence modulates the association of gait speed with falls in older fallers: a prospective cohort study. *J Am Med Direct Asso.* 2023;24(12):2002–2008. doi:10.1016/j.jamda.2023.05.025

51. Adam CE, Fitzpatrick AL, Leary CS, et al. The association between gait speed and falls in community dwelling older adults with and without mild cognitive impairment. *Int J Environ Res Public Health.* 2021;18(7):3712.

52. Verghese J, Lipton RB, Hall CB, Kuslansky G, Katz MJ, H B. Abnormality of gait as a predictor of non-Alzheimer's dementia. *N Engl J Med.* 2002;347(22):1761–1768.

53. Hoogendijk EO, Rijnhart JJM, Skoog J, et al. Gait speed as predictor of transition into cognitive impairment: findings from three longitudinal studies on aging. *Exp Gerontol.* 2020;129:110783. doi:10.1016/j.exger.2019.110783

54. Spenciere B, Alves H, Charchat-Fichman H. Scoring systems for the clock drawing test: a historical review. *Dementia Neuropsychol.* 2017;11(1):6–14. doi:10.1590/1980-57642016dn11-010003

7

Examination of Vision and Vestibular Systems

Chapter Goals

1. Identify which vision/oculomotor tests should be performed
2. List possible central signs observed during an oculomotor examination
3. List contraindications to vestibular testing/treatment

This chapter will outline a bedside-type examination that can be used in many settings, such as inpatient, outpatient, and home health. Generally, very little equipment is required. However, for a more in-depth examination for dizziness or disequilibrium, you may wish to use Frenzel goggles or infrared (IR) goggles.

When performing a neurological assessment of someone complaining of dizziness, falls, or disequilibrium, you need to assess or screen for the following:

1. Vision and oculomotor function
2. Vestibular system
3. Somatosensory system
4. Cerebellum
5. Musculoskeletal system (strength/range of motion [ROM])
6. Blood pressure/cardiovascular
7. Cognition

8. Gait
9. Balance and fall risk

Be thorough! In today's world, we are all under pressure to perform and perform quickly. When you are examining a patient complaining of dizziness, falls, or disequilibrium, you must include each of the items listed above. If you do not, you may miss important clues related to the etiology of the problem. Given the items on the list, there are many tests that may be performed for each; you do not have to do all of them, but you should assess each item. For some patients, the exam may be completed in 30 minutes. For other patients, it may take an hour. It takes as long as it takes! Do not allow yourself to be rushed, or the patient may not get the examination or treatment they deserve. If you do not have time to complete the examination, continue it on your next visit. *Caution*: As you will not be able to bill for two examinations, you will likely need to begin treatment on the second visit for deficits that you have already identified. As you progress in your proficiency, you will be able to complete the examination in one visit for most of your patients.

VISION/OCULOMOTOR EXAMINATION

Assessments of vision differ based on the professional performing the exam, as well as the setting in which the assessment is occurring. Here, a bedside

DOI: 10.1201/9781003524441-7

examination that may be performed without much equipment is described. Such an exam may be performed by a physician, optometrist, or therapist in any setting. The examination of vision and the oculomotor systems includes the following tests/screenings. The following tests, once proficient, take a total of about 5 minutes or less to perform:

- Fixation
- Range of motion
- Pursuits
- Volitional saccades
- Ocular alignment for near and distant targets
- Nystagmus

Other tests may be used when warranted:

- Visual acuity (near and distance)
- Visual fields (moving confrontation, finger counting confrontation)
- Optokinetic reflex testing
- Near point of convergence
- Contrast sensitivity
- Color vision
- Suppression
- Visual midline/egocentric location
- Visual processing (finger counting confrontation)
- Parks–Bielschowsky three-step test (isolates a paretic extraocular muscle)
- Various tests for unilateral inattention

Before beginning the exam, ask the patient if they can see out of each eye and if they have and use prescription spectacles (glasses) or over-the-counter reading glasses. If they use prescription spectacles to see distant objects, have them wear them during the examination for all but the near-vision exam. If they use reading glasses or prescription spectacles for near vision, have them wear them during the near-vision examination. Take note if the patient wears progressive lenses or other multifocal (bifocal, trifocal) lenses. A study in 2022[1] established that multifocal glasses wearers were more than twice as likely to fall. Multifocal glasses impair contrast sensitivity, depth perception, and the ability to negotiate obstacles, all of which increase the risk for falls.[2]

🎥 FIXATION

We use saccades, smooth pursuit, and vergence movements to find our target. However, once we find what we want to see, we need to keep our eyes on it. To do this, we use fixation (aka gaze holding), the vestibulo-ocular reflex (VOR), and optokinetics (OPK). Visual fixation is the patient's ability to hold their eyes steady on a target. Another way to say this is that it is our ability to hold an image steady on our fovea.

Fixation is tested not just in the primary positions of the eyes (looking straight ahead) but also at or near endpoints around the ocular ROM. During the assessment of fixation at these various eye positions, you may also assess the alignment of the eyes by asking the patient to report if they have diplopia (double vision). During fixation at each test point, the examiner watches the patient's eyes to see if they are relatively held still on the target or if they are unable to remain on the target. During tests of fixation, assess the following:

- Can the patient maintain visual fixation on a target? When a patient lacks fixation, the eyes constantly move in a saccadic fashion around the target in a circular motion and frequently change directions, never quite keeping still on it.
- When fixating on a target, does the patient develop nystagmus or suppress existing nystagmus?
- Does the patient complain of diplopia?

Visual Fixation Testing Instructions

When visual fixation with a near target is being tested, the patient fixates for about 5 to 15 seconds on a target (such as a Wolff wand, fingertip, or the end of a pen) that is 12 to 15 inches (30–38 cm) away from the patient's eyes. Avoid giving the patient a visual target that is too large. For example, avoid holding the pen vertically and asking the patient to look at the pen, or similarly holding a finger vertically as a target. Hold the pen, pencil, or finger so only one end (usually the tip) is visible to the patient. In this way the patient directs gaze at a single, discrete point. Alternatively, if you prefer to hold the pen vertically, instruct the patient to "look at the *end* of my pen/pencil/finger." Illuminating your fingertip by placing it on the tip of a penlight is another great way to present a visual target and may hold the attention of younger patients or those with attention deficits.

If you are using an ophthalmoscope during the exam, have the patient fixate on a visual target with the contralateral eye. When using an oph-thalmoscope you will see some normal eye move-ments while looking at the optic nerve while the patient fixates with the contralateral eye. These motions include microsaccades, continuous drift, and microtremor.[3] Square wave jerks are a type of saccadic intrusion to fixation and is considered normal if the frequency is <9 per minute with an amplitude of <5 degrees.[3,4]

OCULAR RANGE OF MOTION

How far can the eyes move? A slight loss of upgaze is normal with aging. However, the patient should be able to demonstrate all ranges of motion. Except for vergence when the eyes are moving in oppo-site directions, the eyes should move in the same direction and speed. When they do not, the patient may complain of diplopia, headaches, and diffi-culty reading. A lack of ocular range will interfere with someone's vision. It is important to determine whether the patient has normal gross ocular ROM in each eye, as well as whether there is any diffi-culty maintaining certain ranges in one or both eyes.

▶ Ocular Range of Motion Testing Instructions

Use Figure 7.1 as a reference for ROM testing. The circle represents the patient's face. There are nine circles at points (three rows of three dots) representing the cardinal positions as well as the primary position. There are two lighter dots at 45 degrees to either side of the primary position. These points represent the gaze and fixation targets (your fingertip, pen tip, etc.). Direct the patient to gaze toward each of these positions and hold the gaze between 5 and 10 seconds. Have the patient inform you if they have diplopia at any of the gaze points.

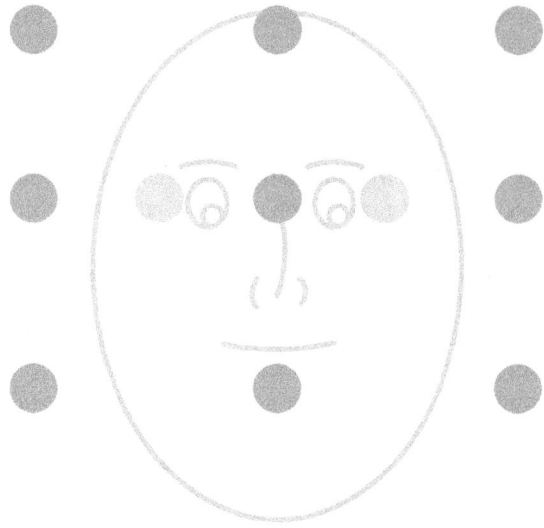

Figure 7.1 Ocular Fixation Points

First, let's discuss testing the middle row of the chart we just reviewed. Start in the primary posi-tion of centered gaze (the center dot) and observe the patient's ability to fixate. Another important observation, if it occurs, is the development of nys-tagmus while the patient is fixating on the visual target; this would be a central finding.

Now, move your pen until the patient's eyes are 45 degrees laterally from primary gaze (the light gray dots). In our example, we first have the patient gaze left. After holding this position, the target is moved almost to the patient's end-range laterally on the same side. After testing the left gaze, observe the patient's gaze on their right at 45 degrees and near end-range.

Once you have tested the primary position, each 45-degree position laterally, and near end-ranges laterally, the middle line of the chart is completed. There is no reason to bring the visual target back to any of these points unless you wish to retest it.

Next, with the head still, move the visual target up as far as the patient can visually track. You will place the visual target in three places, as depicted on the top line of the chart: up + left end-range, straight up (center), and up + right end-range. Remember to hold each position. Again, we are using extreme upward gaze, so you may see nys-tagmus at any of these test points, with more than 3 beats being abnormal. Keep in mind that a lack of upward gaze is a central sign. Patients who lack upward gaze will compensate by extending the head, neck, trunk, or a combination. Do not allow the patient to move the head, neck, or trunk during testing.

Now that you have examined the first two lines of the chart, we will test the bottom line, which includes end-ranges down + left, straight down (center), and down + right.

While the patient is in downgaze, it is sometimes difficult to see the eyes. When this occurs, you will need to lift the eyelids (remember to inform the patient you will be doing this before you pull on their eyelid). There are pathologies that will cause one eye to have nystagmus but not the other, so check both eyes for a downward gaze. Since this is an extreme downward gaze, you may see nystagmus of 3 beats or less in any of these positions. Any observation of nystagmus greater than 3 beats may represent pathology.

Interpretation of Tests for Fixation and Range of Motion

Negative test results are as follows:

- There is no nystagmus while fixating on a visual target.
- The patient is able to move both eyes to each indicated point of the visual field and maintain gaze.
- No nystagmus is noted in less than near-end-range motions.
- There are 3 beats or fewer at extreme endpoints or near end-ranges.
- The patient does not complain of diplopia.

Positive test results are as follows:

- The patient has limited range/motion into certain ocular ranges with one or both eyes.
- Any nystagmus at 45 degrees indicates possible pathology.
- More than 3 beats of nystagmus at near-end-range positions.
- Nystagmus that are direction-changing.
- The patient complains of diplopia.

For some, more than three beats of nystagmus may still be a normal finding. However, as a screening

technique, it is a good practice to report more than three beats as an abnormal finding and request further examination by neurology. Remember, *at no time* should nystagmus be seen at 45 degrees of gaze. If you do observe this, it is an abnormal finding. If horizontal nystagmus is seen at 45 degrees of gaze, document the direction they are beating (remember, you name the nystagmus for the fast-phase direction). When you assess the contralateral 45 degrees of gaze, if there are nystagmus beating in the same direction, consider vestibulopathy as the cause, although you will need to rule out central pathology as well. If there are nystagmus bilaterally but in opposite directions (i.e., direction-changing), this is a central finding (typically stroke).

When testing ocular ROM, you are examining cranial nerves and eye muscles. Upward gaze may decrease somewhat (but not completely) with advanced age. Disruption of the ability to maintain fixation in general may be due to central or peripheral dysfunction. Examples of central lesions that may disrupt fixation include seizures, occipital lobe infarct,[5] infranuclear (below the oculomotor nuclei) and supranuclear lesions (above the oculomotor nuclei),[6] and certain brainstem and cerebellar syndromes.[7]

PURSUIT

Questions to ask yourself:

- Do the eyes move conjugately (together)?
- Are the motions smooth or saccadic while following a slow-moving target?
- Does the patient lose fixation during pursuit (and in which direction)?

🎥 Smooth Pursuit Testing Instructions

Pursuit testing should be performed both monocularly and binocularly.

1. The examiner sits directly in front of the patient holding a visual target ~15 inches (40 cm) from the patient. The patient is instructed to maintain fixation on the target.

2. The examiner slowly moves the target at a constant speed ~2.5 inches (~6 cm) past the patient's midline from left to right, and then back (this is one cycle). Do two cycles at 2 seconds/cycle.

3. Repeat two cycles with vertical motions in midline 2.5 inches (~6 cm) past the primary position of the eyes.

4. Instruct the patient to pursue clockwise and counterclockwise circles (two each).

Interpretation of Impaired Smooth Pursuit Examination

There are numerous central anatomical structures involved in smooth pursuit. Causes of impaired smooth pursuit include:

- Neurologic disorders
- Vestibular disorders
- Medication side effects
- Developmental disorders
- Aging

Because there are so many causes of impaired pursuit, abnormal findings during testing are nonlocalizing.

VOLITIONAL SACCADES

🎥 Saccades Testing Instructions

There are different types of saccades with different instructions for testing each type. We will only be discussing how to assess voluntary (volitional) saccades. You should test both horizontal and vertical saccades.

1. The examiner sits directly in front of the patient, holding up two visual targets (e.g., examiner's finger and nose, or two fingers held about 45 degrees to each side of patient's nose) ~15 inches (40 cm) from the patient. The patient is instructed to maintain fixation on one of the targets.

2. The patient is then instructed to look horizontally between the two targets on command (one motion per command).

3. Repeat the test to assess vertical motions with targets ~45 degrees above the patient's eye level, and one 45 degrees below the patient's eye level, so the patient will need to use vertical saccades to look between them.

Interpretation of Saccades Testing

Common terms used to describe saccades include *hypometric* and *hypermetric*. If we break down the word *hypometric*, we see *hypo* (less than) and *metric* (referring to distance). A hypometric saccade would be one that moves a shorter distance than normal. If your eye movements fall short of the normal distance while performing a saccade, you will need more saccades to get from point A to point B. While examining saccades, if the patient consistently uses more than two saccades to look between targets no more than 90 degrees apart, describe these saccades as being hypometric.

If we break down the word *hypermetric*, we see *hyper* (more than) and *metric* (distance). A hypermetric saccade moves too far and overshoots the target. When this happens, the patient needs to make a corrective saccade in the opposite direction to go back to the target. It is not uncommon to see a hypermetric saccade during the first saccade that is tested (i.e., the first command you give the patient to look at the other target). However, if the patient consistently presents hypermetric (overshooting) saccades, the test would be considered positive for a hypermetric deficit (aka hypermetria).

While testing saccades, we look to see if the patient can perform accurate saccades and are careful to observe how many saccades are required to move between two targets. Positive findings of saccades testing include the following:

- *Hypometric saccades*, which consistently undershoot the target, requiring more than two saccades to reach the target. Causes include:[8]
  - Medications that increase the risk of hyponatremia (diluted sodium in the body)
  - Syndrome of inappropriate antidiuretic hormone
  - Chronic and severe vomiting or diarrhea (dehydration)

- Drinking too much water, hormonal changes, recreational drug Ecstasy use

- *Hypermetric saccades* consistently overshooting the visual target. The saccades move too far and miss the target, and the patient must add a corrective saccade in the opposite direction to reach the target. Causes include[9]:
  - Injury
  - Diseases
  - Genetic disorders
  - Lesions to the cerebellum, diencephalon, or brainstem.

- *Velocity of saccades.* Remember, saccades are the quickest eye motions. If a patient cannot generate saccades of sufficient speed, it appears as if the patient were performing smooth pursuit. Slow saccades are caused by:[10]
  - Illicit drug use
  - Fatigue
  - Basal ganglia syndromes (e.g., Huntington's chorea)
  - Oculomotor weakness (myopathy, third and sixth nerve palsy)
  - White matter diseases
  - Miscellaneous disorders

- *Initiation of saccades.* Delayed initiation of saccades occurs with some metabolic and degenerative disorders, such as Parkinson's disease.[11]

Repeat tests when you observe positive findings. As with the example of the first saccade, which may overshoot, we may see some hyper- or hypometric saccades as the patient tries to locate the target. However, after a few repetitions, the majority of saccades should be accurate and on target.[11]

OCULAR ALIGNMENT

Are the eyes pointing at the same target? There are three common bedside tests used to check for ocular alignment. These include the unilateral cover test (aka cover–uncover test), the alternate (or alternating) cover test, and Maddox rod test. The first two do not require equipment.

Cover Tests

The cover test is composed of two tests commonly used as screens for ocular alignment: the *unilateral cover test* and the *alternate cover test* (also known as the *cross-cover test*). Always perform the unilateral cover test first. These tests should be done for both a near and distant target.

UNILATERAL COVER TEST

The first test, the *unilateral cover test*, also known as the *cover–uncover test,* tests the patient for heterotropia (also known as *manifest strabismus*), which is an abnormal eye deviation. This test answers the question, "Are the eyes consistently pointing at the same object?" In Figure 7.2 we are looking down on top of our patient, and the dark pointed lines show the direction in which each eye is pointing. Ideally both eyes would be pointing at the same object.

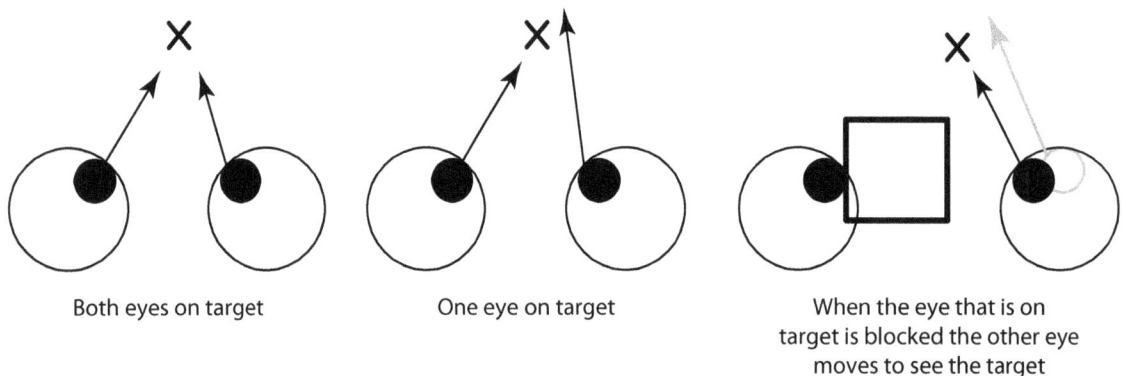

Both eyes on target

One eye on target

When the eye that is on target is blocked the other eye moves to see the target

Figure 7.2 Cover Test, Line of Sight

During the test, we cover one of the patient's eyes while observing the uncovered eye. If the observed uncovered eye is already pointing at the target, it will not move during the test. As an example, if we cover the patient's left eye (which is pointed at the target), the patient will be able to look at the target only with the right eye. If the right eye is deviated and not pointing at the target, as the left eye is covered, the patient must move the right eye to see the target. It is this motion, called a *corrective saccade*, that indicates a positive test for heterotropia.

Unilateral Cover Test Instructions (For Near Targets)

1. The examiner sits ~15 inches (40 cm) away from and directly in front of the patient.
2. Instruct the patient to visually fixate (with both eyes) on the end of the examiner's nose. If the examiner is wearing a mask, simply point to the end of their nose and ask the patient to fixate there. Alternatively, using a pen, place a mark on the mask to represent the location of their nose.
3. The examiner covers the patient's left eye (using a paddle occluder or the palm of the hand) for 10 seconds while watching the right eye, noting any motions and direction of motion if it occurs.
4. The examiner completely removes the occluder, and after 10 seconds repeats the procedure by occluding the patient's right eye.

Interpretation of the Unilateral Cover Test

If the uncovered eye moves to acquire the visual target after the contralateral eye is covered, the test is positive for *heterotropia*. Note the direction of the uncovered eye's motion as it fixates on the target.

- If no eye motion occurs, the test is negative (normal).
- If the eye moves inward (nasally), we name the deviation *exotropia*.
  - Causes include craniofacial anomalies, ocular albinism, cerebral palsy, mechanical factors (shape of orbit, interpupillary distance, extraocular muscle characteristics), overcorrection of an esotropia, or poor visual acuity in one eye.[12]

- If the eye moves outward (temporally), we name the deviation *esotropia*.
  - Esotropia is normal up to about 6 months of age, otherwise, causes include a lack of coordination of eye muscles, genetics, neurological conditions (stroke, nerve damage/palsy), thyroid conditions, or eye injuries.[13]

- If the eye moves downward, we name the deviation *hypertropia*.
  - Causes in children include third or fourth cranial nerve palsy, Brown syndrome, and Duane syndrome.[14] Causes in adults include stroke, Graves' disease, thyroid disease, myasthenia gravis, eye injuries, trauma, and brain tumors.[15]

- If the eye moves upward, we name the deviation *hypotropia*.
  - Causes in adults are associated with thyroid disease, fourth nerve palsy, intracranial and intraorbital lesions, ocular myasthenia gravis, third nerve palsy, Brown syndrome, Parkinson's disease, carotid-cavernous fistula, superior oblique myokymia, meningitis, Lyme disease, and trauma.[16]

An observation of vertical eye movements indicates a more serious finding; in these cases, the clinician should refer the patients for tests to rule out central pathologies.

ALTERNATE COVER TEST

The alternate cover test is a test of heterophoria (also known as *latent strabismus*). This condition allows for binocular fusion, but when the fusion is broken, as when one eye is covered for at least 10 seconds, the eyes lose alignment (i.e., the covered eye moves away from the target and instead moves to a resting position). During the test, the examiner observes the eye that they uncover. This test always follows the unilateral cover test.

Alternate Cover Test (Cross-Cover Test) Instructions

1. The examiner sits ~15 inches (40 cm) away from and directly in front of the patient in a dimly lit room.

2. Instruct the patient to visually fixate (with both eyes) on the end of the examiner's nose. If the examiner is wearing a mask, simply point to the end of their nose and ask the patient to fixate there. Alternatively, using a pen, place a mark on the mask to represent the location of the nose.

3. The examiner covers the patient's left eye (using a paddle occluder or the palm of the hand) for 10 seconds. There is no need to observe the uncovered eye at this point.

4. Next, the examiner moves the occluder to cover the patient's right eye. As the examiner moves the occluder, they should observe the eye that they just uncovered (in this case, the patient's left eye) and observe any motion and direction of motion the eye makes to reacquire the target.

5. The examiner then moves the occluder back to the patient's left eye, while observing the patient's right eye.

Interpretation of the Alternate Cover Test

Movement of the eye *just after* it is uncovered is a positive test for heterophoria. Observations of vertical eye movements may indicate a more serious finding; in such a case, the clinician should refer the patient to neurology to rule out central pathologies.

- If the eye moves inward, an *exophoria* is present. When the eye was covered, it drifted outward; when uncovered, a correction was needed to reacquire the target.
- If the eye moves outward, an *esophoria* is present. When the eye was covered, it drifted inward; when uncovered, a correction was needed to reacquire the target.
- If the eye moves downward, a *hyperphoria* is present. When the eye was covered, it drifted upward; when uncovered, it had to make a correcting downward saccade to reacquire the target. This is a vertical skew deviation and is indicative of possible stroke.
- If the eye moves upward, a *hypophoria* is present. When the eye was covered, it drifted downward. When uncovered, it had to make

a correcting upward saccade to reacquire the target. This is a vertical skew deviation and is indicative of possible stroke.

Single Maddox Rod Test

The Maddox rod test uses the principle of "diplopic projection," or the "perception of the image of each eye simultaneously." Images of a red line from one eye and a dot of light from the other are used to test ocular alignment. This test detects phorias and tropias but *does not differentiate* between them. For this reason, the cover tests should be performed prior *to* the Maddox rod test. It is not a suitable test for those with large (obvious) deviations. Place the lens over the fixating (nondeviating) eye. In cases of an alternating phoria or tropia, you will be unable to measure the deviation using horizontal or vertical prism bars.

The Maddox rod has a red prism lens comprised of rows of glass or plastic rods (a series of plano-convex lenses) with the centers of each prism being 3 mm apart that produce the image of a line that is oriented 90 degrees from the orientation of the rods when light is shining through it. Depending on how the lens is held (the direction of the rods vertically or horizontally in front of the eye) the red line will appear to be either horizontal or vertical. When the rows of rods are oriented horizontally in from of the patient's eye, they should see a vertical line. When the rows of rods are oriented vertically in front of the patient's eye, they should see a horizontal line. From the uncovered eye, the patient will see a dot of light from a penlight held by the examiner. The patient reports where the white dot of light is with regard to the red line. When testing at a near distance the light source should be ~15–16 inches (40 cm) from the patient and held at eye level. When testing distance, they light source should be ~20 feet from the patient (~6 m). During the test, the eye that is covered by the lens is called the fixating eye, while the uncovered eye is the test eye. When testing at a distance, a Maddox tangent scale (which basically are two rulers that are marked in either diopters or degrees that cross to make a plus sign, with the light source at the center) is used to measure the deviation, with the number on the Maddox tangent scale where the red line falls being the amount of heterophoria (or misalignment). Trained clinicians can also use a prism bar at both near and far distances to measure the deviation in diopters.

MADDOX ROD INSTRUCTIONS

1. The patient is sitting in a dimly lit room with the examiner sitting directly in front of them. There should only be one light source in the room (e.g., the penlight).
2. Instruct the patient to keep both eyes open and fixed on a light source (penlight) held in front of them.
3. The examiner places the Maddox rod lens over the patient's right eye with the rows of the lens oriented horizontally. This produces a vertical line that the patient sees and is used to measure horizontal deviations.
4. The patient is asked to describe the dot of light in relation to the red line. Is it left of, on top of, or to the right of the line?
5. Next, the Maddox rod lens is held so that the rows are vertical and producing a horizontal red line that the patient sees. This is used to measure vertical deviations, and the patient reports if the light is above, on top of, or below the red line.
6. Repeat the test on the left eye.

INTERPRETATION OF THE MADDOX ROD TEST

Each of these interpretations (Figure 7.3) describe a right eye that is covered by the Maddox rod lens. In this case, the right eye is the fixating eye. For each interpretation, the description is that of the patient's perception. The patient judges where the line is with regard to the light source (not the other way around). As an example, imagine the lens covers the patient's right eye, and that eye is turned inward (esotropic), the image of the line will fall on the nasal retina and will be perceived as being temporal (with the light source falling to the left side of the line from the patient's perception). Thus, the patient would have a right esodeviation.

What the patient sees (Figure 7.3):

- The white dot (light source) is superimposed on the line; there is no deviation.
- The vertical line is to the right of the white dot (A); a right *esodeviation* is present.
- The vertical line is to the left of the white dot (B); a right *exodeviation* is present.
- The horizontal line is above the white dot (C); a right *hypodeviation* is present.
- The horizontal line is below the white dot (D); a right *hyperdeviation* is present.

OTHER VISION/OCULOMOTOR TESTS (AS NEEDED)

While these tests are not included in the list of a "minimal" exam, they still are fairly frequently used when examining patients who have a suspected stroke.

VISUAL ACUITY

Visual acuity (VA) is a measure of the resolving power of the eye (in other words, how sharply someone can see). Several tests may be used to test VA:

1. Recognition acuity tests ask the patient to "recognize" and identify a series of targets.
   - *Examples*: Snellen acuity chart (ages 6+), ETDRS chart (developed to detect diabetic retinopathy).
2. Resolution acuity test: Requires the patient to resolve a difference between two targets.
   - *Examples*: Preferential looking (used for young infants and toddlers).
3. Alternative VA tests use pictograms (pictures/drawings) or have the patient point.

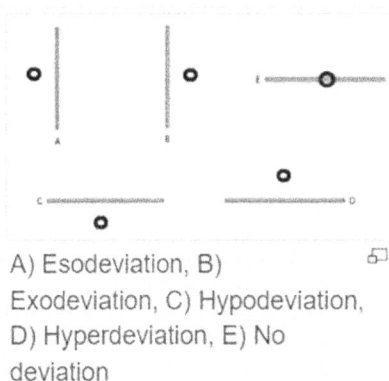

A) Esodeviation, B) Exodeviation, C) Hypodeviation, D) Hyperdeviation, E) No deviation

Figure 7.3 Maddox Rod Test Interpretation

• *Examples*: Tumbling E test, or tests used in the preschool population (Broken Wheel Test for ages 3+ and the LEA Symbols test for ages 4+).

Snellen Charts

The *Snellen chart* (aka the big E chart) is probably the most widely known and was developed by Hermann Snellen in the 1860s. It is the chart with a very large letter *E* at the top. People or children who cannot read might use the *tumbling E chart* or a chart utilizing pictures/drawings. The letters on the Snellen chart are called *optotypes*. There are 11 lines of optotypes, with increasing numbers of optotypes on each line that get progressively smaller as you move down the chart. Each line is numbered, with the line number to the right of the optotypes. To the right of the line number is the visual acuity level for that line. The patient is asked to stand at a distance away from the eye chart that is printed on it (the standard is 20 feet for those using the imperial system of measurement and 6 m for those using the metric system). Some eye charts have the patient stand closer than 20 feet, but the visual acuity is still referenced to the 20-foot standard. Patients are asked to identify the optotypes, reading from the top of the chart down and from left to right. As they read the chart, they are allowed to miss up to two optotypes per line and continue. If they miss three optotypes, the previous line will be recorded as their VA. You may write the VA as the chart distance over the lowest line read minus the number of optotypes they missed on that line.

Imperial system example: 20/20 –2

• This indicates the patient was able to read the line corresponding to 20/20 (standing 20 feet away from the chart) missing two optotypes, but was unable to read the next smaller line or missed three or more optotypes on the next smaller line.

Metric system example: 6/6 –2

• This indicates the patient was able to read the line corresponding to 20/20 (standing 6 m away from the chart) missing two optotypes, but was unable to read the next smaller line or missed three or more optotypes on the next smaller line.

To interpret the visual acuity, you will read a fraction such as 20/20 (or 6/6). The first number (or top number) represents the equivalent of the distance the person is standing from the eye chart. The second number (or bottom) represents the distance at which a person with normal or average vision can read the line. Another way to think of this is the distance the patient can see the line (first number) over the distance at which a person with normal vision can see the line. For example, using the eye chart in Figure 7.4, if the last line a patient can read and only miss up to two optotypes is line 8, they have 20/20 VA. There is a thick light gray line below row 6, as row 6 is the minimum vision required to drive in the USA. There is a thick dark gray line below row 8, as row 8 indicates normal or average vision.

INSTRUCTIONS FOR VISUAL ACUITY TESTING

Test the patient without wearing their prescription spectacles (if they have them). This will be recorded as "uncorrected VA." If you are not an optometrist or ophthalmologist, you may wish to test the patient with and without their spectacles to get an idea if their VA has changed since they last were given their prescription. If testing while wearing their prescription spectacles, you will record this as "best corrected VA." When documenting a patient's VA, you will indicate the VA of the right eye (oculus dexter, OD), the VA of the left eye (oculus sinister, OS), and the VA while using both eyes (oculus uterque, OU). The test procedure is as follows:

1. Have the patient stand at the distance indicated by the eye chart.
2. Cover the patient's left eye and have them read the chart using only their right eye (OD). Record the OD VA.
3. Cover the patient's right eye and have them read the chart only using their left eye (OS). Again, record the OS VA.
4. Read the chart using both eyes (OU), and record the OU VA.

Snellen

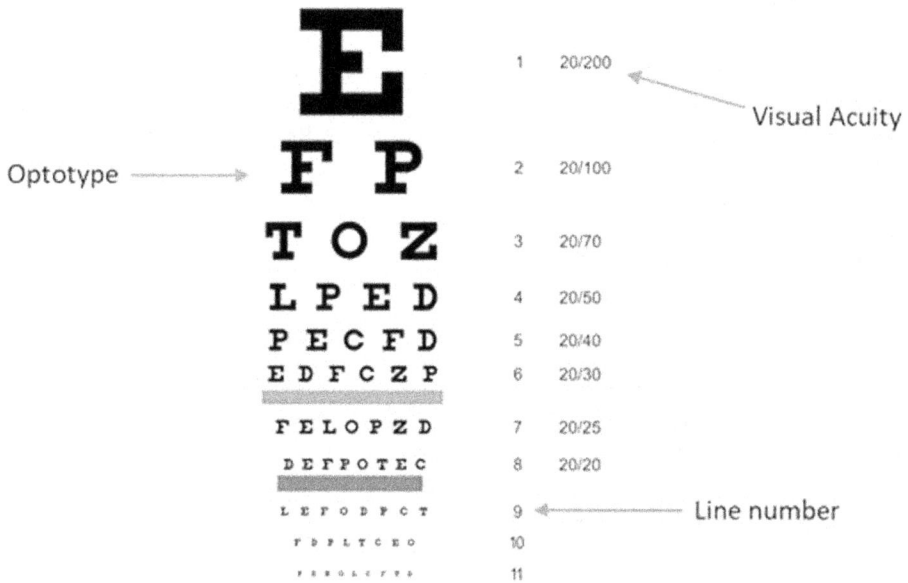

Figure 7.4 Snellen Eye Chart

For near vision, you test in the same way. The differences between a near chart and a distance chart are that the patient can hold the eye chart in their hand at a normal reading distance (~35.5 cm, or 14 inches), and they are only allowed to miss one optotype per line to continue.

Instructions for Counting Fingers Test

What can you do if you do not have an eye chart? If you do not have an eye chart available, you may use a counting fingers test by holding up one to four fingers on one hand at different distances from the patient. The farthest distance the patient correctly reports the finger count is recorded as CF (count fingers) at (distance).

- For example, a patient reports the correct number of fingers the examiner is holding up at 3 feet (~1 m) away, but cannot correctly identify how many are held up at 4 feet. The examiner would document:
  - Imperial: CF at 3 feet
  - Metric: CF at 1 m

GEEK STUFF

Hold the pointer finger of each hand close to your face on the edges of your peripheral vision. Now move the fingers straight in front of you about 6 inches (~15 cm) without bringing them medially. You will notice that your visual field has expanded. If you want your fingers on the edge of your peripheral vision, you will now need to move each finger laterally. This is because you see in a visual cone that expands the farther away the visual target is from your eyes. How do you know you are in the patient's peripheral vision? Sit in front of a patient and close one of your eyes and have the patient cover the eye directly across from it. Place the visual target equidistant between yourselves on the edge of your peripheral vision. If the target is equidistant, and your visual fields are intact, the target should also be on the edge of the patient's peripheral vision.

VISUAL FIELDS

Visual fields are important to check if your patient has had (or you suspect) a stroke or head injury, complains of walking into objects on one side, or reports reading difficulties. In a retrospective study of 220 patients (160 traumatic brain injury [TBI] patients, 60 cerebrovascular accident [CVA] patients), Suchoff et al. found 46% had visual field defects on perimetry testing (39% of TBI and 60% of CVA patients).[17] There are numerous ways to test visual fields: confrontation tests, Amsler grid, static automated perimetry, kinetic perimetry, and frequency doubling perimetry. Some are "screening" in nature, others are data-driven. Typical bedside confrontation tests include the *moving confrontation test* and sometimes the *finger counting confrontation test*. As the names imply, the moving confrontation test will assess the patient's ability to detect a moving object (e.g., a finger or pen), while the finger counting confrontation test assesses the patient's ability to visually process what they see using their peripheral vision (i.e., distinguish how many fingers the examiner is holding up). Make sure visual targets are equidistant between the examiner and the patient so that the visual fields are the same.

Instructions for the Moving Confrontation Test

1. The patient sits directly in front of the examiner and is instructed to cover their left eye with their left palm and visually fixate with their right eye on the examiner's left eye (which is directly across from them).
2. The examiner closes their right eye and places their hand equidistant between themselves and the patient (about 20 inches or 51 cm distant from the patient).
3. Since one of the examiner's eyes are closed and the hand is equidistant between the examiner and the patient, the visual fields of the examiner and patient should be the same. The examiner holds a visual target (finger, pen, or Wolff wand) just outside of the visual field and slowly moves it into the visual field on a diagonal

toward the eye. Instruct the patient to tell the examiner when the target is first seen.
4. This is done for each quadrant (upper and lower), testing one quadrant at a time.
5. Repeat the test for the left eye while having the patient cover their right eye and the examiner closes their left eye.
6. Note any quadrants (or parts of quadrants) that cannot be seen.

Instructions for the Finger Counting Confrontation Test

1. The patient sits directly in front of the examiner and is instructed to cover their left eye with their left palm and visually fixate with their right eye on the examiner's left eye (which is directly across from them).
2. The examiner closes their right eye and places their hand equidistant between themself and the patient (about 20 inches or 51 cm distant from the patient).
3. Because one of the examiner's eyes is closed and the hand is equidistant between themself and the patient, the visual fields of the examiner and patient should be the same. The examiner holds a hand on the edge of one of the four quadrants of the eye and holds up varying amounts of fingers (one, two, or three) asking the patient to say how many fingers are being held up while maintaining fixation on the examiner's eye.
4. This is done for each quadrant (upper and lower), testing one quadrant at a time.
5. Repeat the test for the left eye by having the patient cover their right eye, while the examiner closes their left eye.
6. Next, the patient is asked to fixate on the examiner's nose with both eyes open. Fingers are held up on each hand simultaneously on the edges of vision while testing upper quadrants and then lower quadrants. The patient must report the total number of fingers held up (adding those from the left and right hands) while maintaining fixation on the examiner's nose.
7. Note any quadrants that cannot be seen at all.

Interpretation and Documentation of Confrontation Tests

MOVING CONFRONTATION

The examiner will record if the patient can detect the moving object as it enters the visual field. If the patient cannot see the moving object, it is recorded as either a *quadrantanopia* if only one quadrant is missing or a *hemianopia* if both quadrants on one side (left or right) are missing.

When documenting finger counting confrontations, use a box showing four quadrants for each eye. There is no standard way to document moving confrontation, so you may use the strategy used for finger counting confrontation, only use an *M* (moving) for an intact quadrant and place an *X* in the box if it is not. An example is listed in Figure 7.5.

FINGER COUNTING CONFRONTATION

- Visual inattention (visual neglect) is recorded if the patient can see the hand(s) but cannot correctly report the number of fingers held up (on one hand for a quadrant).
- Visual loss is recorded if the patient cannot see the hand(s).
- If the patient can correctly identify the number of fingers held up in each upper or lower quadrant (when the quadrant is tested individually) but is unable to report the correct number of fingers held up on both hands simultaneously, this is recorded as *visual extinction* and indicates a visual processing problem.
- You may document your examination for each eye by crossing two lines, making four quadrants, and indicating *CF* for an accurate count of the fingers, and an *X* for visual extinction (Figure 7.6).

🎥 NEAR POINT OF CONVERGENCE (NPC) TEST

The NPC is the closest point that the patient can converge the eyes and still maintain fusion on a visual target (see only one image). There are many recommendations for normal NPC distance that ranges from 5 cm to >17.5 cm. NPC recovery is the point at which fusion is recovered after it has been lost by convergence; published values range from 7.5 cm to 11 cm.[18] Testing procedures and visual targets likewise vary. If you are using

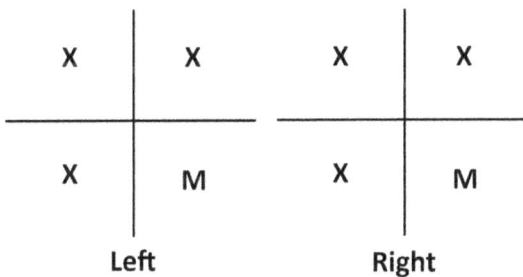

Figure 7.5 Moving Confrontation Documentation

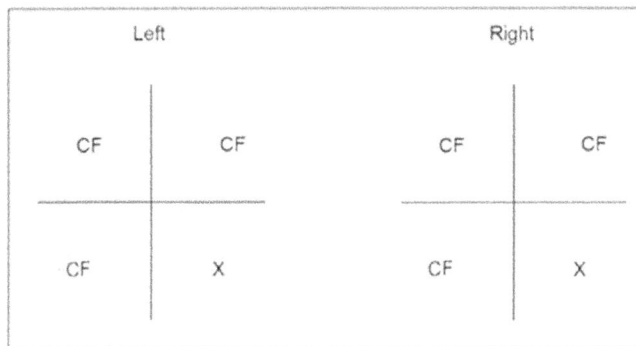

Figure 7.6 Finger Counting Documentation

an accommodative target, you will need to assess visual acuity first, so that you may pick a target that is just above their level of acuity (one line easier). For example, if the patient has 20/20 (6/6) vision, you want to choose a target that is 20/25 (6/7.5).

NPC Test Instructions (Using an Accommodative Rule)

Using the method provided by Scheiman et al.[18]

1. With the patient sitting, the accommodative rule is placed just above the nose at the brow between the two eyes.
2. The target is moved toward the patient at a rate of about 1 to 2 cm/s.
3. Patients are encouraged to try to keep the target single.
4. The subjective "break" and "recovery" values are measured and recorded in centimeters. If there is no subjective report of diplopia, the points at which the patient objectively lost and regained ocular alignment are recorded as the break and recovery.

If you do not have an accommodative rule, use the non-shiny end of a pen/pencil or your finger as a visual target while holding the end of a tape measure to the patient's head placed just above the nose at the brow between the two eyes; the tape measure roll is in the hand with the visual target. While this is not ideal, it will give you a rough estimation of NPC.

Interpretation of NPC Testing

A study took place designed to determine the most appropriate target(s) to be used and to establish normative data for NPC break and recovery. It found the following for adults:[18]

- *NPC normal values*: 0.5 to 5.0 cm
- *Recommended clinical cutoff for NPC break*: 5 cm
- *Recommended NPC recovery*: 7 cm
- *Maximum break*: 7 cm for the accommodative target
- *Convergence insufficiency subjects*: Average NPC break 12.1 cm, increasing with repeated measures

- *Recommended visual target for NPC measure*: An accommodative target provides the best precision
- *Recommended visual target to discriminate convergence insufficiency*: Penlight and red/green glasses; you may still use an accommodative target if you do not have a penlight and reg/green glasses

Hayes et al. established normative values for NPC for school children (kindergarten, third and sixth grades), and suggested a clinical cutoff of 6 cm for NPC break using an accommodative target.[19]

CONTRAST SENSITIVITY TESTING

To evaluate contrast sensitivity (CS), you need a special chart. The chart shows a line of blocks of alternating striped bars of light and dark bands, with the width of the bars defining the spatial frequency (pairs of dark and light bars that subtend an angle of 1 degree at the eye).[20] High spatial frequencies have narrow bars, whereas low spatial frequencies have wide bars. The blocks are numbered, and the patient reports the last block in which they can distinguish the bars.

There are three types of CS deficits:

- *High frequency*, characterized by an increased loss at high frequencies.
- *Level loss*, where the patient demonstrates the same loss at all kinds of spatial frequencies.
- *Selective loss*, where the patient demonstrates a loss in a narrow band of spatial frequencies.

Yellow or copper-tinted spectacles help to improve contrast in low ambient light, but should be avoided while driving due to glare. But they can have an antireflective coating to reduce glare.[20]

COLOR VISION TESTING

The most common method of testing color vision is with pseudoisochromatic plates. Other tools that are used to test color vision include ordering tests, in which patients must sort discs based on color progression, and matching tests.[21]

VESTIBULAR FUNCTION EXAMINATIONS

Clearly document any sedating medications the patient is taking or has taken within the prior 48 hours. If possible, have sedating medications held with a medical order at least 24 to 48 hours prior to testing, as they may hide signs and symptoms. Some medications require a weaning schedule (e.g., antipsychotics); this needs to be planned in advance. You may *not* instruct a patient to withhold *any* medication without a physician's order, even when the medication orders are "as needed" or over the counter. Prior to performing bedside tests of the vestibular system, you should know the patient's active cervical ROM and be aware of contraindications to testing, such as cervical ROM restrictions, recent cervical fractures, C1–C2 instability, or recent retinal detachment.

VESTIBULO-OCULAR REFLEX (VOR) BEDSIDE TEST

While you can test any of the three semicircular canals in each ear, tests of the lateral vestibular canal are used most often. We assess only the lateral vestibular canals and use the resulting VOR function to give an indication of the general function of the vestibular system. In reality testing, only the lateral canal function does not truly test the entire vestibular system. Remember, the superior vestibular nerve innervates the lateral canal (along with the anterior canal and utricle), while other parts of the vestibular system (the saccule and posterior canal) are innervated by the inferior vestibular nerve.

The VOR is relatively easy to elicit; here are a few testing options:

1. The head impulse test (also known as the *head thrust test*)
2. The head shake test
3. The instrumented dynamic visual acuity (DVA) test

None of these tests localize lesions. That is, if there is pathology interfering with the VOR, these tests do not tell you exactly where the pathology is located. They do grossly indicate a left-sided versus right-sided vestibular weakness, but you cannot tell from these tests if a lesion is *peripheral* (in the inner ear) or *central* (within the brain or central nervous system). If, in using one of these bedside tests, you determine that there is a unilateral vestibular deficit, without instrumented tests all you can really say is that the vestibular system is somehow involved. There are some signs and symptoms that point us in the direction of peripheral versus central pathologies, but without more specific clinical tests, these bedside tests may only *suggest* which is involved. As this is the case, any time a clinician finds a positive bedside test indicating a vestibular weakness, they should recommend further clinical testing. Usually, this means ordering a videonystagmography (VNG) and an audiogram (hearing test). Using a VNG, the audiologist can tell more specifically how much the vestibular apparatus of the ear is involved. Keep in mind that the head impulse test (HIT) is a high-frequency test, while the VNG/caloric is a low-frequency test. There are times when the HIT is positive while the VNG is negative for vestibular loss, and vice-versa. Because some patterns of hearing loss indicate possible central pathology, the hearing test will help point to possible brain or nerve issues that would require further investigation, as with magnetic resonance imaging. When both a VNG and audiogram are ordered, the battery of tests used by the audiologist usually also includes a gross balance screen as well as an oculomotor examination. This battery of tests is extremely helpful in gaining information of vestibular function as well as to screen out more serious central pathologies. As bedside testing is limited in sensitivity, a negative test does not always mean the patient has "normal" vestibular function, but that they do not have a deficit that is bad enough to be detected with a gross screening. If the patient has signs or symptoms that lead you to think that there may be a vestibular problem (e.g., vertigo, loss of balance during head turns, nausea in busy visual environments), it is important to request more in-depth vestibular testing.

Prior to performing vestibular bedside tests, the clinician should first check the integrity of the

C1–C2 ligaments and gauge the patient's active cervical range of motion. This is especially true if there is a history of trauma. Many leaders in the vestibular research realm no longer recommend using the vertebral artery screen.

🎥◀ Head Impulse Test (Lateral Canal)

The head impulse test is a passive test on the patient's part that indicates which vestibular apparatus (left or right) is working well enough to turn on the VOR for the canal that is being tested. The patient should wear their usual eyeglasses for this test.

HEAD IMPULSE TEST (E.G., LATERAL CANAL) INSTRUCTIONS

1. The examiner is at eye level with the patient (sitting or standing while the patient sits on a plinth).
2. The examiner instructs the patient to tip their head down (30 degrees), correcting with their hands.
3. The patient in instructed to visually fixate on the tip of the examiner's nose.
4. The examiner grasps the patient's head at or above the ears, and briskly passively turns the patient's head ~15–30 degrees (or less) toward the patient's left shoulder and keeps it there while observing for a catch-up saccade.
5. The examiner returns the patient's head to midline (still flexed 30 degrees) and retests the left side.
6. Repeat the examination on the right side.

INTERPRETATION OF THE HEAD IMPULSE TEST

When the patient's head is rapidly turned, the eyes should remain on the examiner's nose. If the eyes move with the head and come off the target, you will see a corrective saccade toward the target. This is a positive test and indicates a vestibular weakness for the ear in the direction of the head turn. For example, if the left ear is tested, the head is rapidly turned to the patient's left. If there is a vestibular deficit, the eyes will move with the head, and the clinician will see a corrective saccade to the right in order to reacquire the target. The clinician will document a "positive left head impulse test."

Key things to remember:

- To improve the sensitivity of the test, the head is tilted 30 degrees.[22]

It is a given that the lateral canals are not exactly parallel to the horizontal plane but are actually angled about 30 degrees, with the anterior portions being more orientated and more cephalic. By positioning the patient in 30 degrees head/neck flexion, the lateral canals will roughly be level with the ground.

- Unpredictable tests have better sensitivity.[22]

For this test, *unpredictably* indicates that while prior to the test we instruct the patient that we will be turning their head, the patient does not know in which direction (left or right) we will turn it or exactly when. We *do not* say, "On three ... 1, 2 ..." By moving the head unpredictably, we can be sure that the patient is not anticipating the motion and using that information for motor planning.

- The side to which you rotate the patient's head is the side you are testing. For example, if you rotate the patient's head to their left, you are testing the left vestibular apparatus. If you rotate the head to their right, you are testing the right vestibular apparatus.
- In performing this test, do not turn the patient's head while holding the jaw. Remember, the jaw has joints holding it to the skull (temporomandibular joints [TMJs]). These joints move: you may inadvertently strain them by turning the head rapidly while applying force to them. While you are performing the test, be sure to keep your hands high on the patient's head (ear level or higher).
- A common error that clinicians can make while performing it is to turn the head away from midline and then immediately bring it back to center. Remember, turn the head and *stop it in the turned position*. Do not immediately bring it back to midline.
- If the patient is unable to keep their eyes on your nose while the head is being turned, they will have to make a corrective saccade (by moving their eyes) to look for your nose after the head is turned. If you observe a

corrective eye motion, the test is positive and indicates a likely vestibular weakness (loss) on the side in the direction of the head turn.

- Test each side.
- Always take the patient's subjective complaints into account. Should the patient complain of dizziness, especially while turning, while in darkness, or in busy visual environments such as grocery stores or shopping malls, a VNG/audiogram may be revealing even if the head impulse test is negative.
- To test the anterior or posterior canals, perform the head impulse test in the plane and direction of the canal you wish to test.

HEAD IMPULSE TEST SENSITIVITY

- 88% for complete unilateral vestibular loss (UVL)[22]
- 84% for bilateral vestibular hypofunction (BVH)[22]
- 100% for complete bilateral vestibular loss[22]

🎥◀ Head Shaking Test

The head shaking test assesses vestibular symmetry. The results indicate whether one vestibular organ (left or right) is stronger than the other. How does this test work? While the clinician is shaking the patient's head, the vestibular system is stimulated. Part of the cerebellum that deals with vestibular information, called the *velocity storage system*, gathers information about this repetitive head motion and stores it. It "is a multisensory element whose function is to compute an accurate estimate of rotation velocity using multiple sensory cues, e.g., canal signals, otolith signals, and vision" and improves "the temporal response of the canals by compensating for their dynamics."[23]

HEAD SHAKING TEST INSTRUCTIONS

1. The examiner sits across from the patient.
2. The patient is instructed to tip the head down 30 degrees (corrected by the examiner for position).
3. The patient is instructed to close their eyes (or wear Frenzel or IR goggles).
4. Quickly rotate the patient's head back and forth horizontally (as if the patient were

shaking their head no) at 2 Hz of motion 20–30 times (20–30 seconds).
5. Ask the patient to open their eyes, and then stop shaking their head.
6. Observe the patient's eyes for nystagmus.

Key things to remember:

- If you stop shaking the patient's head before you ask them to open their eyes, you may miss detecting nystagmus.
- If the patient's head is still flexed when they open their eyes, and your head is higher than theirs, they will look up to find you. This may be misinterpreted as vertical nystagmus. If you bring the patient's head out of the 30 degrees of tilt during the final five head shakes, and you place your face in front of theirs, this is avoided. Alternatively, you can have the patient sitting on a plinth higher than yourself, so that when they open their eyes, they are looking directly at you even though their head is tilted down 30 degrees.

INTERPRETATION OF THE HEAD SHAKING TEST

- If no nystagmus is observed post-head shaking, the test is negative (normal).
- If ≥3 nystagmus beats are observed, the test is positive for vestibular asymmetry. Note the direction of the quick phases (they will beat toward the more active ear).
- Central signs for this test include post-horizontal head shake nystagmus that is beating vertically (cerebellar lesions, and ~25% for migraine[24]) or dysconjugately.

Sensitivity

- Ménière's disease: 58.1%
- Acoustic neuroma: 47.6%
- Vestibular neuronitis: 50%
- Recurrent vestibulopathy: 30.8%

Here is a simple explanation of how this test works: The brain keeps track of head motions. For example, say, you are sitting in a chair that swivels and are turning clockwise. As you turn, you need to use the VOR in order to see clearly. As you are turning and accelerating, the vestibulocerebellum buffers information about the direction and speed of turning and uses that information to drive the VOR. This makes it easier and more efficient to turn on and use this reflex. *Think of it this way*: Imagine that you have a watch spring in your right ear, which provides the power to turn on the nystagmus (VOR) that are needed for seeing while turning to the right and another watch spring in the left ear to activate the VOR needed for seeing while turning left. As you spin clockwise (right), you "wind up the right watch spring" and store energy, then use it to turn on the nystagmus needed to see clearly. If you were turning left, you would store energy to turn on the VOR with quick phases to the left. When you stopped turning, you would continue to expend this buffered energy in the form of nystagmus until the watch spring unwound—the vestibulocerebellum buffer would be empty.

If we spin to the right, while we are spinning and accelerating, we will get quick-phase nystagmus to the right. The changes in velocity stimulate the lateral canals of the vestibular system, but we also get some optokinetic stimulation through the eyes owing to the constantly moving environment. If we spin to the left, while we are spinning, we will get quick-phase nystagmus to the left. When we are spinning at a constant velocity, the endolymph and cupulae are relatively still, as they are moving at the same speed, but now the optokinetic system is driving the nystagmus. When we decelerate or stop moving, the nystagmus will change direction owing to the inertia of the endolymph pushing on the cupula. That is to say, we stop moving, but the liquid endolymph in our ears does not. It pushes against the cupula and the vestibular system is once again excited. In one ear the flow of endolymph will be toward the cupula, while in the other ear it will be away from the cupula. A simple way to imagine fluid motion once we stop is to use a bucket of water. Using full shoulder motion, swing the bucket in a circle. What happens if you stop swinging and suddenly stop the bucket? The water will continue moving and slosh over the sides of the bucket, even though the bucket has stopped moving.

Now take your understanding of stored energy and apply it to our head shake test. What would happen if you *repeatedly and alternately* turned the patient's head left and right at a velocity of about 2 Hz? While you are shaking the patient's head, the head is accelerating to 2 Hz and then suddenly stopping, then reversing direction and accelerating again to 2 Hz (over and over). The vestibular system is excited by the lag of endolymph pushing on the cupulae because of these repeated changes in velocity in each direction. Would nystagmus be present if you stopped shaking the head after turning it alternately left and right for 20 to 30 seconds, as when shaking the head horizontally? The vestibulocerebellum will still be buffering information (winding our watch springs) while the head is moving. If each inner ear is working and equally strong, the vestibulocerebellum will buffer information about the head shake for *each* direction. Would you see nystagmus after stopping the head shake? The answer is no; you should not see any nystagmus after stopping the head. There is still stored energy, but when both ears are working, there are *equal amounts* of stored energy regarding each direction of spin. This is different from nystagmus observed after having a subject spin in one direction while their eyes are open. When spun in only one direction, only one ear is excited. When the subject stops spinning, one ear has buffered energy to expend, and nystagmus will beat toward that ear. During the head shake test, however, the clinician moves the head in both directions (left and right). It is like a tug-of-war with Team Left and Team Right each trying to elicit nystagmus in its direction. In keeping with our tug-of-war analogy, if one ear is stronger than the other, it will be able to pull the flag (nystagmus) in its direction. If one ear's watch spring (vestibular system) is working and storing energy while the other ear's watch spring is not working, there will be asymmetry between the systems. Once the head stops shaking, the vestibulocerebellum will discharge energy. If there is more information regarding a healthy ear versus a damaged one, you will see quick-phase nystagmus in the direction of the stronger (or more stimulated) ear. If both ears are working well enough, you should not observe any nystagmus.

Dynamic Visual Acuity Test (DVA)

This test determines the patient's visual acuity (sharpness of vision) while the head is still (static) or moving (dynamic), with the difference between the two tests helping determine whether the vestibular system is working properly. There are two types of dynamic visual acuity tests: dynamic-object (head still, moving target) and static-object DVA (head moving, still target).[25] There are many different types of static-object DVA examinations. The most common is the clinical DVA (or bedside DVA). This test is performed by the patient reading a Snellen chart, and then again while their head is passively rotated at ~2 Hz. However, in a study by Cochrane et al., subjects involuntarily slowed their head movements to see the optotypes clearly, and instead of using the VOR, they use smooth pursuit. Because of this, the reliability of the examiner and intra-examiner was poor for assessing vestibular hypofunction.[26] A computerized DVA uses a rate sensor to detect head speed and only presents an optotype when the head is moving fast enough to use the VOR. This increases the test's validity.[27]

If the VOR is not working properly, the patient will have at least a three-line difference between static and dynamic visual acuity.

Computerized (Instrumented) Dynamic Visual Acuity

SENSITIVITY AND SPECIFICITY: COMPUTERIZED DYNAMIC VISUAL ACUITY

- Sensitivity: 94.5%
- Specificity: 95.2%[27]

Key things to remember:

- The clinical (non-instrumented) DVA has poor reliability.
- The computerized DVA is valid and reliable, and has been studied in the vestibular hypofunction population.

📹 VOR Cancellation Test (VOR-C)

Do not be fooled by the name of this test. It is not a test of the VOR but instead assesses the cerebellum's ability to suppress the VOR. Remember, the VOR causes the eyes to move in the *opposite direction* to that of the head motion. For example, if you turn your head to the right, your eyes will reflexively move to the left. However, there are times when we don't want our eyes to move in the opposite direction as our heads. When we watch a plane or bird fly across the sky or watch a tennis match, we need to have our heads and eyes moving in the same direction in order to keep the image of those objects on our retinas (foveae). To do this, we need to suppress (cancel) the VOR. This test is actually a cerebellar screening test.

VOR Function Examinations Summary

There are a variety of options to test vestibular function. You should use at least one bedside test of vestibular function (e.g., head impulse, head shake, or computerized DVA) to assess a patient who complains of disequilibrium or dizziness, unless you have more sophisticated equipment to do so. You do not have to use all of these VOR function tests, but you may choose to use more than one if you suspect vestibular involvement but get a negative test using just one of them. Remember, if you find a positive test, the wise course is to recommend further testing, such as a VNG/audiogram. This may help to confirm a vestibular issue as well and to rule out central involvement.

Keep in mind that a negative bedside test does not necessarily indicate normal function. Take test results into consideration with current complaints as well as other signs and symptoms. Use more sophisticated tests to confirm or rule out pathology.

PRESSURE TESTING OF THE EAR

Clinicians use pressure tests to detect possible perilymphatic fistulas and occasionally hypermobile stapes. Pressure testing may also produce symptoms in patients with Arnold–Chiari malformations or canal dehiscence syndromes.[28] The various tests put either positive or negative pressure on the vestibular system or external auditory canal. If nystagmus or eye drifting is noted during testing, the test is considered positive. These pressure tests include tragal compression, the Valsalva maneuver, and pneumatic otoscopy. When possible, use Frenzel or IR goggles during testing.

Interpretation of Pressure Tests of the Ear

In tests of pressure, consistent eye deviation or nystagmus movement imply abnormal coupling (connection) between either the outside atmosphere with the inner ear or the intracranial space and the inner ear. Likely locations of abnormalities include the following:

- Oval window (fistula, excessive footplate movement)
- Round window (fistula)
- Lateral semicircular canal (dehiscence)
- Eye elevation and intorsion with loud sounds or during a nose-pinch Valsalva, suggesting superior canal dehiscence[29]
- Vertical downbeating nystagmus with any maneuver that increases intracranial pressure, suggesting an abnormality of the craniocervical junction (e.g., Arnold–Chiari malformation)[30]

Tragal Compression Test

During this test, the examiner changes intracranial pressure by pushing on the patient's tragus (part of the external ear). During the test, the patient is in a sitting position. Testing in other positions may change the intracranial pressure and affect the test results.

TRAGAL COMPRESSION TEST INSTRUCTIONS

1. The patient is in a sitting position. The test is preferably performed with the patient's vision blocked by Frenzel or IR goggles.
2. With the patient sitting, the examiner firmly and steadily presses the tragus in toward the patient's external auditory canal for about 3 seconds while observing for tonic eye drift or nystagmus. During the test, sufficient pressure should be applied against the tragus (using fingers or thumb); this will be uncomfortable for the patient but not sharply painful. Each ear should be tested separately.

INTERPRETATION OF THE TRAGAL COMPRESSION TEST

Observed nystagmus or tonic deviation of eye position during the test indicates possible deficits to the test side, such as perilymph fistulas and canal dehiscence.

Valsalva Maneuver (Nose-Pinch Valsalva)

The Valsalva maneuver is another test in which the clinician observes the patient's eyes for nystagmus or tonic deviation. Here, pressure is placed on the inner ear during forced expiration while pinching the nose and against a closed glottis (closed airway). You may use it to assess pressure sensitivity and superior canal dehiscence/fistula. It may be performed sitting, supine, or in a recumbent position. According to Shuman et al.,

> Valsalva against a closed glottis causes increased intracranial pressure, which exerts a downward force at the site of dehiscence. This results in ampullopetal endolymph flow in the canal, and the patient develops an inhibitory nystagmus with a slow phase that moves down and rotates toward the affected ear.[29]

While there are no contraindications, caution should be taken for patients with preexisting coronary artery disease, valvular disease, or congenital heart disease.[31,32]

VALSALVA MANEUVER INSTRUCTIONS

1. The patient is in a sitting position, keeping their eyes open (they may wear Frenzel or IR goggles).
2. Instruct the patient to either pinch their nose and glottis (airway) closed and to bear down for 10 seconds while attempting to exhale with moderate force while keeping the eyes open.

Key thing to remember:

- Patients may become lightheaded or have body/head shakes while performing this test

INTERPRETATION OF THE VALSALVA MANEUVER

- During the Valsalva maneuver, the examiner observes the patient's eyes for nystagmus or eye drifting. This test may produce signs and symptoms in patients with craniocervical abnormalities, perilymph fistula, or canal dehiscence syndrome.
- A change in the direction of nystagmus during a nose-pinch Valsalva maneuver versus a closed glottis is characteristic of a superior canal dehiscence syndrome.[14]
- Make sure the patient closes the glottis during the test if the patient has complaints of dizziness.[33]
- In superior canal dehiscence, the test may produce upbeating nystagmus and nystagmus beating with torsional. Although rare, a horizontal canal fistula (from cholesteatoma or fenestration surgery) may produce horizontal nystagmus.[33]
- For patients with Arnold–Chiari malformation, and also in some normal subjects, the test may induce a low-amplitude downbeating nystagmus.[30]

Pneumatic Otoscopy

A pneumatic otoscopy tests the mobility of the tympanic membrane and is typically performed by an otorhinolaryngologist. It is frequently used for diagnosing otitis media with effusion. It may also be a useful tool to screen for perilymphatic fistula and superior semicircular canal dehiscence syndrome (SSCD).[34]

PNEUMATIC OTOSCOPY INSTRUCTIONS

1. The patient should be sitting in a brightly lit room and asked to look at a stationary target.
2. Gently squeeze the rubber bulb and then release (positive/negative pressure), instructing the patient to tell you when they perceive movement of the target or symptoms of vertigo/disequilibrium.
3. If the test is repeated with the same results, it is positive.

Key things to remember:

- You may modify this test with the patient's vision blocked, using VNG monitoring to improve sensitivity of the test. Another variation of the test is to monitor postural sway using computerized dynamic platform posturography while applying pressure to the ear.[35]
- Eye movements in Hennebert's sign consist of two or three small-amplitude horizontal (not torsional) jerks that are away from the ear on positive pressure and toward the ear on negative pressure (which will elicit stronger responses). Other conditions that can cause Hennebert's sign include congenital syphilis, Ménière's disease, stapes surgery, footplate fractures, and sudden deafness.[35]

INTERPRETATION OF THE PNEUMATIC OTOSCOPY TEST (FOR SSCD)

- When positive, it indicates an abnormal coupling between the external canal and the labyrinth, which is referred to as *Hennebert's sign.*[36]

STAGING A VESTIBULAR NEURITIS/LABYRINTHITIS USING NYSTAGMUS

Spontaneous nystagmus is often observed following acute vestibular loss, due to a neuritis/labyrinthitis. These constant unidirectional nystagmus movements typically last between 12 and 36 hours. Following Alexander's law, they are often diminished when looking in the direction of the affected ear and more robust while gazing toward the healthy ear. While spontaneous nystagmus may not be present, the patient may have nystagmus beginning at 45 degrees of gaze toward the intact ear during the early subacute phase, and later only near end-range toward the intact ear. During the late subacute phase, unidirectional gaze nystagmus are difficult to see in room light. However, they are often observable by removing fixation using Frenzel goggles or IR goggles; the patient is no longer able to override the nystagmus by using fixation. If a fixation light is turned on inside the goggles and the patient fixates on it, the nystagmus will diminish or stop during fixation. For chronic vestibular loss, nystagmus is usually not observable with or without fixation.

POSITIONAL VERTIGO ASSESSMENT/BENIGN PAROXYSMAL POSITIONAL VERTIGO

Prior to performing bedside tests of benign paroxysmal positional vertigo (BPPV) and the vestibular system, you should know the patient's active cervical ROM. Be aware of contraindications to testing, such as cervical ROM restrictions, recent cervical fractures, C1–C2 instability, history of aneurysm clipping, Arnold–Chiari malformation, vertebrobasilar insufficiency, new onset subarachnoid or subdural hematoma, presence of a ventriculoperitoneal (VP) shunt, cervical spondylosis, blood pressure >145/90,[37] or recent retinal detachment. If you believe you can safely perform testing/repositioning maneuvers with modifications, have a physician's approval and obtain a prescription for the maneuver.

Canals affected by BPPV are different, likely because of their anatomical positions. One study found the posterior semicircular canal was affected 88.4% of the time, whereas the lateral canal was affected 6.4%, and the superior canal was only affected 5.2%.[38]

Observing nystagmus during positioning tests can assist in determining if the patient has BPPV caused by displaced otoconia in the vestibular apparatus or centrally caused positioning nystagmus. As two of the semicircular canals are oriented vertically, you may use the modified Dix–Hallpike test to assess both as the same time, with the eye motion indicating which canal (anterior or posterior) is involved. As the lateral canal is situated ~30 degrees off the horizontal plane, a different test is needed to assess it, such as the roll test. Prior to vestibular testing or treatment, the integrity of the transverse and alar ligaments should be assessed. Also consider test modifications for other conditions. If the patient has a positive Sharp–Purser test, stop your examination, immobilize the patient's neck, and have them taken to the emergency department of a hospital for further assessment.

Factors predisposing patients to BPPV include inactivity, acute alcoholism, major surgeries, and central nervous system disease.[39]

🎥◀ MODIFIED DIX–HALLPIKE TEST

The modified Dix–Hallpike test is a gravity-driven test; however, if the patient progresses through the test too slowly, you will not likely see nystagmus. The test is "modified" from the originally described test due to the instructions and position of the examiner.

Modified Dix–Hallpike Instructions

1. Instruct the patient to long-sit on a bed or plinth.
2. Ask the patient to turn their head 45 degrees toward the side being tested as you tap the shoulder of the direction you wish the patient to turn their head. Instruct the patient that the head should remain turned as they lie back as quickly as possible, allowing their head to extend off the plinth by 30 degrees. Correct the head position as needed, but try to remain hands off as much as possible.
3. Hold the uppermost eyelid open using your thumb, if needed, and observe for nystagmus.
4. The patient should stay in the test position until 45 seconds have passed, nystagmus stops before 45 seconds, nystagmus continues more than 1 minute, or the patient cannot tolerate the test position.

Key things to remember:

- The clinician's hand placement is really a matter of personal preference and patient safety.
- The clinician may use Frenzel goggles or IR goggles if they choose.
- The head and face are very intimate areas for people; most do not like a stranger grabbing, twisting, and turning their heads. By limiting

how much you touch the patient's head and face, and by giving them more control over the test, the patient may be more comfortable and relaxed during the test. For example, we know that ultimately the patient's head is in 45 degrees of rotation to the testing side and extended 30 degrees. Many clinicians grab the patient's head and turn and extend it for them. However, aren't most patients capable of turning their own heads? Do they *really* need us to do that for them? The simple instruction to "turn your head halfway" while tapping the patient's shoulder on that side as a tactile cue will accomplish the goal of placing the patient's head in the correct position of rotation for testing.

- If needed, touch a patient's head only long enough to move it to the correct position and then ask the patient to maintain that position. When the patient moves into supine and naturally goes into cervical extension, then you may use one hand as a support and guide.
- When the patient returns to sitting, keep your hands off their head unless they need support.
- Make modifications to accommodate patients who are restricted from neck extension or rotation, or can't tolerate it. For example, clinicians in a hospital setting can use a tilt table or hospital bed to position the patient's head down 30 degrees (with the neck in neutral) instead of requiring cervical extension. In the home health or clinic setting, clinicians may have the patient move from sitting into a supine position without any cervical extension. In this position, you will likely still get a good response to elicit nystagmus, but without cervical extension; the likelihood of moving the crystals into a different canal during your test or treatment interventions increases. While this may necessitate more maneuvers, ultimately the clinician can still clear the canals of debris.
- If the patient cannot rotate their neck, position the head toward the side you wish to test while keeping the head and neck neutral by positioning/rotating the entire body *en bloc*. Remember, it is the position of the head with respect to the ground that is important. You can achieve the same positions of the head with respect to the ground by moving and turning the neck, by keeping the head and neck

neutral, and instead moving the entire body or using a combination of head rotation and body positioning.
- There is a side-lying version of the test if the patient cannot or does not wish to lie supine.

Dix–Hallpike Sensitivity

Published estimates of the Dix–Hallpike test's sensitivity range from 48% to 88%.[40]

Interpretation of the Modified Dix–Hallpike (mDH)

1. If nystagmus is observed after positioning, the test is positive.
2. If positive, while testing the left ear, the clinician will see torsion toward the stimulated ear (in most cases toward the ear being tested), and either an up- or downbeating.
3. Use Table 7.1 to interpret nystagmus after the mDH:

LATERAL CANAL TESTS

There are different BPPV tests of the lateral canal, such as the roll test, which detects BPPV, and the bow-and-lean test, which is useful to help lateralize the condition to help you determine which ear is involved once lateral canal involvement has been identified. When the patient has BPPV of a lateral canal, the test will be positive when each ear is tested, so we need to distinguish the quick-phase direction of the nystagmus to determine which ear is involved.

Before we discuss the test procedure, we need to learn some new terminology that will describe the nystagmus that occurs in lateral canal BPPV. When the patient is in the roll-test position, one ear will be toward the ground and the other toward the ceiling. Nystagmus seen during BPPV of the lateral canal beats laterally, with quick phases either beating toward the ground or away from it. We use the following names to describe this:

- *Geotropic*: Quick phases toward the ground (or earth).

Table 7.1 Interpretation of the Modified Dix–Hallpike

Side Being Tested	Torsion Noted and Direction	Vertical Beating Up/ Down?	Duration of Nystagmus	Interpretation
Left	Yes, left	Yes	<1 minute	• Left posterior canalithiasis for upbeating/torsional nystagmus • Left anterior canalithiasis for downbeating/torsional nystagmus*
Left	Yes, left	Yes	>1 minute	• Left posterior cupulolithiasis for upbeating/torsional nystagmus • Left anterior cupulolithiasis for downbeating/torsional nystagmus*
Left	Yes, left	No	Any	• Possible central sign
Left	No	Yes, any	Any	• Possible central sign
Right	Yes, right	Yes	<1 minute	• Right posterior canalithiasis for upbeating/torsional nystagmus • Right anterior canalithiasis for downbeating/torsional nystagmus*
Right	Yes, right	Yes	>1 minute	• Right posterior cupulolithiasis for upbeating/torsional nystagmus • Right anterior cupulolithiasis for downbeating/torsional nystagmus*
Right	Yes, right	No	Any	• Possible central sign
Right	No	Yes, any	Any	• Possible central sign

*As anterior canal BPPV is the least likely to occur, central pathology may also be considered.

 ◦ Remember, *geo* means "earth" (as in the word *geography*). This is theoretically a canalithiasis variant with loose crystals.
• *Apogeotropic*: Quick phases beating away from the ground.
 ◦ This is theoretically a cupulolithiasis variant with otoconia that are adhered to the cupula, or a canalith jam of otoconia that are trapped in the short arm (closer to the cupula) of the canal.

For lateral canal BPPV, the quick phases of the nystagmus of each ear should present in the same way. That is, if they are geotropic when the right side is being tested, they should *also* be geotropic on testing the left.

In cases of cupulolithiasis, the onset of nystagmus is immediate when the patient is placed into the test position, with nystagmus lasting a minute or longer. Geotropic BPPV (canalithiasis) is easier to correct using repositioning maneuvers. Geotropic nystagmus has quick phases that beat toward the *ground* and are *good* because the crystals are easy to fix. Remember: G=Ground=Good.

With apogeotropic nystagmus the crystals are either "stuck" on the cupula or otherwise trapped in the short arm of the canal. You will probably have to treat the patient more than once (*again* and *again*) and may feel that you want to *apologize* for the apogeotropic nystagmus. *Remember*: A=Away=Again and again.

Although *light cupula syndrome* is uncommon, it can resemble horizontal canal BPPV and should be taken into account. This syndrome presents with a constant sense of imbalance and positional vertigo that lasts >1 minute and is geotropic. It has no latency and is non-fatiguing. There is a null point when the head is rotated 20–30 degrees toward the affected ear where nystagmus subside.[41]

Roll Test (Pagnini–McClure Maneuver)

During the roll test, the patient's head is "rolled" into left rotation for 45 seconds, and the clinician assesses if the patient develops nystagmus. After a brief break, the patient's head is rolled into right rotation. Once again, the clinician assesses for nystagmus. The lateral canals are pitched approximately 30 degrees from the horizontal plane, so the Dix–Hallpike maneuver will not sufficiently place them in a position to be tested for loose crystals. Therefore, the clinician needs to place the head in a different position with respect to the ground, using the roll test to accomplish this. A few variations exist in performing this test. The first variation is the starting supine position, where some clinicians have the patient's neck in neutral, whereas other clinicians start with the patient in supine and neck flexed 30 degrees to better position the lateral canals perpendicular to the ground. Because the flexed position better places the lateral canals vertically, anatomically speaking, this should be ideal. However, studies have cited both methods and either method is valid. The other portion of the test that has variations is regarding how the clinician moves the patient from position to position during testing. Some advocate having the clinician move the passive patient's head into the test positions in rapid thrusting motions. Given that this is a gravity-driven test (that is, gravity is pulling the crystals), quick head-thrusting motions are not required. However, as in the mDH, if you move the patient too slowly, you may not see nystagmus. You may give the patient more control by asking them to briskly turn their head to one side as far as possible.

If the nystagmus are *apogeotropic* on one test, they should *also* be *apogeotropic* when testing the contralateral side. If nystagmus movements are *geotropic* on one test, they should *also* be *geotropic* when testing the contralateral side.

ROLL TEST INSTRUCTIONS

1. From a long-sitting position, the patient is assisted in slowly lying supine.

2. With the patient supine and the head in a neutral position (nose to ceiling), the patient is instructed to turn their head briskly to the left as far as possible. Ideally, the patient's head should be turned 90 degrees. If they are unable to turn the head this far, have them roll toward the test side until the head is nose-horizontal with the ground.
3. The clinician assesses the uppermost eye for nystagmus, noting direction of quick phases (geotropic or apogeotropic), holding the eyelid open with one thumb if needed.
4. After 30–45 seconds, the patient is instructed to turn the head briskly to the opposite side. (Again, nose-horizontal to the ground.)

Key things to remember:

- The position of the canal versus the ground is what is important. Not the position of the head versus the neck. If needed, keep the patient's head/neck in neutral and roll their entire body to position them nose-horizontal to the ground.
- For lateral canal BPPV, both ears should be tested, with nystagmus for each ear being either geotropic or apogeotropic.

INTERPRETATION OF THE ROLL TEST

1. *Each ear demonstrates geotropic nystagmus*: This indicates free-floating (loose) otoconia, with the ear demonstrating the stronger, more robust nystagmus as the involved ear. The nystagmus is typically brief.
2. *Each ear demonstrates apogeotropic nystagmus*: Otoconia are adhered to the cupula or a canalith jam of otoconia are trapped in the short arm (closer to the cupula) of the canal. The nystagmus movements are typically prolonged.
3. *Atypical presentation*: One ear demonstrates geotropic nystagmus, while the other demonstrates apogeotropic nystagmus. There is possibly the presence of otoconia particles of different sizes and densities in the same canal, with the larger ones trapped in the narrow area of the canal.[41]

4. Nystagmus movements that are geotropic but prolonged are atypical and possibly secondary to a migraine.[42]

Bow and Lean Test

The bow and lean test (also known as *Choung's test*) is useful when the patient presents with a lateral-canal BPPV and the involved side has not been determined. This test determines which ear is affected. When performing the roll test, it is sometimes difficult to determine which ear is involved. The bow and lean test helps you decide which side to treat. During the bow and lean test, you compare the direction of the quick-phase nystagmus when the patient is sitting and in a head bow (head flexion) or lean (head extension). As the patient bows and leans, the crystals will move either toward or away from the cupula of the affected ear. This migration of otoconia will activate nystagmus. Using the direction of the quick phases and the patient's test position, you can determine which ear is involved.

BOW AND LEAN TEST INSTRUCTIONS

Choung et al. described the bow and lean test to determine which ear is affected by horizontal canal BPPV.[43] The execution and interpretation of this test was modified by Marcelli to improve test tolerance (e.g., the patient does not need to bow 90 degrees) and is named the nystagmus intensity and direction bow and lean test (NID-BLT).[44]

1. Instruct the sitting patient to drop their chin (flex the head) ~30 degrees and find the null point (a position of forward head tilt where pseudo-spontaneous nystagmus or nystagmus generated by bow/lean disappears). This positions the lateral canals horizontal with the ground.
2. Next, bow the head 30 degrees from the null point. The patient should remain in this position for ~30 seconds while being observed for nystagmus.
3. Return the patient to an erect sitting (null position) and instruct 60 degrees extension of the head/neck. Hold the position for 30 seconds while observing for nystagmus.
4. Bow the head ~60 degrees once more and assess intensity again (Table 7.2).

Key things to remember:

- Nystagmus intensity[44] is used to interpret the type of BPPV (canalithiasis or cupulolithiasis):
  1. After locating the null point, more intense nystagmus in the bow position compared to the lean position is indicative of the geotropic form (canalithiasis).
  2. More intense nystagmus in the lean compared to the bow position is indicative of the apogeotropic form (cupulolithiasis).
- Nystagmus direction[44] is used to interpret which ear is involved:
  1. If canalithiasis, quick phases in the bow beat toward the affected ear.
  2. If cupulolithiasis, quick phases in the lean beat toward the affected ear.
- Frenzel or infrared goggles will assist the examination by removing fixation and making it easier for the clinician to see the eyes.

CENTRAL POSITIONAL VERTIGO

Signs associated with centrally caused positional vertigo include:[41,45,46]

Table 7.2 Interpretation of the Bow and Lean Test

	Bow Nystagmus Intensity	Bow Nystagmus Direction	Lean Nystagmus Intensity	Lean Nystagmus Direction
Canalithiasis	More intense brief nystagmus	Toward affected ear	Less intense	Away from affected ear
Cupulolithiasis	Less intense prolonged nystagmus	Away from affected ear	More intense prolonged nystagmus	Towards the affected ear

- Nystagmus without vertigo in positional maneuvers
- Atypical direction nystagmus (especially downbeating)
- Direction-changing nystagmus during positional tests
- Poor response to canalith repositioning maneuvers
- Recurrence on more than three occasions, confirmed by positional tests

REFERENCES

1. Lord SR, Dayhew J, Howland A. Multifocal glasses impair edge-contrast sensitivity and depth perception and increase the risk of falls in older people. *J Am Geriatr Soc.* Nov 2002;50(11):1760–1766. doi:10.1046/j.1532-5415.2002.50502.x
2. Lord SR, Smith ST, Menant JC. Vision and falls in older people: risk factors and intervention strategies. *Clin Geriat Med.* 1020;24(4):569–581. doi:10.1016/j.cger.2010.06.002. PMID: 20934611
3. Lemos J, Eggenberger E. Saccadic intrusions, review and update. *Curr Opin Neurol.* 2013;26(1):59–66. doi:10.1097/WCO.0b013e32835c5e1d
4. Kassavetis P, Kaski D, Anderson T, Hallett M. Eye movement disorders in movement disorders. *Movement Disorder Clin Pract.* 2022;9(3):284–595. doi:10.1002/mdc3.13413
5. Wong A. *Eye Movement Disorders.* Oxford University Press; 2008.
6. Borchert MS. Principles and techniques of the examination of ocular motility and alignment. *Walsh & Hoyt's Clinical Neuro-Ophthalmology.* 6th ed. Lippincott Williams & Wilkins; 2005:887–905.
7. Brandt T, Dieterich M, Strupp M. *Vertigo and Dizziness.* Springer; 2005.
8. Mayo clinic contributors. *Hyponatremia.* Mayo Clinic; 2024. https://www.mayoclinic.org/diseases-conditions/hyponatremia/symptoms-causes/syc-20373711
9. Abbas M. *Hypermetria: Causes and Effects of Neurological Movement Disorder.* Senioritis; 2023. https://senioritis.io/science/anatomy/hypermetria-causes-and-effects-of-neurological-movement-disorder/#:~:text=Hypermetria%20is%20a%20neurological%20condition%20characterized%20by%20an,disorders%20affecting%20the%20cerebellum%2C%20cerebrum%2C%20diencephalon%2C%20or%20brainstem.
10. Hain TC. Slow saccades. Dizziness-and-balance.com; 2023. https://dizziness-and-balance.com/practice/saccades/slow.html#:~:text=Table%20%3A%20Causes%20of%20slow%20saccades%201%20Drug,White%20matter%20diseases%20...%207%20Miscellaneous%20disorders%20
11. Walker H, Hall W, Hurst J editors. *Clinical Methods: The History, Physical, and Laboratory Examinations.* 3rd ed. Butterworths; 1990.
12. Kaur K, Gurnani B. *Exotropia.* StatPearls Publishing; Updated 2023. https://www.ncbi.nlm.nih.gov/books/NBK578185/
13. Cleveland clinic contributors. *Esotropia.* Cleveland Clinic; 2024. https://my.clevelandclinic.org/health/diseases/23145-esotropia
14. Christiano D. *What is hypertropia?* Healthline Media; 2024. https://www.healthline.com/health/eye-health/20-20-20-rule#outlook
15. Cleveland Clinic Contributors. *Hypertropia.* Cleveland Clinic; 2024. https://my.clevelandclinic.org/health/diseases/24307-hypertropia
16. Tamhankar MA, Kim JH, Ying GS, Volpe NJ. Adult hypertropia: a guide to diagnostic evaluation based on review of 300 patients. *Eye (Lond).* 2011;25(1):91–96. doi:10.1038/eye.2010.160
17. Rutner D, Kapoor N, Ciuffreda KJ, Shoshana C, Han ME, Suchoff I. Occurrence of ocular disease in traumatic brain injury in a selected sample: a retrospective analysis. *Brain Injury.* 2006;20(10):1079–1086. doi:10.1080/02699050600909904

18. Scheiman M, Gallaway M, Frantz KA, *et al.* Nearpoint of convergence: test procedure, target selection, and normative data. *Optometry Vision Sci.* 2003;80(3):214–225. doi:10.1097/00006324-200303000-00011

19. Hayes GJ, Cohen BE, Rouse MW, De Land PN. Normative values for the nearpoint of convergence of elementary schoolchildren. *Optom Vis Sci.* Jul 1998;75(7):506–512. doi:10.1097/00006324-199807000-00019

20. Kaur K, Gurnani B. *Contrast Sensitivity.* StatPearls Publishing; Updated 2023. https://www.ncbi.nlm.nih.gov/books/NBK580542/

21. Pasmanter N, Munakomi S. *Physiology, Color Perception.* StatPearls Publishing; Updated 2022. https://www.ncbi.nlm.nih.gov/books/NBK544355/

22. Schubert MC, Tusa RJ, Grine LE, Herdam SJ. Optimizing the sensitivity of the head thrust test for identifying vestibular hypofunction. *Phy Therapy Rehabilitat J.* 2004;84(2):151–158.

23. Laurens J, Angelaki DE. The functional significance of velocity storage and its dependence on gravity. *Exp Brain Res.* 2011;210(3–4):407–422. doi:10.1007/s00221-011-2568-4

24. Hain TC, Cherchi M. *Head Shaking Nystagmus.* Dizziness-and-balance.com; 2024. https://dizziness-and-balance.com/research/hsn/index.htm#:~:text=Head-shaking%20nystagmus%20in%20the%20horizontal%20and

25. Chen G, Zhang J, Qiao Q, *et al.* Advances in dynamic visual acuity test research. *Front Neurol.* 2023;13:1047876. doi:10.3389/fneur.2022.1047876

26. Cochrane GD, Christy JB, Kicker ET, Kailey RP, England BK. Inter-rater and test-retest reliability of computerized clinical vestibular tools. *J Vestibular Res.* 2021;31:365–373. doi:10.3233/VES-201522

27. Herdman SJ, Tusa RJ, Blatt P, Suzuki A, Venuto PJ, Roberts D. Computerized dynamic visual acuity test in the assessment of vestibular deficits. *Am J Otolaryngol.* 1998;19:790–796.

28. Rambold H, Deide W, Sprenger A, Haendler G, Helmchen C. Perilymph fistula associated with pulse-synchronous eye oscillations. *Neurology.* 2001;56:1769–1771.

29. Shuman AG, Rizvi SS, Pirouet CW, Heidenreich KD. Hennebert's sign in superior semicircular canal dehiscence syndrome: a video case report. *Laryngoscope.* 2012;122(2):412–414. doi:10.1002/lary.22413

30. Russell GE, Wick B, Tang RA. Arnold-Chiari malformation. *Optometry Vision Sci.* 1992;69:242–247.

31. Pstras L, Thomaseth K, Waniewski J, Balzani I, Bellavere F. The Valsalva manoeuvre: physiology and clinical examples. *Acta Physiol.* 2016;217(2):103–119. doi:10.1111/apha.12639

32. Junqueira LF Jr. Teaching cardiac autonomic function dynamics employing the Valsalva (Valsalva-Weber) maneuver. *Adv Physiol Edu.* 2008;32(1):100–106. doi:10.1152/advan.00057.2007

33. Hain TC. *Valsalva Maneuver for Dizziness.* Dizziness-and-balance.com; 2024. https://dizziness-and-balance.com/practice/valsalva.html

34. Thompson TL, Amedee R. Vertigo: a review of common peripheral and central vestibular disorders. *Oschsner J.* 2009;9(1):20–26.

35. Merchant S, Nadol J. *Schuknecht's Pathology of the Ear.* 3rd ed. McGraw-Hill Education; 2010.

36. Shepard N, Telian S. *Practical Management of the Balance Disorder Patient.* Singular Publishing Group; 1996.

37. Kelley K. *BPPV Background and Contraindications to Testing.* Physicaltherapy.com; 2024. https://www.physicaltherapy.com/ask-the-experts/bppv-background-and-contraindication-to-4261#:~:text=Contraindications%20to%20Testing%201%20OA%20instability%202%20History,7%20BP%20greater%20than%20145%2F90%208%20cervical%20spondylosis

38. Soto-Varela A, Santos-Perez S, Rossi-Izquierdo M, Sanchez-Sellero I. Are the three canals equally susceptible to

benign paroxysmal positional vertigo? *Audiol Neurootol*. 2013;18(5):327–334. doi:10.1159/000354649

39. Li JC. *Benign Paroxysmal Positional Vertigo Clinical Presentation*. Medscape; Updated 2024. https://emedicine.medscape.com/article/884261-clinical#b5?_gl=1*1csjx70*_gcl_au*MTA2NjE0OTc5Ny4xNzI5ODc4NjE2&form=fpf

40. Halker RB, Barris DM, Wellik KE, Wingerchuk DM, Demaerschalk BM. Establishing a diagnosis of benign paroxysmal positional vertigo through the dix-hallpike and side-lying maneuvers: a critically appraised topic. *Neurologist*. 2008;2008(3)(14):201–204. doi:10.1097/NRL.0b013e31816f2820

41. Carmona S, Zalazar GJ, Fernández M, Grinstein G, Lemos J. Atypical positional vertigo: definition, causes, and mechanisms. *Audiol Res*. 2022;12(2):152–161. doi:10.3390/audiolres12020018

42. American physical therapy association contributors. *Bow and Lean Test*. American Physical Therapy Association; 2024. https://www.apta.org/patient-care/evidence-based-practice-resources/test-measures/bow-and-lean-test

43. Choung YH, Shin YR, Kahng H, Park K, Choi SJ. 'Bow and lean test' to determine the affected ear of horizontal canal benign paroxysmal positional vertigo. *Laryngoscope*. 2006;116(10):1776–1781. doi:10.1097/01.mlg.0000231291.44818.be

44. Marcelli V. Nystagmus intensity and direction in bow and lean test: an aid to diagnosis of lateral semicircular canal benign paroxysmal positional vertigo. *Acta Otorhinolaryngol Italica*. 2016;36(6):520–526. doi:10.14639/0392-100X-795

45. Büttner U, Helmchen C, Brandt T. Diagnostic criteria for central versus peripheral positioning nystagmus and vertigo: A review. *Acta Otolaryngol*. 1999;119:1–5. doi:10.1080/00016489950181855

46. Soto-Varela A, Rossi-Izquierdo M, Sánchez-Sellero I, Santos-Pérez S. Revised criteria for suspicion of non-benign positional vertigo. *QJM*. 2013;106:317–321. doi:10.1093/qjmed/hct006

8

Examination of Somatosensory and Musculoskeletal Systems

Chapter Goals

1. Describe a somatosensory examination
2. Discuss muscle strength testing
3. Discuss joint range of motion testing

SOMATOSENSORY SYSTEM EXAMINATION

Somatosensation should be tested for every patient complaining of disequilibrium. Always explain the test and gain permission prior to beginning the examination. Before the examination, ask the patient whether they are experiencing abnormal sensations, numbness, or pain in any part of their body.[1] Since the somatosensory system is responsible for a variety of sensory inputs, many tests are possible. The somatosensory system includes sensations of different types of touch (light, fluttering, vibration, and coarse), temperature, pain, pressure, joint position (proprioception), and movement (kinesthesia). These sensations are carried to the brain via the dorsal column–medial lemniscus (DCML). During the examination, you should note any involuntary movements, fasciculations, tremors, and muscle wasting. Signs of DCML lesions include impaired sensations of soft touch, vibration,

proprioception, discrimination sense, and a positive Romberg test.[1]

When documenting sensation, you may use the following terminology:

Touch sensations[1]

- *Analgesia*: Numbness/loss of sensation
- *Hypoesthesia*: Decreased sensation reported during testing
- *Hyperesthesia*: Increased sensation reported during testing

Pain sensations (algesia)[1]

- *Analgesia*: Absence of pain appreciation
- *Hypoalgesia*: Decrease in pain appreciation
- *Hyperalgesia*: Exaggeration of pain appreciation

LIGHT TOUCH

To evaluate light touch, you may first do a quick screen by running your fingers along the face, neck, and limb dermatomes bilaterally, asking the patient if they feel the touch sensation equally. A more methodical examination is performed when the screen indicates diminished light touch sensations. For spinal cord injury, the trunk is also assessed. Use the ASIA examination for new spinal cord injuries (see Figure 8.1).

DOI: 10.1201/9781003524441-8

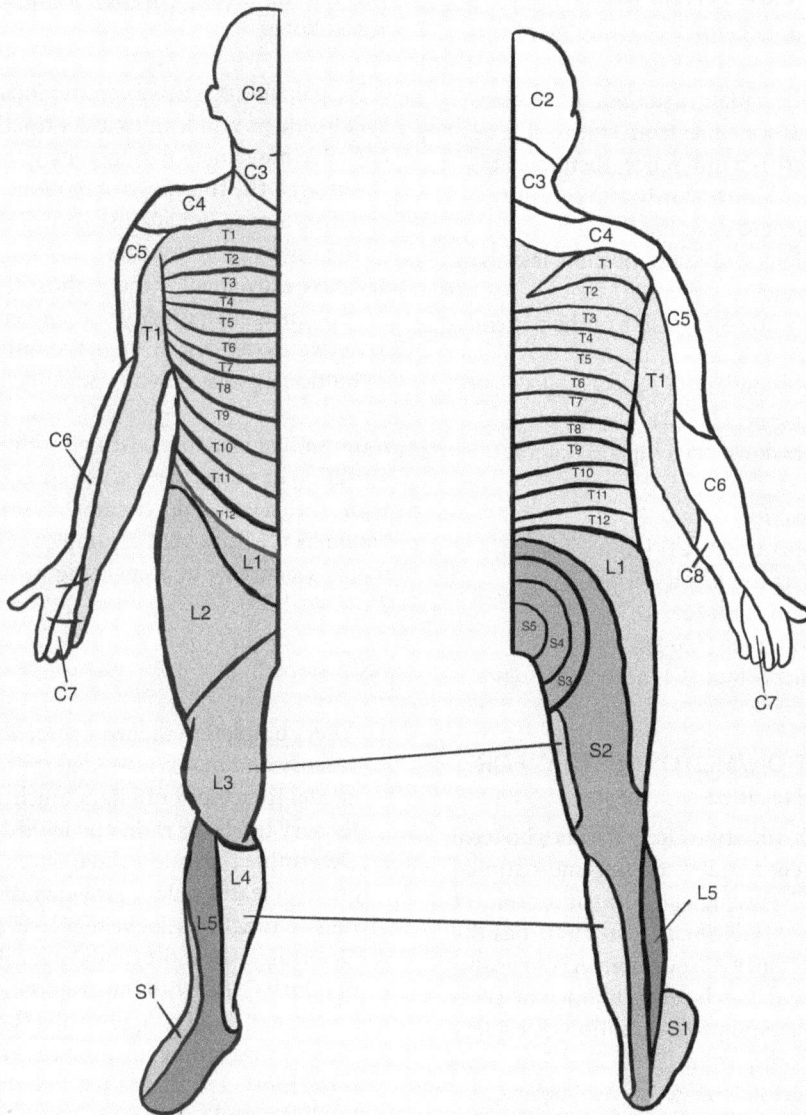

Figure 8.1 Dermatome Map

Light Touch Examination Instructions

FACE

1. The patient is seated.
2. The examiner may use a finger or cotton swab to touch both sides of the patient's forehead (V1), cheeks (V2), and chin simultaneously, asking the patient if sensations are equal bilaterally. This tests the three divisions of the trigeminal nerve.

3. If the patient indicates a presence of diminished sensations, more slowly and deliberately check each dermatome.
4. You may wish to check for gross sensation or have the patient close their eyes and report where they feel being touched by the examiner. This is also a good way to make sure that the patient is not inaccurately reporting intact sensation.

LIGHT TOUCH: REST OF THE BODY

1. The patient is seated with their eyes kept closed.
2. As you touch the patient, ask them to indicate if the sensations are equal from side to side or different. If there is a difference, then repeat the dermatome(s) more slowly and carefully, asking the patient to describe the difference. Are the sensations more than normal, less than normal, or absent?
3. Run two fingers down each side of the patient's neck (C3–C4).
4. Run two fingers down each arm (radial aspect C5–C6, ulnar aspect C8–T1).
5. Run two fingers down each hip/LE (lateral aspect):
   a. Lateral hips (L1)
   b. Lateral upper thigh (L1–L2)
   c. Lateral lower thigh/knee (L2–L3)
   d. Lateral calf (L5, S1, S2)
   e. Anterior lower leg (L3–L4)
   f. Anterior ankle/foot (L4–L5)

TOUCH SENSATION/MOTOR TESTING FOR SPINAL CORD INJURIES

To examine touch sensations for patients who have suffered a spinal cord injury, use the International Standards for Neurological Classification of Spinal Cord Injury (ISNCSCI), also known as the American Spinal Injury Association (ASIA) examination. This test assesses both light touch to a cotton swab as well as a pinprick sensation of a safety pin to 28 dermatomes from C2 to S4–S5 on each side. The worksheet for this test is available at asia-spinalinjury.org.[2]

Key sensory points for this test are available in diagrams by the ASIA (asia-spinalinjury.org) (also see Table 8.1).[3]

The ASIA exam also tests motor function of the key muscles listed in Table 8.2 (also see Figure 8.2).

The scoring method for dermatomes is as follows:

0: Absent sensation to the dermatome
1: Altered sensation when compared with the face (reference point)
2: Normal sensation (same as the face)

The scoring method for motor scores (myotomes) is as follows:

0: No palpable or visible contraction of muscle
1: Palpable or visible muscle contraction
2: Active movement with gravity eliminated through the full range of motion
3: Active movement against gravity throughout the full range of motion
4: Active movement through the full range of motion against gravity and moderate resistance
5: Active movement through the full range of motion against gravity and sufficient resistance

If the patient has a preexisting condition impairing sensation or motor scores, use an asterisk (*) along with the score. For example, sensation testing would be 0*, 1*, or NT*. Examples of motor testing scores secondary to preexisting conditions: 0*, 1*, 2*, 3*, 4*, NT*.

ASIA steps:[4]

1. After completing the worksheet with all the sensory and motor tests, determine the most caudal intact for both light touch and pinprick sensory levels for right and left sides.
2. Determine the most caudal motor levels that are of at least grade 3, provided that all key muscle functions above that level are grade 5.
3. Determine the most caudal neurological level of injury (NLI) with intact sensation (grade 2) and motor score of 3, provided there is normal sensory and motor function rostrally. The NLI is the most cephalad of sensory and motor levels determined in steps 1 and 2.
4. Anal sensation/motor function determines if the injury is complete or incomplete. "The examiner inserts a finger into the patient's rectum and asks them to squeeze like they are holding in a bowl movement." If the patient has voluntary muscle contraction, the injury is "incomplete." Make sure to differentiate between voluntary and reflex contractions. If the patient consistently perceives pressure on the anal wall from the examiner's finger, the patient has a "sensory incomplete" injury. If the patient had pinprick sensation at S4–S5 dermatome levels, anal pressure does not need to be

Table 8.1 Key ASIA Exam Sensory Points

Dermatome	Key Sensory Point
C2	At least 1 cm lateral to the occipital protuberance at the base of the skull; or at least 3 cm behind the ear
C3	In the supraclavicular fossa, at the midclavicular line
C4	Over the acromioclavicular joint
C5	On the lateral (radial) side of the antecubital fossa, just proximal to the elbow
C6	On the dorsal surface of the proximal phalanx of the thumb
C7	On the dorsal surface of the proximal phalanx of the middle finger
C8	On the dorsal surface of the proximal phalanx of the little finger
T1	On the medial (ulnar) side of the antecubital fossa, just proximal to the medial epicondyle of the humerus
T2	At the apex of the axilla
T3	At the midclavicular line and the third intercostal space, found by palpating the anterior chest to locate the third rib and the corresponding third intercostal space below it
T4	At the midclavicular line and the fourth intercostal space, located at the level of the nipples
T5	At the midclavicular line and the fifth intercostal space, located midway between the level of the nipples and the level of the xiphisternum
T6	At the midclavicular line, located at the level of the xiphisternum
T7	At the midclavicular line, one-quarter the distance between the level of the xiphisternum and the level of the umbilicus
T8	At the midclavicular line, one-half the distance between the level of the xiphisternum and the level of the umbilicus
T9	At the midclavicular line, three-quarters of the distance between the level of the xiphisternum and the level of the umbilicus
T10	At the midclavicular line, located at the level of the umbilicus
T11	At the midclavicular line, midway between the level of the umbilicus and the inguinal ligament
T12	At the midclavicular line, over the midpoint of the inguinal ligament
L1	Midway between the key sensory points for T12 and L2
L2	On the anterior–medial thigh, at the midpoint drawn on an imaginary line connecting the midpoint of the inguinal ligament and the medial femoral condyle
L3	At the medial femoral condyle above the knee
L4	Over the medial malleolus
L5	On the dorsum of the foot at the third metatarsal phalangeal joint
S1	On the lateral aspect of the calcaneus
S2	At the midpoint of the popliteal fossa
S3	Over the ischial tuberosity or infragluteal fold (depending on the patient, their skin can move up, down, or laterally over the ischii)
S4/5	In the perianal area, less than 1 cm lateral to the mucocutaneous junction

Table 8.2 ASIA Exam Myotome Testing

Myotome	Description
C5	Elbow flexors
C6	Wrist extensors
C7	Elbow extensors
C8	Finger flexors
T1	Finger abductors (little finger)
L2	Hip flexors
L3	Knee extensors
L4	Ankle dorsiflexors
L5	Long toe extensors
S2	Ankle plantar flexors
S3–S4	External anal sphincter (determines complete vs. incomplete SCI)

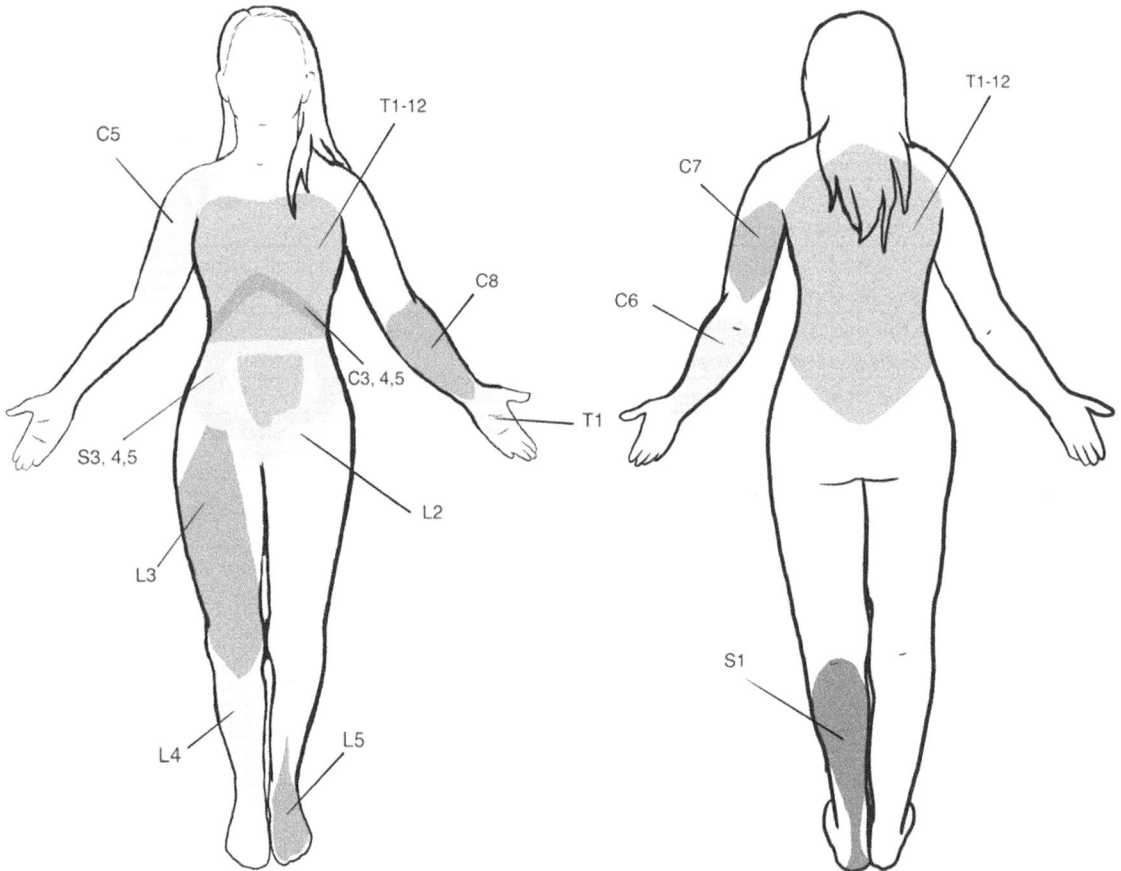

FIGURE 8.2 Myotome Map

assessed, but the examiner still needs to assess the motor component.

5. Determine the ASIA Impairment Scale grade.

Semmes–Weinstein Monofilament Test

The Semmes–Weinstein monofilament test requires the purchase of monofilaments (2.83–6.65), which are similar to a piece of fishing line, to test light touch and pressure sensations of the foot. This test is frequently used for diabetic patients who are at risk of foot ulcers. Test sites over the bare plantar surface of the first, third, and fifth metatarsal heads; medial and lateral sides of the arch and heel; and plantar surface of the big toe (toe pad).[1]

Semmes–Weinstein Monofilament Test Instructions

1. The patient should be supine (for ease of access to plantar feet).
2. Demonstrate the monofilament on your hand first, and then the upper arm of the patient.
3. Instruct the patient to say yes when they feel the pressure/touch of the monofilament.
4. With the patient's eyes closed, push the monofilament onto the test sites until it bends, and hold for 1–2 seconds, then remove the contact. If the patient does not respond, repeat the test over the same site, reminding them that they should say yes when they feel the touch/pressure of the monofilament.

Key things to remember:

- Avoid areas of callus or thickened skin when testing pressure sensations.
- Do not ask the patient, "Did you feel that?" when testing.

Interpretation of the Semmes–Weinstein Monofilament Test

- The inability to sense 3.84 monofilament (equal to 0.6 g of linear force) indicates "diminished light touch."
- The inability to sense monofilaments of ≥4.17 monofilaments (equal to 1.0 g of linear force) is consistent with neuropathy.

- The inability to sense 4.56 monofilaments (equal to 4 g of linear force) indicates "diminished protective sensation."
- The inability to sense a 5.07 monofilament (equal to 10 g of linear force) is consistent with severe neuropathy and loss of protective sensation.[1]

VIBRATION SENSATION TESTING

Use a standard 128 Hz tuning fork to produce the vibration stimulus.[5] Test distally to proximally. If vibration is not sensed at distal joints, test proximally over bony prominences until it is perceived. Bilateral test sites include the big toes, metatarsal heads, malleoli, tibia, anterior superior iliac spine, sacrum, spinous processes of the vertebrae, sternum, clavicle, styloid processes of the radius and ulna, and finger joints.[6]

Instructions for Vibration Sense Testing

1. Patient is supine.
2. Testing proceeds from distal sites to proximal ones.
3. Place the struck tuning fork 90 degrees to the surface of the bony prominence and hold there until the patient no longer feels the vibration.
4. Document all sites tested, and those where the patient cannot sense vibration or has diminished vibration.

Interpretation of Vibration Sense Testing

If you wish to conduct a quantitative vibration sense test, you need to purchase a Rydel–Seiffer tuning fork that can discriminate various vibration intensities.

WEBER TWO-POINT DISCRIMINATION (STATIC) TEST

To perform this test, you will need to obtain a circular two-point discriminator or a baseline aesthesiometer. Testing whether the patient can identify two close points in a small skin area

Table 8.3 Weber Two-Point Discrimination Test Norms

Weber Two-Point Discrimination (Static) Test (Sharp Point)	Mean Normal Discrimination (in Millimeters)	
Test Site	Men	Women
Forehead	13.3	10.8
Cheek	10.4	9.3
Upper lip	2.9	2.8
Tongue tip	2.0	1.9
Index finger	2.1	1.9

simultaneously, the Weber two-point discrimination (static) test can measure how fine the patient's ability is to discriminate.[6]

Weber Two-Point Discrimination (Static) Test Instructions

1. With the patient's eyes closed, randomly touch test sites with one or two points, avoiding pressing on the caliper and increasing the delivered pressure.
2. Instruct the patient to indicate if they feel one or two points.

Key things to remember:

- When applying two points, they should be in a longitudinal direction (perpendicular to the long axis of the fingers).
- The hand must be immobile on a hard surface.

Weber Two-Point Discrimination (Static) Test Interpretation

The minimal distance the patient can distinguish between two stimuli is called the *two-point threshold*.

Testing points and the smallest "normal" distance that should be perceived are as listed in Table 8.3.[7]

PROPRIOCEPTION AND KINESTHESIA

Proprioception is the ability to use somatosensory input using the following mechanoreceptors:

Merkel discs, Ruffini endings, Meissner corpuscles, muscle spindles, and Golgi tendon organs to know joint positions.[8] We use proprioception (as well as kinesthesia that detects joint motion) to help us determine whether we are swaying while standing. This allows us to correct body position around the ankle joint. In the following, two methods are reviewed: threshold to detect passive movement and joint position reproduction (aka joint position matching). Even though these tests are widely used, existing tests of thresholds to detect passive motion lack evidence for reliability, validity, and responsiveness.[9]

Threshold to Detect Passive Movement (TTDPM)

TTDPM determines if the patient can sense the movement and direction of a limb/joint.

TTDPM INSTRUCTIONS

1. The patient is seated and instructed to close their eyes.
2. The joint being tested is moved in one direction.
3. Instruct the patient to indicate *when they first detect* passive movement of the joint and the direction (up/down).
4. The clinician records either the time taken to report the limb movement or the degrees moved prior to the patient's report of movement. They also record the direction of movement and the patient's report of direction.
5. If the patient incorrectly reports the direction, attempt up to three trials.

Joint Position Reproduction (JPR) or Joint Matching

There are two methods of testing joint position matching: ipsilateral matching and contralateral matching.

IPSILATERAL MATCHING INSTRUCTIONS

1. The patient is sitting and instructed to close their eyes.
2. The clinician passively moves a limb to the desired joint-angle test position and returns it to the starting point.

3. Instruct the patient to actively move the same limb to the same joint-angle test position.

CONTRALATERAL MATCHING INSTRUCTIONS

1. The patient is sitting and instructed to close their eyes.
2. The clinician passively moves one limb to a desired joint-angle test position.
3. Instruct the patient to actively move the contralateral limb to the same joint angle.

Key things to remember:

• You should do this a number of times on the same limb, each time choosing a different joint position.
• Repeat the test on the contralateral limb.

JPR TEST INTERPRETATION

The difference between the two joint positions indicates the patient's proprioceptive acuity.

ROMBERG TEST (A TEST OF THE POSTERIOR COLUMN)

The Romberg test assesses balance under two conditions: standing on a firm surface with eyes open and with eyes closed. According to Forbes et al., "Often the Romberg test can be confused as a sign of cerebellar disease, but this test demonstrates the effects of posterior column disease."[10] When positive, the findings are referred to as a Romberg sign and occur due to:[10]

• Loss of proprioception for those with myelopathies and sensory neuropathies
• Uncompensated vestibular dysfunction
• Anterior vermis and paravermis pathology of the anterior cerebellar lobe[11]

Romberg Instructions

1. Instruct the patient to remove their shoes and stand with feet together.
2. Next, instruct the patient to either cross their arms across their chest or hold them next to the body for 1 minute.

3. The patient is instructed to close their eyes and stand in the same position (feet together, arms next to or crossed over the body).

Interpretation of the Romberg Test

The test is deemed positive when a patient cannot stand on a firm surface with their eyes closed and arms next to (or crossed) the body.

Key things to remember:

• You can increase the sensitivity of the test by having the patient stand heel-to-toe (called a sharpened Romberg test) or stand on foam.[10]

MODIFIED CLINICAL TEST OF SENSORY INTERACTION AND BALANCE (mCTSIB)

The mCTSIB assesses the patient's balance under four different conditions: eyes open, eyes closed, standing on a firm surface, and standing on a compliant foam surface. The mCTSIB was "modified" from the original Clinical Test of Sensory Interaction and Balance,[12] which had six conditions. In this original study, the authors found that all subjects could stand under the "eyes open and closed on a firm surface" conditions for 30 seconds. They suggest that standing on foam (eyes open and closed) for at least 20 seconds is within normal limits for older subjects.[12] Another study similarly found that "with eyes closed, on foam, some significant differences were found between patients and controls, especially for subjects older than 59 years."[13]

Under each condition, our brain gives weight (importance) to the systems that are giving us information used for balance (vision, vestibular, somatosensory) differently. According to one author:

> The contributions of the somatosensory, vestibular, and visual systems on balance control are not given the same weight under different sensory situations.[14,15] For example, on firm surfaces, balance is somatosensory feedback is given more weight by the cerebellum,

with vestibular and visual inputs also playing important roles. In contrast, when standing on surfaces that are complaint (such as thick carpet or grass), the system prioritizes vestibular input and relies more on visual cues, while the contribution from somatosensory signals is reduced. Often in research and academia, 70% somatosensory–20% vestibular–10% visual scheme is listed as the contribution to balance under normal conditions. Unfortunately, this is highly oversimplified, and these exact values have not been discovered in any research.[16]

The mCTSIB can help you figure out if a patient has weighted these sensory inputs correctly or perhaps give a clue to systems that are not functioning properly.

The mCTSIB is basically a Romberg test on a firm surface and also on foam. The patient is timed for 30 seconds under each condition with feet together and arms either by their sides or crossed. The timer is stopped if the patient opens their eyes (while testing in a closed position), moves their arms, or loses balance. Sway may be rated using the following rating method:

1: Minimal sway
2: Mild sway
3: Moderate sway
4: Fall

Whitney and Wrisley found the mCTSIB could be performed with or without shoes.[17] When choosing a foam pad, the Airex™ and Neurocom™ foam pads led to the accurate identification of fallers among older persons.[18]

mCTSIB Interpretation

Longer stance times up to 30 seconds for each of the four conditions (or up to a total of 120 seconds for a combined score) are interpreted as "better balance and sensory integration," while shorter durations indicate potential deficits. You may also take the mean value of the sway scores and track improvement.

Another way to use information gained from the mCTSIB is to look at the conditions under which patients are struggling to balance. If a patient cannot stand 30 seconds on a firm surface with their eyes open, then they likely need an assistive device. If someone cannot stand on a firm surface with eyes closed, then they likely will also have difficulty balancing in low-lighted environments. If they cannot stand for 30 seconds on foam with their eyes open, then they will likely also have difficulty while standing on other soft, compliant surfaces such as thick carpet or grass, or standing on gravel that may also shift under their feet. A clinician may use this information to plan intervention strategies.

MUSCLE STRENGTH TESTING

There are several methods available to test muscle strength including the following:

- Handheld dynamometry
  - Measures peak strength and rate of torque development (RTD)[19]
  - Good reliability
- Isometric dynamometry
  - Measures torque exerted by muscle groups on the static skeleton in a single plane[20]
  - *Examples*: Handheld dynamometry, fixed dynamometry, sphygmomanometry
  - Sensitive for all muscle grades
  - Good reliability
- Isokinetic dynamometry
  - Measures maximal force production against constant speed
  - *Examples*: Biodex®, Cybex®
  - Not recommended for strength below 3/5
  - Good reliability
- Isotonic testing
  - Tests muscle strength against constant load, but velocity may vary
  - *Examples*: Free weights
  - May be more applicable to evaluations in sports science, rehabilitation medicine, and human factors engineering[21]
- Manual muscle testing
  - Most commonly used method to evaluate strength

- Reliability ranges from poor to good
- Uses a rating scale from 0 to 5:[22]
  - 0: No muscle activation
  - 1: Trace muscle activation, such as a twitch, without achieving full range of motion
  - 2: Muscle activation with gravity eliminated, achieving full range of motion
  - 3: Muscle activation against gravity, full range of motion
  - 4: Muscle activation against some resistance, full range of motion
  - 5: Muscle activation against examiner's full resistance, full range of motion

There are different types of manual muscle tests, including the following:

- *Break test (passive strength)*: Gradual resistance is applied at the end of the tested range.
- *Make test (active strength)*: Similar to maximum voluntary isometric contraction, the examiner acts as a fixed point against which the patient pushes. It may be graded on the 0–5 scale or by using a handheld dynamometer to measure peak force.[23]

RANGE OF MOTION (ROM)

The measurement of joint angles is called *goniometry*. The tools used to measure the joint angles are called goniometers, and there are a couple different types.

- The goniometer[24]
  - Consists of either a half circle (180 degrees) or full circle (360 degrees), called the body, with degrees marked along the circle. A stationary arm is attached to the body. A moving arm is attached to the center of the goniometer body (fulcrum). This moving arm aligns with the moving limb or segment.
  - Measures flexion, extension, abduction, adduction, and rotation.
  - Long-armed goniometers are used to measure long bone joints, while short-arm goniometers measure shorter joint ranges.

- The bubble inclinometer[24]
  - Has a fluid-filled 360-degree rotating dial and scale with degrees marked along the dial edge. The dial has a visible bubble inside that indicates the angular position of the targeted body part and the ROM as it moves.
  - Measures flexion, extension, abduction, adduction, and rotation.
  - A tape measure may be used to identify lumbar ROM if an inclinometer is not available (measuring fingertips to floor with a standing and flexed patient).

REFERENCES

1. Khoo YH, Abdullah JM, Idris Z, Ghani ARI, Halim SA. Dorsal column bedside examination test: tips for the neurosurgical resident. *Malaysian Journal of Medical Sciences*. 2023;30(2):172–179. doi:10.21315/mjms2023.30.2.16
2. Rupp R, Biering-Sørensen F, Burns SP, Graves DE, Guest J, Jones L, Schmidt Read M, Rodriguez GM, Schuld C, Tansey KE, Walden K, Kirshblum S. International standards for neurological classification of spinal cord injury. *Topics in Spinal Cord Injury Rehabilitation: Revised 2019*. 2021;27(2):1–22. doi:10.46292/sci2702-1
3. American Spinal Cord Association Contributors. *ISNCSCI Resources: Key Sensory Points*. American Spinal Cord Association; 2024. https://asia-spinalinjury.org/wp-content/uploads/2016/02/Key_Sensory_Points.pdf
4. Yu T, PM, Mendelson S, Wilhelm M. Neurological examination and classification of SCI. *PM&R: The Journal of Injury, Function and Rehabilitation*. 2024. https://now.aapmr.org/neurological-examination-and-classification-of-sci/#:~:text=The%20ISNCSCI%20exam%2C%20also%20known%20as%20the%20ASIA,sensation%20compose%20the%20sensory%20portion%20of%20the%20examination.
5. Prabhakar AT, Suresh T, Kurian DS, Mathew V, Shaik AIA, Aaron S, Sivadasan A, Benjamin RN, Alexander M. Timed vibration

sense and joint position sense testing in the diagnosis of distal sensory polyneuropathy. *Journal of Neurosciences in Rural Practice.* 2019;10(2):273–277. doi:10.4103/jnrp.jnrp_241_18

6. Campbell WW, Barohn RJ. *DeJong's the Neurologic Examination.* 8th ed. Wolters Kluwer; 2020.

7. Won SY, Kim HK , Kim ME, Kim KS. Two-point discrimination values vary depending on test site, sex and test modality in the orofacial region: a preliminary study. *Journal of Applied Oral Science.* 2017;4:427–435. doi:10.1590/1678-7757-2016-0462

8. Gadhvi M, Moore MJ, Waseem M. *Physiology, Sensory System.* StatPearls Publishing; Updated 2023. https://www.ncbi.nlm.nih.gov/books/NBK547656/

9. Strong A, Arumugam A , Tengman E, Röijezon U, Häger CK. Properties of tests for knee joint threshold to detect passive motion following anterior cruciate ligament injury: a systematic review and meta-analysis. *Journal of Orthopaedic Surgery and Research.* 2022;17(1):134. doi:10.1186/s13018-022-03033-4

10. Forbes J, Munakomi S , Cronovich H. *Romberg Test.* StatPearls Publishing; Updated 2023. doi:https://www.ncbi.nlm.nih.gov/books/NBK563187/

11. Lanska DJ, Goetz CG. Romberg's sign: development, adoption, and adaptation in the 19th century. *Neurology.* 2000;55(8):1201–1206. doi:10.1212/wnl.55.8.1201

12. Cohen H, Blatchly CA, Gombash LL. A study of the clinical test of sensory interaction and balance. *Physical Therapy.* Jun 1993;73(6):346–351; discussion 351–354. doi:10.1093/ptj/73.6.346

13. Cohen HS, Mulavara AP, Peters BT, Sangi-Haghpeykar H, Bloomberg JJ. Standing balance tests for screening people with vestibular impairments. *Laryngoscope.* Feb 2014;124(2):545–550.

14. Peterka RJ. Sensorimotor integration in human postural control. *Journal of Neurophysiology.* Sep 2002;88(3):1097–1118. doi:10.1152/jn.2002.88.3.1097

15. Peterka RJ, Loughlin PJ. Dynamic regulation of sensorimotor integration in human postural control. *Journal of Neurophysiology.* Jan 2004;91(1):410–423. doi:10.1152/jn.00516.2003

16. Pritt B. *Modified Clinical Test of Sensory Interaction in Balance (CTSIB-M).* Science of Falling: 2025. Accessed March 3, 2025. https://scienceoffalling.com/articles/modified-clinical-test-of-sensory-interaction-in-balance%20trials%20of%20that%20condition

17. Whitney SL, Wrisley D. The influence of footwear on timed balance scores of the modified clinical test of sensory interaction and balance. *Archives of Physical Medicine and Rehabilitation.* 2004;85(3):439–443. doi:10.1016/j.apmr.2003.05.005

18. Boonsinsukh R, Khumnonchai B, Saengsirisuwan V, Chaikeeree N. The effect of the type of foam pad used in the modified Clinical Test of Sensory Interaction and Balance (mCTSIB) on the accuracy in identifying older adults with fall history. *Hong Kong Physiotherapy Journal.* Dec 2020;40(2):133–143. doi:10.1142/s1013702520500134

19. Lesnak J, AD, Farmer B, Katsavelis D, Grindstaff TL,. Validity of hand-held dynamometry in measuring quadriceps strength and rate of torque development. *International Journal of Sports Physical Therapy.* 2019;14(2):180–487.

20. O'Leary SP, VB, Jull GA,. A new method of isometric dynamometry for the craniocervical flexor muscles. *Physical Therapy.* 2005;85(6):556–564. doi:10.1093/ptj/85.6.556

21. Xu HQ, XY, Zhou ZJ, Koh KT, Xu X, Shi JP, Zhang SW, Zhang X, Cai J,. Xu HQ, Xue YT, Zhou ZJ, Koh KT, Xu X, Shi JP, Zhang SW, Zhang X, Cai J. Retentive capacity of power output and linear versus non-linear mapping of power loss in the isotonic muscular endurance test *Scientific Reports.* 2021;11(1):22677. doi:10.1038/s41598-021-02116-2

22. Naqvi U, SA. *Muscle Strength Grading.* StatPearls Publishing; Updated 2023. https://www.ncbi.nlm.nih.gov/books/NBK436008/

23. Conable KM, RA. A narrative review of manual muscle testing and implications for muscle testing research. *Journal of Chiropractic Medicine.* 2011;10(3):157–165. doi:10.1016/j.jcm.2011.04.001

24. Shultz S, HP, Perrin D,. *Examination of Musculoskeletal Injuries.* 4th ed. Human Kinetics; 2015.

9

Neurologic Bedside Examination

Chapter Goals

1. Describe the HINTS examination
2. List cerebellar tests
3. Discuss muscle tone
4. Explain deep tendon reflex testing
5. Discuss other corticospinal tract tests
6. List tests of memory and cognition
7. Explain functional tests linked to cognition

While neurologic signs may be present in oculomotor and vestibular testing, this chapter will explain neurologic-specific bedside tests, as well as cardiovascular examinations.

HINTS EXAMINATION

The HINTS exam is a group of three tests that, when the results of each are analyzed, are used to assist in the differential diagnosis of stroke versus a peripheral vestibular disorder (Table 9.1).

INTERPRETATION OF THE HINTS PROTOCOL

- If the head impulse test is positive (in one direction), this is a likely indicator of a peripheral vestibular issue. If it is positive bilaterally, this is a possible central sign.
- If there are nystagmus present, you need to determine:
  1. Is the nystagmus present at rest? If they are new, present at rest, and not congenital, this indicates an acute condition.
  2. Does the nystagmus only beat in one direction with gazes? If they do, the cause may be central or peripheral; however, in most cases it is peripheral. If the quick phases of the nystagmus changes direction with the direction of gaze, or are vertical, this indicates a central pathology.
  3. Are there any *vertical* skew deviations with the alternating cover test (test of skew)? If there are, this indicates a central pathology. Keep in mind that many people have exophorias (when the eye is uncovered, the eye moves laterally toward the target). This is not considered an important central finding for most patients.

Even if the patient has a positive head impulse test, if the patient has either direction-changing nystagmus or a vertical skew, refer them for an MRI. Although not discussed in the original author's article regarding the HINTS exam, if the patient has a positive bilateral head impulse test, refer them for an MRI.

The HINTS+ (HINTS plus) protocol adds screening for the detection of sound (rubbing your fingers next to each of the patient's ears). If the patient has a decreased or new hearing loss, it may indicate either peripheral labyrinthitis or a

DOI: 10.1201/9781003524441-9

Table 9.1 HINTS Test Explanation

	HINTS Meaning	Test Used	Indications of a Positive Test
HI	Head impulse	Head impulse test	A catch-up saccade
N	Nystagmus	Oculomotor ROM test	• Unidirectional gaze nystagmus may be central or peripheral • Direction-changing nystagmus is a central finding
TS	Test of skew	Alternating cover test	Hypo- or hypertropia or phoria, indicating possible central finding

Note: Nystagmus is discussed in Chapter 3; and the head impulse test, alternate cover test (a test of skew), and ocular ROM test are discussed in Chapter 7.

Table 9.2 HINTS Test Interpretations

HINTS	Result 1	Result 2	Result 3	Result 4	Result 5
Head impulse (aka head thrust)	Negative	Negative	Negative	Positive (1 ear)	Positive bilaterally
Direction-changing nystagmus	Positive	Negative	Positive	Negative	Negative
Tests of skew (alternate cover test)	Negative	Positive	Positive	Negative	Negative
Suspected finding	Stroke	Stroke	Stroke	Peripheral (infection)	Possible central finding

stroke. Remember, acute bilateral vestibular loss is rare and typically found after aminoglycoside toxicity, following cisplatin chemotherapy, with autoimmune ear diseases, later stages of Ménière's disease, and meningitis.[1] It is also a sign of a large unilateral cerebellopontine angle tumor.[2]

Table 9.2 may be read in columns and is a visual representation of possible HINTS outcomes.

NYSTAGMUS

Pathologic nystagmus may be caused by peripheral vestibular or central deficits. Following is a list of nystagmus caused by central deficits:[3,4]

• *Epileptic nystagmus*
• *Rebound nystagmus* caused by cerebellar deficits,[5] pontine lesions, or congenital defects. To be considered rebound nystagmus, the eyes must reverse direction from both left and right sides following gaze holding[6]
• *See-saw nystagmus* caused by lesions in the mesodiencephalic junction, optic chiasm

lesions, thalamic lesions, lower brainstem lesions, congenital anomalies, and multiple sclerosis
• *Spontaneous nystagmus*
• *Central vestibular nystagmus* (downbeat, upbeat, torsional, or horizontal) caused by vestibulocerebellar or vestibular pathway conditions (degeneration, stroke, congenital, multiple sclerosis, and drugs [e.g., lithium and anticonvulsants, alcohol])
• *Vertical nystagmus* caused by posterior fossa lesions, medication side effects, vitamin deficiencies, inflammatory and autoimmune/paraneoplastic conditions, hereditary/degenerative cerebellar ataxias

CEREBELLAR TESTS

The cerebellum assists us with coordinated and accurate movements for balance, functional movements, eye movements, and speech. Screening tests of the cerebellum include accuracy and coordination of limb movements, clear speech, assessment of eye motions and nystagmus (see Chapter 7), deep tendon reflexes (DTRs), tests of rebound, balance, and gait. When assessing a patient complaining of dizziness or disequilibrium, testing the cerebellum is a priority. There are many different screening tests, and you will not be able to do them all. However, most take very little time. When testing limbs, you should try to include both upper and lower extremities. Positive tests indicate cerebellar dysfunction. Each test is first demonstrated by the clinician.

COORDINATION/ACCURACY TESTS

There are many tests of coordination to assess the cerebellum. When a lack of coordinated movement is observed, it is recorded as *dysmetria* for the limb being tested. Intention tremors are also a sign of cerebellar dysfunction and occur when a patient's hand/finger gets closer to the target that they are attempting to touch. It is a course, low-frequency tremor. This tremor does not occur throughout the entire movement, as this would be named an intention tremor (*action tremor*), but occurs as the hand/finger approaches the target. Dysmetria and intention tremor are both suggestive of ipsilateral cerebellar pathology.

Upper Extremity Tests

FINGER-TO-NOSE (POINT-TO-POINT)

The patient is tasked with touching the pad of their index finger to the tip of their nose (Figures 9.1 and 9.2).

Finger-to-Nose Instructions

1. Patient is sitting and instructed to close their eyes.
2. Instruct the patient to extend their arm to the side with shoulder abduction to 90 degrees, and then touch the tip of their nose using the pad of the index finger.
3. After each touch of the target (nose tip), the patient returns to the starting position with the arm abducted to 90 degrees. Repeat this several times using each hand and arm. (Alternatively,

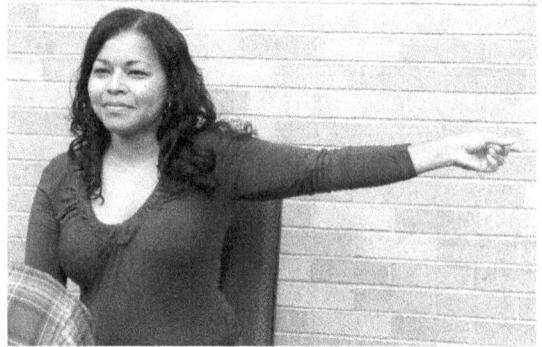

Figure 9.1 Finger-to-Nose 1

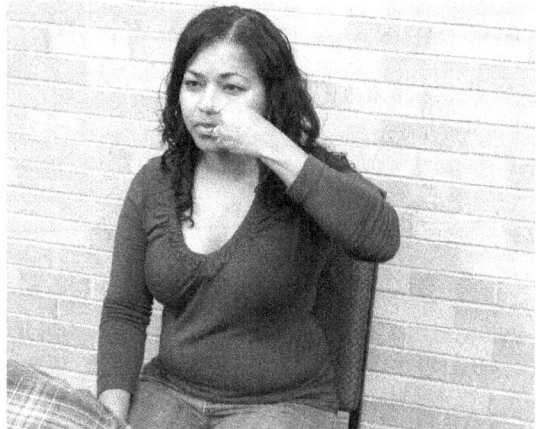

Figure 9.2 Finger-to-Nose 2

the patient may be instructed to extend their arms out to the sides [90 degrees of abduction], then, keeping their eyes closed, alternately touch the tip of the nose with each hand, returning the arms to full extension to the sides after each touch.)
4. Repeat this test of accuracy several times with the eyes open and closed.

Key things to remember:

- The patient should not need to use vision to accomplish this task.
- This test should be performed slowly and carefully, as the clinician may miss early cerebellar signs when it is performed rapidly.[7]

Interpretation of the Finger-to-Nose Test

- When a patient is unable to accurately touch the tip of their nose, this is recorded as *dysmetria*.
- Document if the patient demonstrates an intention tremor. Intention tremors increase as the finger approaches the target.

FINGER–NOSE–FINGER

The patient is tasked with touching the pad of their index finger to the tip of their nose, and then the tip of the examiner's index finger. Sometimes the examiner keeps their finger stationary, other times they move it to different locations during testing.

Finger–Nose–Finger Instructions

1. The patient is sitting with their eyes open.
2. Instruct the patient to touch the tip of the nose using the pad of their index finger (as described in the Finger to Nose test above, and then reach in front of them at arm's length to touch the examiner's index fingertip.
3. The examiner moves the target after the patient touches the fingertip, and the patient repeats the sequence.
4. Test each arm.

Key things to remember:

- The patient should fully extend their arm (elbow/shoulder) in order to reach the target (i.e., the examiner's fingertip), as you are testing the coordination of each joint to reach the target.

Interpretation of the Finger–Nose–Finger Test

Tests are positive when the patient consistently misses the target or has intention tremors.

RAPID-ALTERNATING HANDS/FEET

This test is typically performed with hands, but the examiner may also test feet (Figures 9.3 and 9.4).

Rapid-Alternating Hands/Feet Instructions

1. The patient is sitting with their hands on their lap.

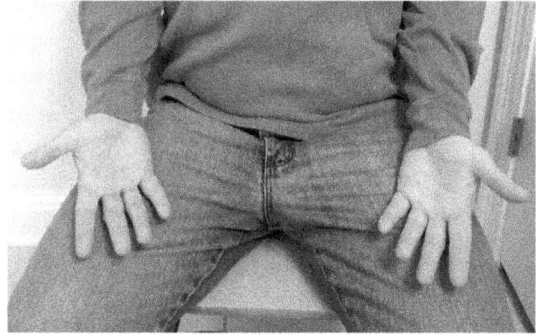

Figure 9.3 Diadochokinesia 1

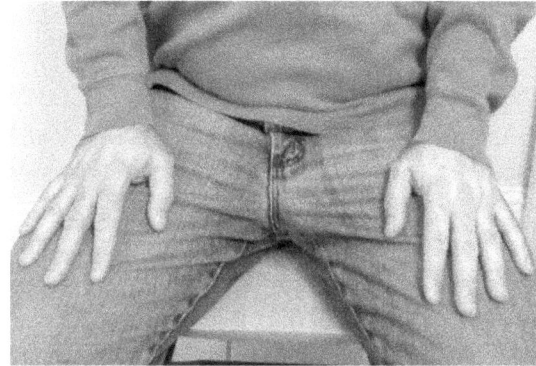

Figure 9.4 Diadochokinesia 2

2. Instruct the patient to flip their hands palms up/palms down on their lap as quickly as possible.
3. Repeat this several times.

Key things to remember:

- You may also ask the patient to alternately tap the toes of each foot against the floor as quickly as possible.

Interpretation of the Rapid-Alternating Hands/Feet Test

- Compare the quality of movement of each hand. Do they smoothly flip each hand? Is the timing correct, or is one hand not sequenced with the contralateral one?
- If the patient is unable to perform rapid-alternating movements, report *dysdiadochokinesia*.

HAND CLAPPING

The quality, timing, and motions of each hand are observed as the patient claps.

Hand Clapping Instructions

1. The patient is seated.
2. Instruct the patient to clap both hands together with equal motion, distance, speed, and force.
3. The clinician demonstrates and then asks the patient to replicate the hand clapping.
4. The clinician observes symmetry and coordination of motions.
5. If needed, repeat the demonstration, and ask the patient to replicate it.

Interpretation of the Hand Clapping Test

If the patient is unable to clap hands with equal motion, distance, speed, or force, the test is positive for *cerebellar dysfunction*.

Lower Extremities

PATELLAR TAPPING

The patient is tasked with tapping the heel of one foot on the contralateral patella gently and repetitively.

Patellar Tapping Instructions

1. The patient is seated.
2. Instruct the patient to tap the contralateral patella with the heel of the foot three to five times. Each leg swing toward and away from the patella should be large (about 2 feet, or 60 cm).
3. Repeat with each foot.

Key things to remember:

- Patients need to have adequate hip and knee range of motion to perform this test.

Interpretation of the Patellar Tapping Test

Any abnormalities of force, rhythm, or accuracy are considered to be secondary to *cerebellar dysfunction*.

HEEL–SHIN SLIDE

The patient is tasked to slide the heel of one foot down the shin of the contralateral leg (Figures 9.5 and 9.6).

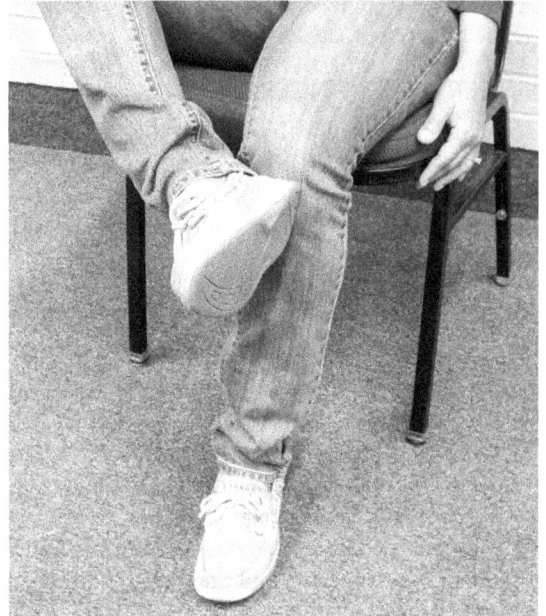

Figure 9.5 Heel-to-Shin 1

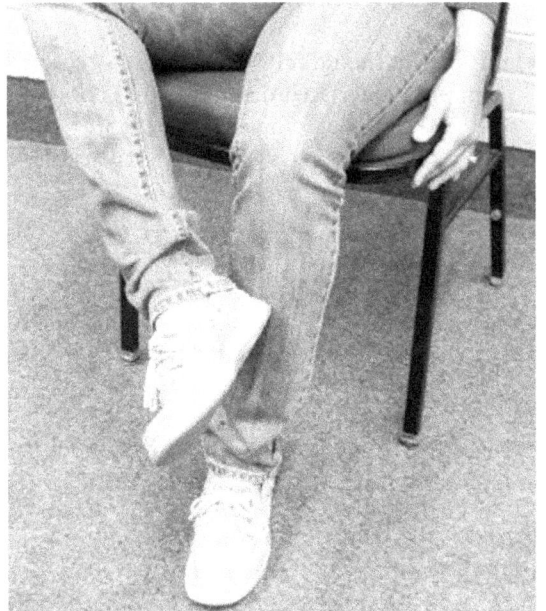

Figure 9.6 Heel-to-Shin 2

Heel–Shin Slide Instructions

1. Patient is positioned supine.
2. Instruct the patient to place the heel of the right foot on top of the shin just below the patella of the left leg.
3. Instruct the patient to slide the heel of one foot down the shin to the ankle.
4. Repeat with the left heel on the right shin.

Key things to remember:

- The heel should stay exactly on top of the shin (midline) and move in a slow and controlled manner down to the shin.
- Observe and report any side-to-side (mediolateral) leg tremors during the slide.
- Patients should have the available hip/knee ROM to perform the test.

Interpretation of the Heel–Shin Slide

If the patient is unable to keep the heel on the shin as it slides down the leg, it is a positive sign of *cerebellar dysfunction*.

Speech Test

SPEECH TEST INSTRUCTIONS

Instruct the patient to repeat the phrases: "The American Constitution" and "baby hippopotamus."

INTERPRETATION OF THE SPEECH TEST

Staccato speech, where the patient accentuates the separate syllables, and slurred speech are signs of possible cerebellar impairment. When observed, it is documented as *scanning speech* or *ataxic dysarthria*. Most patients with this phenomenon have an injury to the left cerebellar hemisphere.[8]

Rebound Test

Rebound phenomenon is a reflex that occurs when a patient is given resistance against a moving limb and that resistance is suddenly removed. The reflex prevents an exaggerated movement of the arm once the resistance is removed.

REBOUND TEST INSTRUCTIONS

1. The patient is in a seated position with eyes closed and one arm stretched in front of them (shoulder at 90 degrees).
2. Instruct the patient to maintain their arm position as you apply downward resistance.
3. Push downward on the arm and immediately remove resistance.
4. Observe the movement of the tested arm.
5. Repeat on the contralateral limb.

INTERPRETATION OF THE REBOUND TEST

- If the patient's arm only moves a short distance after resistance is removed, this is a normal test.
- If the patient's arm makes an exaggerated upward movement, **this is a positive test of cerebellar dysfunction and spasticity**.

Oculomotor Signs of Cerebellar Dysfunction

Oculomotor testing is described in Chapter 7. Abnormal signs indicating possible cerebellar dysfunction include unidirectional nystagmus (>3 beats), direction-changing nystagmus, vertically beating nystagmus, rebound nystagmus, periodic alternating nystagmus, hyper- or hypometric saccades, post-saccadic drift, impaired initiation of pursuit, impaired smooth pursuit, and vertical skew deviations. Care must be taken to examine the vestibular system when unidirectional nystagmus is noted.

Localization of injury causing impairments is as follows:[9,10]

- *Flocculus/paraflocculus*: Gaze-evoked nystagmus, rebound nystagmus, downbeat nystagmus, post-saccadic drift, and saccadic pursuit (lack of smooth pursuit), spontaneous nystagmus, geotropic horizontal nystagmus
- *Nodulus/ventral uvula*: Loss of tilt suppression of post-rotational nystagmus (after rapid shaking or rotation), periodic alternating nystagmus, apogeotropic horizontal nystagmus
- *Dorsal vermis/posterior fastigial nucleus*: Saccadic hypometria (bilateral vermis),

saccadic hypermetria (bilateral fastigial nucleus), impairment of pursuit initiation

Gait

GAIT INSTRUCTIONS

Instruct the patient to ambulate while looking straight ahead about 15 feet (~5 m), turn/pivot, and walk back to you, under the following conditions:

a. Normal ambulation
b. Ambulating on toes (~15 feet or 5 m)
c. Ambulating on heels (~15 feet or 5 m)

INTERPRETATION OF GAIT[8]

- Slower gait speed (gait speed varies by age, comorbidities such as stroke, and setting).
- Abnormalities include shuffling, loss of balance, veering to one side, short step lengths, jerky or ataxic movements, excessively slow gait speed (<0.7 m/s).[11]
- *A midline cerebellar lesion* presents with a wide-based and lumbering truncal gait.
- *Unilateral cerebellar lesion* presents with the gait veering to one side. As vestibular dysfunction may also give this presentation, care must be taken to assess the vestibular system.
- *Anterior vermis lesions* present with poor balance during ambulation. This is often seen in patients with alcoholic cerebellar degeneration.

Pronator Drift Test

This tests the patient's ability to remain in position with extended arms, palms up.

PRONATOR DRIFT TEST INSTRUCTIONS

1. The patient is sitting or standing.
2. Instruct the patient to fully extend their arms in front of themself with shoulder flexion at 90 degrees with palms facing upward.
3. The patient holds this position for 30 seconds as the clinician observes the hand positions.
4. Repeat the test with eyes closed.

INTERPRETATION OF THE PRONATOR DRIFT TEST

If pronation is observed, the test is positive and suggests a lesion in the ipsilateral cerebellum or ipsilateral dorsal column.[8]

Muscle Tone

Instruct the patient to relax completely as you passively move the joint to be tested slowly through the full ROM, and then quickly through partial ROM.

Interpretation of Muscle Tone Testing

Hypertonia is secondary to upper motor neuron injury, brain tumors, birth injuries, and conditions that affect nerve communication.

Hypotonia is secondary to lower motor neuron injury, brain damage during birth, Down syndrome, muscular dystrophy, cerebral palsy, Prader–Willi syndrome, Tay–Sachs disease, hypothyroidism, spinal cord injury or atrophy, or inherited disorders.

The patient will present as normal tone, hypertonic, or hypotonic. When the patient is hypertonic, you may use the Modified Ashworth Scale to document spasticity (Table 9.3).[12]

Deep Tendon Reflexes (DTRs)

According to Rodriguez-Beato and De Jesus, there are five primary DTRs that include the biceps (C5–C6), brachioradialis (C5–C6), triceps (C7–C8), patellar reflex (L2–L4), and the Achilles reflex (S1–S2).[13] What is considered "normal" depends on the patient's history and previously documented reflex grades.[13]

Typically, clinicians test the L2–L4 myotome in each of the patient's lower limbs while assessing the cerebellum using a deep tendon reflex. When documenting reflexes, you may use the following terms: absent, present, brisk, or hyperactive. If the reflexes are hyperactive, also check for clonus. If you need a scale, the National Institute of Neurological Disorders and Stroke (NINDS) created the following validated scale:[13]

Table 9.3 Modified Ashworth Scale

Modified Ashworth Scale Score	Definition
0	No increase in muscle tone
1	Slight increase in muscle tone, with a catch and release or minimal resistance at the end of the range of motion when an affected part(s) is moved in flexion or extension
1+	Slight increase in muscle tone, manifested as a catch, followed by minimal resistance through the remainder (less than half) of the range of motion
2	A marked increase in muscle tone throughout most of the range of motion, but affected part(s) are still easily moved
3	Considerable increase in muscle tone, passive movement difficult
4	Affected part(s) rigid in flexion or extension

0: Reflex absent
- Reflex small, less than normal, includes a trace response or a response brought out only with reinforcement
- Reflex in the lower half of a normal range
- Reflex in the upper half of a normal range
- Reflex enhanced, more than normal, includes clonus if present, which optionally can be noted in an added verbal description of the reflex

Deep Tendon Reflex Instructions

BICEPS REFLEX

1. Support the patient's forearm on the forearm of the examiner with the patient's arm midway between flexion and extension.
2. The examiner should firmly place their thumb on the patient's bicep tendon with fingers curled around the elbow.
3. The examiner taps on their thumb (and thereby stretching the biceps tendon).
4. The forearm should flex at the elbow.

TRICEPS REFLEX

1. Support the patient's forearm on the forearm of the examiner with the patient's arm midway between flexion and extension.
2. Tap just above the olecranon on the insertion of the triceps.
3. The forearm should extend.

BRACHIORADIALIS REFLEX

1. Support the patient's arm at the elbow with the thumb of the supporting hand on the biceps tendon.
2. With your other hand, tap the brachioradialis tendon, which inserts at the base of the styloid process of the radius, ~1 cm lateral to the radial artery.
3. The forearm should flex and supinate. You may also see finger flexion.

KNEE JERK REFLEX

1. The patient is seated with their legs hanging off the treatment table/plinth, so the limb is unweighted and completely relaxed.
2. Place one hand on the quads, while the other taps the patellar tendon (just distal to the patella) and observe for a reflexive quadriceps contraction.
3. The knee should extend.

ANKLE JERK REFLEX

1. The patient is seated with their legs hanging off the treatment table/plinth, so the limb is unweighted and completely relaxed.
2. The examiner places one hand under the sole of the patient's foot (to be tested) and slightly dorsiflexes it.
3. Tap the Achilles tendon just above the insertion on the calcaneus.
4. The foot should be plantarflex.

INTERPRETATION OF DEEP TENDON REFLEX TESTING

- Hyperactive DTRs indicate an upper motor neuron lesion. This may be an early sign of corticospinal tract abnormalities, or descending pathways influencing the reflex arc due to a suprasegmental lesion (a lesion above the level of the spinal reflex pathway).[13]
- Hypoactive DTRs indicate lower motor neuron lesions and are seen in hypothyroidism, hypothermia, cerebellar dysfunction, or beta-blockade.
- Absent DTRs indicate lesions within the reflex arc.[13]
- Bilaterally absent ankle jerk usually indicates peripheral neuropathy, or cauda equina syndrome.[13]
- Specific peripheral nerve injuries can cause absent or decreased DTRs.[13]

CORTICOSPINAL TRACT (PYRAMIDAL TRACT)

Often used when testing for strokes and spinal cord injuries, the Babinski reflex test is a corticospinal tract integrity and is also used when assessing patients for brain tumors, multiple sclerosis, meningitis, cerebral palsy, and amyotrophic lateral sclerosis.[14]

Babinski Reflex Test (Test of the Corticospinal Tract)

1. The patient is lying supine with bare feet.
2. The clinician uses a blunt instrument (e.g., tongue depressor, edge of a key, or the end of a reflex hammer's handle)[15] and firmly strokes the plantar surface of the foot from the heel along the lateral aspect from the heel toward the metatarsal head of the fifth toe, and then along the metatarsal heads of all toes toward the first toe in a curved path.

INTERPRETATION OF THE BABINSKI REFLEX TEST

- Used for patients 2 years of age and older.[15]
- *Positive test*: The hallux (first toe) extends, and the other toes abduct. This indicates a corticospinal tract injury or deficit.

- *Negative test*: The toes curl, or there is no response. This indicates an intact corticospinal tract.

Clonus

Clonus is a rhythmic oscillating stretch reflex that occurs in the presence of an upper motor neuron lesion and is often accompanied by hyperreflexia.[16] The signals involved with clonus primarily travel the corticospinal tract. While it may be tested in many joints such as the jaw jerk, knee jerk, biceps, and triceps, it is most commonly tested at the ankles. It is also prognostic of seizures in certain drug overdoses.[16]

CLONUS TESTING INSTRUCTIONS

1. The patient is supine.
2. The examiner grasps the dorsum of the foot to be tested and rapidly dorsiflexes the foot briskly and maintains dorsiflexion pressure.
3. When present, the examiner will feel the clonus beats. The initial beat is the longest in duration with the next three beats decreasing in duration, and subsequent beats being the same duration.[16]

INTERPRETATION OF CLONUS TESTING

- When pathological, it is a sign of an upper motor neuron lesion/syndrome.
- While it may be physiologic, in adults it is generally pathological.[16]
- Some term infants can be hyperreflexic, and a few beats of clonus is a normal finding.[16]
- Most infants who will go on to demonstrate cerebral palsy will not exhibit clonus.[17]
- May be the result of stroke, encephalopathy, cerebral palsy, MS, spinal cord injury, or serotonin syndrome (from psychiatric or street drugs).[16]

STATIC BALANCE TEST

THE 4-STAGE BALANCE TEST

The 4-Stage Balance Test assesses static balance with the feet in four different positions and is recommended by the US Centers for Disease Control and Prevention.

4-Stage Balance Test Instructions

1. Demonstrate the four test positions:
   - *Position 1*: Feet side by side.
   - *Position 2*: Place the instep of one foot so it is touching the big toe of the other foot. (This has also been called the "semi-tandem" stance.)
   - *Position 3*: Tandem stance. The patient stands with one foot directly in front of the other, with the heel of one foot touching the toes of the other.
   - *Position 4*: Stand on one foot.
2. Instruct the patient to stand in each position upon your command—"Ready, begin"—for up to 10 seconds. You may assist the patient to assume the correct position and let go of them when they are steady. Patients are not allowed to use an assistive device during testing. Patients are allowed to move their hands and body to balance, but not their feet. After 10 seconds say, "Stop." Continue through each position, stopping the test if they fail a position.

Interpretation of the 4-Stage Balance Test

- Older adults who cannot hold each position at least 10 seconds are at increased risk of falling.

REFERENCES

1. Petersen JA, Straumann D, Weber KP. Clinical diagnosis of bilateral vestibular loss: three simple bedside tests. *Ther Adv Neurol Disord*. Jan 2013;6(1):41–45. doi:10.1177/1756285612465920
2. Kim HJ, Park SH, Kim JS, et al. Bilaterally abnormal head impulse tests indicate a large cerebellopontine angle tumor. *J Clin Neurol*. Jan 2016;12(1):65–74. doi:10.3988/jcn.2016.12.1.65
3. Sekhon RK, Rocha Cabrero F, Deibel JP. *Nystagmus Types*. StatPearls Publishing LLC; 2025.
4. Thrutell MJ. Diagnostic approach to abnormal spontaneous eye movements. *Neuro-Ophthalmology*. 2014;20(4):993–1007.
5. Feil K, Rattay TW, Adeyemi AK, Goldschagg N, Strupp ML. What's behind cerebellar dizziness? - News on diagnosis and therapy. *Laryngorhinootologie*. May 2024;103(5):337–343. Zerebellärer Schwindel, was steckt dahinter? doi:10.1055/a-2192-7278
6. Hain TC. *Rebound Nystagmus*. Dizziness-and-balance.com; 2025. https://dizziness-and-balance.com/practice/nystagmus/rebound.htm
7. Ataullah AHM, Singla R, Naqvi IA. *Cerebellar Dysfunction*. StatPearls Publishing; Updated 2024. https://www.ncbi.nlm.nih.gov/books/NBK562317/
8. Nanthakumaran M. *Cerebellar Examination*. OSCE; 2024. https://www.simpleosce.com/examinations/neurological/cerebellar-examination.php
9. Lal V, Truong D. Eye movement abnormalities in movement disorders. *Clin Parkinsonism Related Disorder*. 2019;1:54–63. doi:10.1016/j.prdoa.2019.08.004
10. Shemesh AA, Zee DS. Eye movement disorders and the cerebellum. *J Clin Neurophysiol*. 2019;36(6):405–41410.1097/WNP.0000000000000579
11. Montero-Odasso M, Schapira M, Soriano ER, et al. Gait velocity as a single predictor of adverse events in healthy seniors aged 75 years and older. *J Gerontol Ser A*. 2005;60(10):1304–1309. doi:10.1093/gerona/60.10.1304
12. Harb A, Margetis K, Kishner S. *Modified Ashworth Scale*. StatPearls Publishing; Updated 2025. https://www.ncbi.nlm.nih.gov/books/NBK554572/
13. Rodriguez-Beato FY, De Jesus O. *Physiology, Deep Tendon Reflexes*. StatPearls Publishing; Updated 2023. doi:https://www.ncbi.nlm.nih.gov/books/NBK562238/
14. Johnson J. *The Babinski Reflex: What to Know*. Health Topics; 2024. https://www.medicalnewstoday.com/articles/babinski-reflex

15. Acharya AB, Jamil RT, Dewey JJ. *Babinski Reflex*. StatPearls Publishing; Updated 2023. https://www.ncbi.nlm.nih.gov/books/NBK519009/

16. Zimmerman B, Hubbard JB. *Clonus*. StatPearls Publishing; Updated 2023. https://www.ncbi.nlm.nih.gov/books/NBK534862/

17. Hamer EG, La Bastide-Van Gemert S, Boxum AG, et al. The tonic response to the infant knee jerk as an early sign of cerebral palsy. *Early Human Develop*. 2018;119:38–44. doi:10.1016/j.earlhumdev.2018.03.001

10

Equipment for Evaluation

Chapter Goals

1. List the "bare minimum" equipment needed for assessment of balance/dizziness
2. List the "more ideal" equipment that will enhance the assessment of balance/dizziness
3. List the "dream equipment" that is typically purchased by larger organizations

There is a wide range of equipment available to today's clinician, ranging from a simple pencil costing pennies to an automatic chair used to reposition loose inner-ear crystals that costs thousands of dollars. In this chapter, equipment that will aid in evaluations will be discussed. Some equipment is essential, while others, while being optional, greatly enhance evaluations.

EQUIPMENT USED IN EVALUATIONS

In order to perform a thorough bedside evaluation, you will need to have a bare minimum of equipment. You do not need to have expensive equipment to perform a good evaluation. However, having more expensive equipment can definitely assist you in quantifying your evaluation. Listed next are the "bare minimum" equipment, the "more ideal" equipment that you may choose to purchase, and the "dream equipment" that is more expensive and typically purchased by institutions and researchers, but nice to have.

BARE MINIMUM EQUIPMENT FOR A BEDSIDE EXAM

To be able to perform the examinations outlined in Chapters 7, 8, and 9, you will need to have the following equipment, with pictures of items with which you may not be familiar:

1. Gait belt
   - A gait belt, sometimes called a transfer belt, is used by a clinician or caregiver to assist the patient's balance in case of a near-fall or to assist the patient slowly to the floor in case of complete loss of balance.
2. Visual target (one of the following: finger, Wolff wand, tongue depressor, pencil/pen)
   - As described in the oculomotor testing description, you will need to give the patient a visual target on which to fixate while examining the eyes. Most times, your finger will do. However, at times it may be preferable to use another object, such as a pen tip or the eraser of a pencil. You may also print a letter that is at the patient's level of visual acuity and paste it to the end of a tongue depressor. The Wolff wand is used by optometrists but can be purchased by anyone. A basic Wolff wand set includes two 14-inch (35.6 cm) steel rods: one with a 1/2-inch (13 mm) polished

brass ball and one with a silver nickel-plated ball. The wand allows the examiner/therapist to comfortably move and position the targets in the patient's near visual space while they fixate on either the ball or their own reflection in the ball.

3. High-density foam (Figure 10.1)
   * Used for examination and also treatment, patients stand on the high-density foam, which is compliant and challenges balance. If you do not have foam, you may substitute another compliant material (e.g., thick pillow) as long as the patient's feet do not sink through and contact a firm surface/floor. Care should be taken that the patient does not fall.

4. Treatment plinth (treatment table)
   * The plinth is usually raised such that the patient may sit on it with the feet hanging freely and not supported (e.g., for deep tendon reflex [DTR] testing). If you do not have a surface high enough to allow the legs to dangle, you may hold the leg under the thigh and raise it for DTR testing. More expensive plinths are adjustable for height and have one end that may be angled (higher or lower) than horizontal. While not a necessity, it is nice to have when testing for benign paroxysmal positional vertigo (BPPV), as the patient may rest their head and have it at 30 degrees of extension.

5. Fifteen feet (~5 m) of straight walking space to assess gait.

6. Occluder. Used to block vision, but the clinician may use the palm of their hand if they do not have an occluder (Figure 10.2).

7. A clock with a second hand or stopwatch for timed procedures.

8. Stethoscope and sphygmomanometer for blood pressure measurements.

9. Tape measure for distance measures.

10. A goniometer or bubble inclinometer to measure joint angles (Figure 10.3).

MORE IDEAL EQUIPMENT

1. Eye chart (e.g., Snellen, LEA Symbols chart, ETDRS chart)
   * Used to test visual acuity, there are many types.

Figure 10.1 High-Density Foam

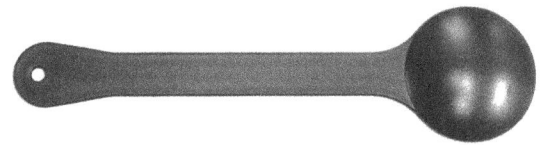

Figure 10.2 Occluder

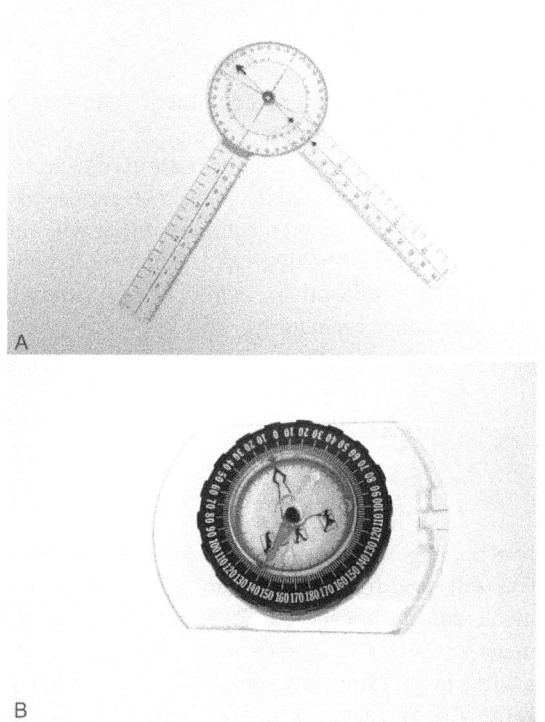

A

B

Figure 10.3 (A and B) Goniometer

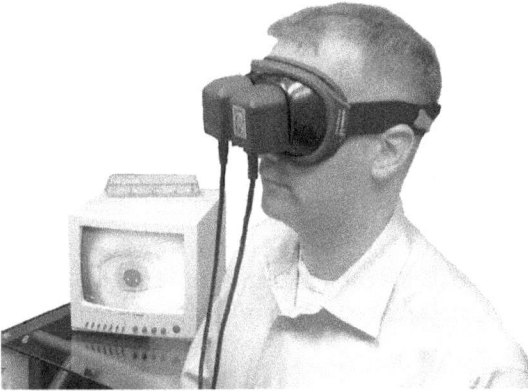

Figure 10.4 Infrared Goggles

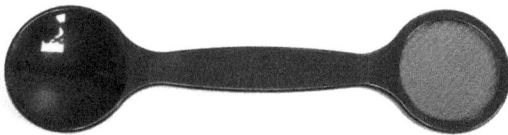

Figure 10.5 Maddox Rod

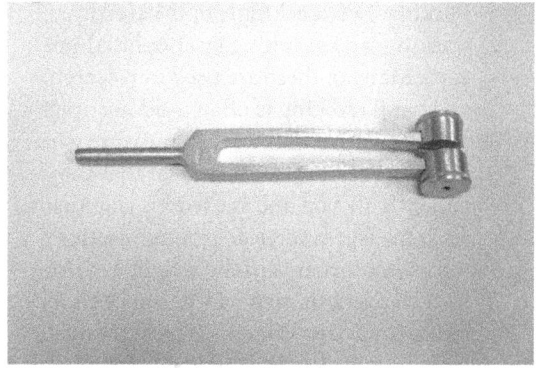

Figure 10.6 Tuning Fork

2. Frenzel or infrared (IR) goggles (Figure 10.4)
   - Frenzel goggles are +20 diopter goggles used to remove fixation. IR goggles remove the patient's vision as no light is allowed to enter, and an infrared camera is pointed at the eyes. Depending on how much money is spent, the software used with the IR goggles may record the exam or even track the eye motion. Both of these usually have a fixation light that may be turned on.
3. Maddox rod and penlight (Figure 10.5)
   - Used to test eye alignment.
4. Accommodative rule
   - Used to measure near point of convergence.
5. Tuning fork (Figure 10.6)
   - Used for testing somatosensation of vibration.
6. Computerized dynamometer (handheld or larger equipment)
   - Measures muscle strength/power in pounds, newtons, and kilograms.
7. Monofilaments (5.07 at a minimum)

DREAM EQUIPMENT

1. Force plate/computerized dynamic posturography
   - There are many types of force plates used to assess balance. Some test/analyze static balance and sway, while others test the patient's ability to balance during dynamic challenges, such as sudden tilting or shifting of the force plate. They range in price from a few thousand US dollars to approximately $100,000. The software may compute the center of pressure and center of gravity of the subject and have various testing protocols.
2. Videonystagmography (VNG) equipment
   - VNG equipment is used to test vestibular function by blowing warm and cold air against the eardrum to change the temperature of the endolymph of the lateral canal, and recording/analyzing the resulting nystagmus. This test is typically performed by an audiologist. This test provides low-frequency information.
3. Video head impulse test (vHIT) equipment
   - This is an instrumented head impulse test, with the software displaying saccades, covert saccades, or the lack of saccades during testing. This test provides high-frequency information. According to Hain, the main use of the vHIT is to detect vestibular neuritis, and is good in combination with VNG, and excellent at diagnosing bilateral vestibular loss.[1]
4. Ocular motion measuring equipment
   - This equipment records and measures eye motions during various tests using different methods: electro-oculography using electrodes placed around the eyes, Dual

Purkinje Eye Tracking, pupil-based eye tracking, and scanning laser ophthalmoscopy. Many of these are used in research, and pupil tracking is often used in clinics.

5. Pressure-sensitive walkways to measure gait
   - This is a pressure-sensitive mat that the patient walks on and is used for gait analysis. It measures vertical ground reaction forces, contact area of the weight-bearing foot, step length, step width, stance time, swing time, step velocity, step time, stride length, stride length, and stride time.

6. Smart insoles
   - Similar to the pressure-sensitive walkways, these are shoe insoles with

pressure-sensitive sensors built in. The benefit of the insoles is that the patient may walk anywhere and does not have to stay on a mat while gait is being analyzed.

REFERENCE

1. Hain, Timothy C. *VHIT Test*. Dizziness-and -balance.com; 2024. https://dizziness-and -balance.com/testing/VHIT/index.html

11

Differential Diagnosis of Diplopia, Dizziness, and Vertigo

Chapter Goals

1. Discuss diplopia and tests of strabismus
2. Explain the Parks three-step test (Parks–Bielschowsky three-step test)
3. List conditions causing unilateral vestibular loss
4. List the signs/symptoms of unilateral vestibular loss
5. List etiologies of bilateral vestibular loss
6. Discuss the positioning tests of BPPV

According to Cook and Décary, "Differential diagnosis is a systematic how process used to identify the proper diagnosis from a set of possible competing diagnoses." They argue that clinicians are required to pay careful attention to (1) how test metrics can be misleading, (2) how a diagnostic label may overcomplicate care, and (3) how using different methods of classifying diagnoses could improve care.[1]

This chapter will discuss the differential diagnosis of diplopia, dizziness, and vertigo. Diplopia is a common complaint, with one study reporting almost 80,500 ambulatory visits and 50,000 emergency department visits in the USA annually.[2] According to Neuhauser, dizziness (including vertigo) affects about 15% to over 20% of adults yearly in large population-based studies.[3]

Vestibular vertigo accounts for about a quarter of dizziness complaints and has a 12-month prevalence of 5% and an annual incidence of 1.4%. Its prevalence rises with age and is about two to three times higher in women than in men.[3] Dizziness and vertigo in grammar school students appear to be as common as in adults.[4] According to Hain, the causes of dizziness are:[5]

- 50%   Otologic dizziness
- 5%   Central dizziness
- 5–10% Medical dizziness
- 15%   Psychological
- 25%   Unknown cause

Clearly, the overwhelming causes are those of the ear. However, because the central pathologies have the potential to cause death, they are extremely important to rule out. Gurley and Edlow note that dizziness and vertigo are the symptoms most tightly linked to missed strokes. They report that almost 10% of strokes are misdiagnosed, with these patients more likely to be under 50 years old, and also women or minorities.[6] In previous chapters, the importance of the oculomotor exam was discussed, and the many signs that point to central pathology that may be discovered. In addition, Hain did not list vision issues as a possible cause of dizziness, and it is possible that a portion of the 25% of "unknown causes" are secondary to vision or oculomotor deficits.

DOI: 10.1201/9781003524441-11

According to Dougherty et al., the first step to narrowing the differential diagnosis is to classify the vestibular dysfunction as peripheral or central.[7] Examples of central pathologies contributing to dizziness/vestibular deficits include posterior fossa strokes or tumors, Chiari malformation, multiple sclerosis, vestibular migraine, mal de débarquement syndrome, and degenerative ataxia disorders such as Parkinson's disease.[7] The most common peripheral conditions are benign paroxysmal positional vertigo (BPPV), Ménière's disease, vestibular neuritis, and labyrinthitis.[7] Less commonly, the following can cause vestibular dysfunction: cerebellopontine angle tumors, such as acoustic neuromas, perilymphatic fistula, semicircular canal dehiscence, vestibular paroxysmia, Cogan syndrome, vestibulotoxic medications, and otitis media.[7] Because the potential etiologies of dizziness are so broad, it exceeds the scope of a single clinical specialty.[7]

In a study of 1,091 patients in emergency departments in the United States of America, physicians used templates to document the presence or absence of nystagmus in 887 of the patients (80%). Nystagmus was said to be present in 185 patients (21%). Of these 185 patients, sufficient information regarding nystagmus to be diagnostically useful was recorded in only 10 patients (5.4%).[6] The misdiagnosis of patients with dizziness results from the following common pitfalls in thinking:[8]

1. "True vertigo" implies an inner ear disorder.
2. If the patient complains of worse dizziness/vertigo with head movements, it implies a peripheral etiology.
3. Auditory symptoms imply a peripheral etiology.
4. The diagnosis of vestibular migraine is the cause when headaches accompany dizziness.
5. Isolated vertigo is not a transient ischemic attack (TIA) symptom.
6. Strokes causing dizziness or vertigo will have limb ataxia or other focal signs.
7. Younger patients have migraines rather than strokes.
8. A CT is needed to rule out cerebellar hemorrhage in those with isolated acute dizziness/vertigo.
9. A CT is useful to search for acute posterior fossa strokes.
10. A negative MRI-DWI rules out posterior fossa stroke.

To address these pitfalls in thinking, Saber Tehrani et al. remind us:[8]

- Dizziness and vertigo may be caused by both central and peripheral causes, presenting similar symptoms.
- While the peripheral causes are more common, central pathology must be ruled out.
- Auditory symptoms of tinnitus or hearing loss may be caused by lateral pontine and inner ear strokes.[9–11]
- Sudden, severe, or sustained headache or neck pain may indicate aneurysm, dissection, or other vascular pathology.[12]
- Isolated vertigo is the most common vertebrobasilar "warning" symptom before stroke.[13,14]
- Fewer than 20% of stroke patients presenting with acute vestibular syndrome have focal neurologic signs.[15,16]
- Vertebral artery dissection closely mimics migraine.[17]
- The sensitivity of CT to detect acute posterior fossa stroke is no higher than 16%.[18,19]
- Labyrinthine strokes are not visible on MRI.
- MRI-DWI in the first 24 hours misses 15–20% of posterior fossa strokes.[20]

Additionally, MRI within the first 24 hours after symptom onset may miss up to 50% of brainstem and cerebellar strokes with a diameter of less than 1 cm.[21] So, if you can't depend on CT to catch posterior fossa strokes, and MRI may miss many posterior fossa strokes in the first 24 hours, or small brainstem and cerebellar strokes, what can you do? You can perform a HINTS examination, which has been shown to outperform MRI within the first 2 days after symptom onset.[11] Conduct a thorough oculomotor examination, record orthostatic blood pressures (not just a sitting or supine pressure), assess gait, and perform as many cerebellar tests as time allows. A more involved vision and vestibular assessment may be performed as needed. If a therapist is performing the assessment, they should also include at least two tests of fall risk/balance.

Stanton and Freeman assert it is important to differentiate vertigo from symptoms of disequilibrium and presyncope. Conditions that may lead to these symptoms include acute and chronic anemia, anxiety disorders, benign positional vertigo, brain neoplasms, giant cell arteritis, herpes simplex encephalitis, labyrinthitis, mastoiditis, Ménière's disease, meningitis, migraine, multiple sclerosis, stroke, vertebrobasilar atherothrombotic disease, vestibular neuronitis, and Wernicke encephalopathy.[22]

DIPLOPIA

Double vision (diplopia) is the separation of images vertically, horizontally, or obliquely, and can be categorized as monocular (one eye) or binocular (both eyes) in origin.[23] Binocular diplopia occurs when both eyes are open and disappears when one is closed and is caused by strabismus, whereas monocular diplopia persists even after closing one eye and is associated with dry eyes, corneal scarring, cataract, retinal membranes, or nonorganic causes.[23,24]

Bedside tests of strabismus include the unilateral cover test, alternate cover test, and Parks three-step test. Ocular examination clues of etiology include:

- *Sixth nerve palsy*: An eye is deviated nasally, and the patient complains of horizontal diplopia.
- *Third nerve palsy*: An eye is deviated down and out, and the patient may complain of either horizontal or vertical diplopia.
- *Fourth nerve palsy*: An eye is deviated higher, especially in medial gaze, and the patient may complain of both horizontal and vertical diplopia.
- *Thyroid eye disease and blowout fractures are associated with vertical diplopia.*
- *Ptosis suggests myasthenia gravis (MG) or third nerve palsy.* An ice pack test may help to diagnose MG. (An ice pack is placed over the eye with ptosis. After 2 minutes, if the eye is open >2 mm than before the ice pack, it is considered a sign of MG.)

PARKS THREE-STEP TEST (PARKS–BIELSCHOWSKY THREE-STEP TEST)

The Parks three-step test is used to diagnose cyclovertical muscle palsy. The extraocular cyclovertical muscles are the superior oblique, superior rectus, inferior oblique, and inferior rectus of each eye. The three steps determine (1) which eye is hypertropic, (2) whether hypertropia is greater during left or right gaze, and (3) whether hypertropia is greater on right or left head tilt. In order to avoid confusion, keep in mind that you are trying to determine *which muscle has a palsy and is not working*, leaving another muscle unopposed.

- *Step 1*: Perform cover tests to determine the hypertropic eye.
- *Step 2*: Instruct the patient to gaze left, and then right to determine in which direction the hypertropia is greater. (With the patient gazing, it is sometimes useful to repeat the alternate cover test to help you determine in which direction the hypertropia is greater.)
- *Step 3*: With the patient looking straight ahead, instruct them to tilt the head left, and then right to determine in which direction of head tilt the hypertropia is greater. (With the patient in head-tilt, it is sometimes useful to repeat the alternate cover test to help you determine in which direction the hypertropia is greater.)

To perform Parks three-step test, you need to recall the muscle actions:

- *Elevator eye muscles:* Superior rectus (SR) and inferior oblique (IO)
- *Elevator of an eye that is abducted:* SR
- *Elevator of an eye that is adducted:* IO
- *Depressor eye muscles:* Inferior rectus (IR) and superior oblique (SO)
- *Depressor of an eye that is abducted:* IR
- *Depressor of an eye that is adducted:* SO
- *During head tilt:*
- *Intortors:* SO and SR
- *Extortors:* IO and IR
- During head tilts in normal situations, the eyes should not elevate as the Intortors oppose each other, and the extorters oppose each other

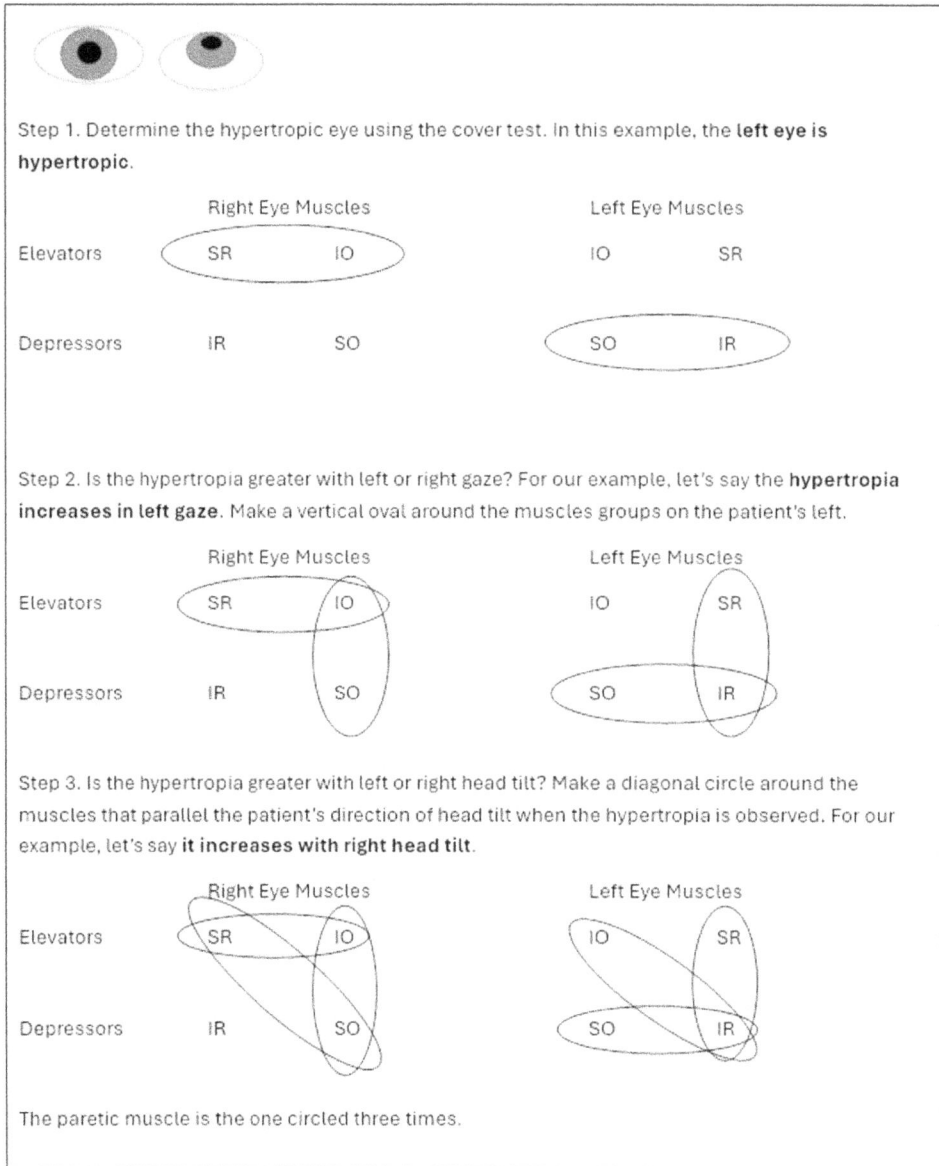

Step 1. Determine the hypertropic eye using the cover test. In this example, the **left eye is hypertropic.**

	Right Eye Muscles		Left Eye Muscles	
Elevators	SR	IO	IO	SR
Depressors	IR	SO	SO	IR

Step 2. Is the hypertropia greater with left or right gaze? For our example, let's say the **hypertropia increases in left gaze.** Make a vertical oval around the muscles groups on the patient's left.

	Right Eye Muscles		Left Eye Muscles	
Elevators	SR	IO	IO	SR
Depressors	IR	SO	SO	IR

Step 3. Is the hypertropia greater with left or right head tilt? Make a diagonal circle around the muscles that parallel the patient's direction of head tilt when the hypertropia is observed. For our example, let's say **it increases with right head tilt.**

	Right Eye Muscles		Left Eye Muscles	
Elevators	SR	IO	IO	SR
Depressors	IR	SO	SO	IR

The paretic muscle is the one circled three times.

Figure 11.1 Parks Three-Step Test

You can use the form in Figure 11.1 to assist in your thinking. In our example:

- *Step 1*: The patient has a left hypertropia as determined by the cover tests. This means that either left depressors or the right elevators are paretic (circle them).
- *Step 2*: The hypertropia increases with left gaze. Place a vertical circle over the muscles on the left side.
- *Step 3*: The hypertropia increases with right head tilt. Draw an oval that parallels the patient's direction of head tilt around the muscles when the hypertropia is seen.

Now, look at the form in Figure 11.1. Which muscle is circled three times? The muscle that is circled three times will be the paretic muscle.

VESTIBULAR CONDITIONS/DISEASES

We classify vestibular pathologies into two categories: *peripheral* and *central*. Peripheral pathologies are those outside of the central nervous system and include conditions like BPPV, labyrinthitis, neuritis, and some tumors that are outside of the central nervous system. If the problem reduces vestibular function and is only on one side (ear), the condition creates a unilateral vestibular loss (UVL). When both ears are affected, it is caused by bilateral vestibular loss (BVL). When UVL occurs, there is an asymmetry of afferent signals from each vestibule and/or semicircular canals causing symptoms of vertigo, nystagmus, nausea, and disequilibrium. For BVL, although vertigo may be present, it is common for the patient to not complain of vertigo or show signs of nystagmus, but they do have oscillopsia (shaky vision) and balance deficits.

The term *vestibular loss* (also called vestibular hypofunction) indicates that the vestibular system is not functioning at 100%. The term should not be associated with only 100% loss, as any percentage of vestibular function loss is termed vestibular loss. Vestibular loss may be caused by many conditions, including acquired brain injuries from strokes, TIA, and trauma, as well as disease and infections such as Parkinson's disease, multiple sclerosis, Ménière's disease, vestibular neuritis, and labyrinthitis. Discussed next are conditions involving the vestibular system, and/or cause vestibular loss, dizziness, and balance deficits.

UNILATERAL VESTIBULAR CONDITIONS

Depending on the difference in function between each inner ear and the level of compensation that has taken place (i.e., how much the brain has learned to modify vestibular signals to restore balance between the ears), you may see any of the following when you are examining a patient with a UVL: spontaneous nystagmus, gaze nystagmus (at 45 degrees of lateral gaze), end-range nystagmus of greater than 3 beats, increased nystagmus with gaze toward the healthy ear, increased gaze with removal of fixation (closed eyelids, darkness,

with Frenzel goggles or infrared goggles), falling or listing toward the lesion side, gaze-holding deficits, and/or imbalance that is worse during turning motions. The patient may complain of balance problems, nausea, and/or dizziness. Patients with peripheral etiologies may have nystagmus that is suppressed when they are fixing on a visual target; they typically feel worse in the dark, when they cannot hold gaze on a visual target. Conversely, patients with central causes of dizziness often feel better in the dark and worse while fixing gaze. They may develop nystagmus while fixating on visual targets and have either unidirectional nystagmus or direction-changing nystagmus.

Compensation is the process whereby the cerebellum "corrects" signals for a weak ear. While the affected patient moves within their environment, the cerebellum will ultimately change the vestibular signals to improve balance and make normal functional movement possible again. This occurs because of the demand placed on the balance system by the patient's activity. If the patient spends most of their time sitting in a chair and not moving, there is not enough stimulus to induce change, and compensation will be limited. If the patient is physically active, the cerebellum will compensate for the damaged side out of necessity and adjust the signals in order to have vestibular signal symmetry again. The cerebellum will boost the signals of the weaker ear and slow signals coming from the stronger, healthier ear in an attempt to get each side to produce the same resting firing rates. The closer the resting firing rates become, the less affected the patient will be by the damage. After compensation occurs, the patient usually does not have symptoms under most everyday conditions and activities. However, if such a patient turns very quickly, they may still experience slight disequilibrium and dizziness (Table 11.1).

Superior Canal Dehiscence Syndrome

The diagnosis of superior canal dehiscence syndrome (SCDS) requires a combination of tests, with patients who meet at least one criterion in each of the three major diagnostic categories are considered to have SCDS:[25]

Table 11.1 UVL Signs/Symptoms by Acuity of Vestibular Loss

Acute	Subacute	Chronic
• Resting nystagmus • Vertigo/dizziness • Nystagmus at 20 degrees–40 degrees of gaze • Nausea • Vomiting • Disequilibrium • Fluctuating hearing loss (labyrinthitis) • Unsteady gait • Symptoms worse with movement	• Dizziness while turning • Disequilibrium while turning • Nausea in busy visual environments (e.g., grocery stores, highways, action movies, near ceiling fans) • Unidirectional gaze nystagmus, sometimes elicited only at end-ranges (more than 3 beats) or in darkness • Unsteady gait • Symptoms worse with movement • Fatigue	• Typically, do not complain of vertigo • Loss of balance if turning quickly • Unsteady, wide-based gait • Decreased spatial awareness • Difficulty with memory and concentrating • Decreased cervical ROM • Depression • Fatigue

- At least one symptom consistent with SCDS and attributable to the "third mobile window":
  - Hyperacusis related to bone-conducted sound
  - Sound-induced vertigo and/or oscillopsia time-locked to the stimulus
  - Pressure-induced vertigo and/or oscillopsia time-locked to the stimulus
  - Pulsatile tinnitus
- At least one physiologic test or sign indicating that a "third mobile window" is transmitting pressure:
  - Eye movements in the plane of the affected superior semicircular canal when sound or pressure is applied to the affected ear
  - Low-frequency negative bone conduction thresholds on pure tone audiometry
  - Enhanced vestibular-evoked myogenic potential (VEMP) responses:
    - Low cervical VEMP thresholds
    - Elevated ocular VEMP amplitudes
- High-resolution CT scan with multiplanar reconstruction in the plane of the superior semicircular canal consistent with dehiscence

Vestibular Neuritis/Labyrinthitis

The difference between vestibular neuritis (VN) and labyrinthitis is that with VN there is swelling of the vestibular branch of the vestibulocochlear nerve, while with labyrinthitis both the vestibular and cochlear branches are swollen, and there may be fluctuating hearing loss.

Vestibular neuritis commonly results from the herpes simplex virus.[26] The superior vestibular nerve is more likely to be involved than the inferior vestibular nerve.[27] A bedside examination gives clues as to whether the issue is peripheral or central, but only diagnostic tests are definitive.

These inflammations cause the vestibular nerve to fire more slowly than usual while the patient is at rest and moving. While at rest, the vestibular nerve from each ear should have the same firing rate. However, due to this inflammation, there is now a difference between the firing rates of each ear, which is interpreted by the brain as movement. As the patient moves, the disparity grows as the intact vestibular system changes its firing rate. This causes vertigo, nausea, and balance problems. Typically, these inflammations are due to viral infections that last about 2 weeks and are treated short term with medications to suppress vestibular function and reduce nausea. If no damage is done to the vestibular system by the infection, the vestibular system typically returns to normal. However, if damage occurs, the patient may experience continued vertigo and balance deficits requiring vestibular therapy.

Acoustic Neuroma

An acoustic neuroma, also known as a schwannoma, develops from the sheath of Schwann cells of the vestibular and cochlear nerves and is a non-malignant tumor of the eighth cranial nerve (the vestibulocochlear nerve). They are most commonly seen on the inferior vestibular nerve, but often compress other cranial nerves (V, VII, IX, and X), and if large can compress the cerebellum or brainstem.[28] The incidence is 2–4 people per 100,000.[29]

Symptoms depend on compression of other nerves and location and may include:[28]

- *Auditory (most common symptom)*: High-frequency retrocochlear sensorineural hearing loss ("cookie bite" pattern of hearing loss referring to the audiogram pattern), tinnitus
- *Vestibular*: Nystagmus, unstable balance
- *Facial nerve (CN VII)*: Twitching, increased lacrimation, facial weakness
- *Trigeminal nerve (CN V)*: Paresthesia of the tongue, corneal reflex impairment, pain mimicking trigeminal neuralgia
- *Glossopharyngeal nerve (CN IX) and vagus nerve (CN X)*: Palatal paresis, hoarseness of the voice, dysphasia
- *Cerebellum*: Unsteady gait, lack of coordination, balance deficits, tremors, fine motor deficits, dysarthria
- *Brainstem*: Pyramidal symptoms (spasticity, hyperactive reflexes, weakness, Babinski sign)
- *Raised intracranial pressure*: Headache, nausea, vomiting, increased blood pressure, confusion and decreased mental abilities, disturbed level of consciousness, papilledema

Diagnosis may be made with ENG/audiography or an auditory brain response test, magnetic resonance imaging with gadolinium enhancement,[28] or computed tomography (CT).[28] Physicians treat this tumor with observation, surgery or radiation. Symptoms are treated with medications and vestibular rehabilitation. Therapy goals are typically to decrease dizziness and oscillopsia and to improve balance.

Perilymphatic Fistula

Also known as perilymph fistula, this lesion is an abnormal opening between the perilymph-filled inner and middle ear cavity, mastoid, or intracranial cavity.[30] When a tear develops in the round window, the liquid perilymph can escape the inner ear, thereby changing the pressure within the inner ear that commonly causes vestibular and cochlear symptoms (e.g., sudden unilateral hearing loss, tinnitus, vertigo, aural fullness, Tullio phenomenon, Hennebert's sign, and disequilibrium).[30] Head injury with a direct blow to the ear is the most common cause,[31] but actual numbers of cases may vary by country. Idiopathic cases range from 24% to 51%.[30] It occurs in children secondary to congenital anomalies and is thought to occur in up to 6% of children with idiopathic sensorineural hearing loss.[32] Other causes include ear surgery, pressure trauma, and infection.

Diagnosis may be made using the patient history of hearing loss, tinnitus, and/or vestibular symptoms immediately preceded by one of the following: internal event or external event barotrauma, or direct inner ear trauma.[30] A bedside test that may detect this condition is the nose-pinch Valsalva. Watch for downbeating nystagmus with a fast torsional phase toward the affected ear.

Diagnosis is made through a thorough history and physical examination. Patients may complain of disequilibrium after an increase in cerebrospinal fluid pressure (Hennebert's sign) or exposure to loud noises (Tullio phenomenon). Physical examination may demonstrate a brief episode of nystagmus with positive pressure applied to the ear through pneumatic otoscopy (fistula test), with external pressure on the tragus (tragus test), or an improvement in the audiogram after lying in the Trendelenburg position for 30 minutes (Fraser test).[33]

Physical therapy is not offered for this condition; it is typically treated with rest, restriction of activity (such as lifting, bending, diving, and loud noises), and in some cases surgery. This is a rare condition with an incidence rate of 1.5/100,000 adults.[30]

BILATERAL VESTIBULAR LOSS (BVL)

In cases of BVL (also called bilateral vestibular hypofunction [BVH]), the vestibular end organ or the eighth cranial nerve is damaged in each ear. Lucieer et al. studied 154 patients diagnosed with BVH and found a definite etiology in 47%, a probable etiology in 22%, and 31% were idiopathic.[34] Reasons of the identified etiologies included genetic disorders (17%), Ménière's disease (16%), ototoxicity (12%), infectious diseases (6%), and neurodegenerative diseases (4%). Migraine seems to play a role in idiopathic BVL, with 50% of subjects in the idiopathic group having a history of migraines, while only 11% in the non-idiopathic group (definite etiology and probable etiology) having a migraine history.

Patients with BVL typically experience disequilibrium, gait ataxia, oscillopsia (shaking visual environment) during head motions. They will present with a wide-based gait pattern and positive tests of vestibular hypofunction (e.g., head impulse tests) bilaterally. Generally, patients with BVL do not complain of vertigo, although they may if there are differences in the percentage of function of each ear.

Even though the vestibular system is deficient bilaterally, vestibular therapy still helps patients with BVL. According to the Clinical Practice Guideline for Peripheral Vestibular Hypofunction from the Academy of Neurologic Physical Therapy of the American Physical Therapy Association, there is strong evidence that clinicians should offer supervised vestibular physical therapy for those with BVL, beginning vestibular therapy as soon as possible.[35]

Goals for patients with BVL include enhancing gait and balance stability by increasing function in whatever is left working in the vestibular systems using gaze stabilization exercises, and using assistive devices (walkers, canes). Patients with BVL improve balance with vestibular rehabilitation but never return to their prior level of function, as ambulation never returns to normal.

BPPV

Positioning tests and patient history are used to diagnose loose crystals (otoconia) in the inner ear, called BPPV, with oculomotor and cerebellar screens being used to exclude central etiologies of vertigo/nystagmus. BPPV causes bouts of vertigo when the head is pitched or turned in such a way as to allow the otoconia to move within the semicircular canals, causing movement of the endolymph, which pushes or pulls on the cupula.

Palmeri and Kumar share these facts about BPPV:[36] It is the most common cause of peripheral vertigo and accounts for over half of all cases. At least 20% of patients presenting with vertigo have BPPV. About 50–70% of BPPV cases are idiopathic. Known causes of BPPV include head trauma, vestibular neuritis, labyrinthitis, Ménière's disease, migraine, ischemia, post-surgery, and iatrogenic causes with the most commonly known reason for BPPV being head trauma (7–17% of BPPV).

In cases of BPPV, the otoconia are no longer adhering to the otolithic membrane in the utricle, and they float/fall within the vestibular canals due to the head position and gravity. As they fall, they push endolymph, which either pushes or pulls against the cupula, changing the vestibular nerve firing rate in the stimulated canal, and thereby causing vertigo. BPPV is typically treated by physicians, physical/occupational therapists, or audiologists with canalith repositioning maneuvers where the clinician moves/rotates the patient's head and "roll" the offending otoconia "crystals" back into place.

We classify BPPV into two groups: loose or stuck. *Canalithiasis* is the term used to describe the loose variety and represents >98% of BPPV cases.[37] If we break this word down, we see *lith*, which is a derivation of *lithos* (Greek for "stone"); we also see the word *canal*. So *canalithiasis* refers to a stone that is loose in the canal. *Cupulolithiasis* describes the stuck variety of BPPV. Again, if we break down the word, we see that there is a stone (*lith*) and *cupulo*, referring to the cupula. The word *cupulolithiasis*, therefore, refers to a stone that is stuck on the cupula. There is some controversy regarding cupulolithiasis,[37] with some contributing symptoms to otoconia that are adhered to the cupula, while others believe that the cause is actually a canalith jam where bunches of displaced otoconia covered with an adhesive substance and fragments of the otolithic membrane clump together and become larger than the canal opening, becoming jammed at the opening. Whatever the cause, in this book, cupulolithiasis will refer to apogeotropic nystagmus on a roll test and will indicate the BPPV is resistant to repositioning. Both types of BPPV can be treated by clinicians.

Here is an easy way to understand the crystal movements. Imagine that you take a tire that is sitting on the ground (as if it were on a car) and drill a hole in it, through which you drop a bunch of pebbles. What happens? The pebbles would fall to wherever the ground was, but inside the tire. If you rolled the tire, the pebbles would move and roll inside the tire, again to lowest point closest to the ground. This is what happens in BPPV with otoconia inside the vestibular system. You have a canal that is almost a complete circle and have a bunch of pebbles loose inside (otoconia) that will fall/roll to wherever the bottom happens to be. Unlike the tire, the vestibular canals are full of endolymph fluid. As the otoconia roll, they push the fluid in front of them and pull (like a plunger) the fluid behind them. Depending on the direction of fluid motion, the cupula will bend either toward or away from the utricle. As the cupula moves, the signals from that canal will either increase or decrease compared with the normal resting rate. The signal change depends on the canal that is being stimulated and in which direction the cupula of that canal deflects. Otoconia rolling in one ear will stimulate only that ear. Since both ears are now firing at different rates, the brain interprets the signal difference (asymmetry) as head motion and activates the VOR.

While it is in the anatomical position, the posterior canal sits the lowest (caudal) in the inner ear compared with the other canals. Most BPPV cases involve the posterior canals, as gravity pulls the crystals to the lowest point. However, you may see cases of BPPV in any canal and sometimes in multiple canals simultaneously.

Common complaints from patients with BPPV are as follows:

- "I get dizzy when I roll or get out of bed."
- "I get dizzy when I wash my hair."
- "I get dizzy when I bend over."
- And in the female patient group, "I get dizzy when I go to the hairdresser!"

Interesting facts about BPPV include:

- It is more likely involve the right ear.[38]
- Most cases affect the posterior canal.
- Nystagmus diminishes/fatigues within a treatment session with repeated testing.

MÉNIÈRE'S DISEASE (PRIMARY ENDOLYMPHATIC HYDROPS)

Ménière's disease symptoms include severe vertigo, ear ringing (tinnitus), a feeling of ear fullness, loss of balance called "drop attacks," and eventual hearing loss. These symptoms are caused by the buildup of endolymph that interferes with vestibular and hearing signals. Typically, symptoms begin between the ages of 40 and 60 years, and the disease seems to run in families.[39] There is no definitive test used to make a diagnosis, and there is currently no cure. Diagnostic criteria include the observation of an episodic vertigo syndrome associated with low- to medium-frequency sensorineural hearing loss, fluctuating aural symptoms in the affected ear, and vertigo episodes limited to a period between 20 minutes and 12 hours.[40] It is a progressive disease, and after it runs its course in one ear, it may begin in the contralateral ear. Treatments include medications to relieve symptoms, salt restriction and dietary/behavioral changes, diuretics, gentamicin injections to damage vestibular hair cells (to reduce vertigo), pressure pulse treatment to the inner ear, surgery, cognitive therapy, and alternative medicine. Physical therapy may assist the patient to learn substitution strategies to balance, as well as to use medical equipment such as walkers. Vestibular exercises may be used between vertigo attacks to address differences between ear functions, although some physicians do not agree with this treatment.

PERSISTENT POSTURAL–PERCEPTUAL DIZZINESS (PPPD OR 3PD)

According to the Bárány Society, persistent postural–perceptual dizziness (PPPD; frequently called 3PD) manifests with one or more symptoms that include dizziness, unsteadiness, or non-spinning vertigo. These symptoms are:

- Present on most days for 3 months or more
- Are exacerbated by upright posture, active or passive movement, and exposure to moving or complex visual stimuli

They further state PPPD may be precipitated by conditions that:

- Disrupt balance
- Cause vertigo, or dizziness
- Cause unsteadiness
- May include peripheral or central vestibular disorders, other medical illnesses, or psychological distress

The symptoms cause significant distress and possibly functional impairment and cannot be better accounted for by another disease or disorder.[41]

PPPD is classified as a chronic functional vestibular disorder and is not a structural or psychiatric condition.[41] In most cases, patients present with acute vertigo/dizziness that fades into a chronic condition without a symptom-free interval.

Diagnostic criteria per the Bárány Society include:[41]

1. One or more symptoms of dizziness, unsteadiness, or non-spinning vertigo are present on most days for 3 months or more.
    a. Symptoms last for prolonged (hours-long) periods of time but may wax and wane in severity.
    b. Symptoms need not be present continuously throughout the entire day.
2. Persistent symptoms occur without specific provocation but are exacerbated by three factors:
    a. Upright posture.
    b. Active or passive motion without regard to direction or position.
    c. Exposure to moving visual stimuli or complex visual patterns.
3. The disorder is precipitated by conditions that cause vertigo, unsteadiness, dizziness, or

problems with balance, including acute, episodic, or chronic vestibular syndromes; other neurologic or medical illnesses; or psychological distress.
    a. When the precipitant is an acute or episodic condition, symptoms settle into the pattern of criterion A as the precipitant resolves, but they may occur intermittently at first and then consolidate into a persistent course.
    b. When the precipitant is a chronic syndrome, symptoms may develop slowly at first and worsen gradually.
4. Symptoms cause significant distress or functional impairment.
5. Symptoms are not better accounted for by another disease or disorder.

A neurological examination is generally unremarkable (HINTS, VEMP, MRI/CT, audiogram).[42] Patients with PPPD have lower amplitude of low-frequency fluctuations and lower regional homogeneity in the lower right precuneus (visuospatial imagery, episodic memory retrieval, and self-processing operations) and cuneus regions (visual processing) of the brain.[42]

Treatments include selective serotonin reuptake inhibitors, serotonin and norepinephrine reuptake inhibitors, vestibular balance rehabilitation therapy, and cognitive behavioral therapy.

VESTIBULAR MIGRAINE

Vestibular migraine (VM) is a neurologic condition causing episodic non-positional vertigo associated with other features of migraine and is thought to be the most common cause of spontaneous, non-positional episodic vertigo.[43] Vertigo may last between 5 minutes and 72 hours[44] and may mimic BPPV.[8] Other symptoms that may present include transient auditory symptoms,[45] nausea, vomiting, prostration, unsteadiness, and susceptibility to motion sickness.[44]

Diagnostic criteria for vestibular migraine per the Bárány Society and the Migraine Classification Subcommittee of the International Headache Society (IHS) include:[46]

Table 11.2 How VM Differs from Other Vestibular Disorders

Disease	How the Listed Disease Differs from VM
PPPD	• Symptoms more often than not are present • Symptoms are continuous and ongoing >3 months; VM is episodic
BPPV	• Associated with crescendo–decrescendo nystagmus pattern • Not associated with neurologic or otologic symptoms • Typically triggered only by active motion
Post-concussive syndrome	Typically, symptoms with a trend of improvement after a traumatic event
Ménière's disease	• Aural symptoms more commonly unilateral; VM symptoms more commonly bilateral • Audiogram evidence of sensorineural hearing loss
Stroke/TIA	• Abnormal MRI

1. At least five episodes with vestibular symptoms of moderate or severe intensity lasting 5 minutes to 72 hours
2. Current or previous history of migraine with or without aura, according to the International Classification of Headache Disorders (ICHD-3)
3. One or more migraine features with at least 50% of the vestibular episodes:
   - Headache with at least two of the following characteristics: one-sided location, pulsating quality, moderate or severe pain intensity, aggravation by routine physical activity
   - Photophobia and phonophobia
   - Visual aura
4. Not better accounted for by another vestibular or International Classification of Headache Disorders (ICHD) diagnosis

Diagnostic criteria for probable vestibular migraine:

1. At least 5 episodes with vestibular symptoms of moderate or severe intensity lasting 5 minutes to 72 hours
2. Only one of the criteria B and C for vestibular migraine is fulfilled (migraine history or migraine features during the episode)
3. Not better accounted for by another vestibular of ICHD diagnosis

According to Hac and Gold,[47] differences between VM and other vestibular etiologies are included in Table 11.2.

MAL DE DÉBARQUEMENT (MDD)

Mal de débarquement is a condition causing self-perceived movement after debarking from prolonged passive motion, such as a long boat or airplane ride. Symptoms include a rocking/bobbing sensation, unsteadiness, and disequilibrium, as if one were still on the boat or plane. Symptoms may persist for hours or years (called MdD syndrome).

Diagnosis is made by patient history and ruling out other conditions.[28] The criteria for diagnosis per the International Classification of Vestibular Disorders include:[48]

1. Non-spinning vertigo characterized by an oscillatory perception (rocking, bobbing, or swaying) present continuously or for most of the day
2. Onset occurs within 48 hours after the end of exposure to passive motion
3. Symptoms temporarily reduce with exposure to passive motion (e.g., driving)
4. Symptoms persist for >48 hours

Treatment consists of medications to manage symptoms, stress relief therapy, transcranial magnetic stimulation, and vestibular therapy.

REFERENCES

1. Cook CE, Décary S. Higher order thinking about differential diagnosis. *Brazilian Journal of Physical Therapy*. 2020;24(1):1–7. doi:10.1016/j.bjpt.2019.01.010

2. Lott LD, Kerber K, Lee P, Brown D, Burke J. Diplopia-related ambulatory and emergency department visits in the United States, 2003–2012. *JAMA Ophthalmology.* Dec 1 2017;135(12):1339–1344. doi:10.1001/jamaophthalmol.2017.4508

3. Neuhauser HK. The epidemiology of dizziness and vertigo. *Handbook of Clinical Neurology.* 2016;137:67–82. doi:10.1016/B978-0-444-63437-5.00005-4

4. Langhagen T, Albers L, Heinen F, et al. Period prevalence of dizziness and vertigo in adolescents. *PLoS One.* 2015;10(9):e0136512. doi:10.1371/journal.pone.0136512. PMID: 26361225

5. Hain TC. Outline of causes of dizziness, imbalance and hearing disorders. March 2023. https://dizziness-and-balance.com/disorders/outline.htm

6. Gurley KL, Edlow JA. Acute dizziness. *Seminars in Neurology.* 2019;39(1):27–40. doi:10.1055/s-0038-1676857

7. Dougherty JM, Carney M, Hohman MH, Emmady PD. *Vestibular Dysfunction.* StatPearls Publishing; Updated 2023. https://www.ncbi.nlm.nih.gov/books/NBK558926/

8. Saber Tehrani AS, Kattah JC, Kerber KA, et al. Diagnosing stroke in acute dizziness and vertigo: Pitfalls and pearls. *Stroke.* 2018;49(3):788–795. doi:10.1161/STROKEAHA.117.016979

9. Hausler R, Levine RA. Auditory dysfunction in stroke. *Acta Oto-Laryngologica.* 2000;120:689–703.

10. Chang TP, Wang Z, Winnick AA, et al. Sudden hearing loss with vertigo portends greater stroke risk than sudden hearing loss or vertigo alone. *Journal of Stroke & Cerebrovascular Diseases.* 2018;27(2):472–478. doi:10.1016/j.jstrokecerebrovasdis.2017.09.033

11. Newman-Toker DE, Kerber KA, Hsieh YH, et al. HINTS outperforms ABCD2 to screen for stroke in acute continuous vertigo and dizziness. *Academic Emergency Medicine.* Oct 2013;20(10):986–996. doi:10.1111/acem.12223

12. Newman-Toker DE. Symptoms and signs of neuro-otologic disorders. *Continuum (Minneap Minn).* Oct 2012;18(5 Neuro-Otology):1016–1040. doi:10.1212/01.CON.0000421618.33654.8a

13. Paul NL, Simoni M, Rothwell PM. Transient isolated brainstem symptoms preceding posterior circulation stroke: A population-based study. *Lancet Neurology.* Jan 2013;12(1):65–71. doi:10.1016/s1474-4422(12)70299-5

14. Hoshino T, Nagao T, Mizuno S, Shimizu S, Uchiyama S. Transient neurological attack before vertebrobasilar stroke. *Journal of the Neurological Sciences.* Feb 15 2013;325(1–2):39–42. doi:10.1016/j.jns.2012.11.012

15. Tarnutzer AA, Berkowitz AL, Robinson KA, Hsieh YH, Newman-Toker DE. Does my dizzy patient have a stroke? A systematic review of bedside diagnosis in acute vestibular syndrome. *CMAJ.* Jun 14 2011;183(9):E571–E592. doi:10.1503/cmaj.100174

16. Kattah JC, Talkad AV, Wang DZ, Hsieh YH, Newman-Toker DE. HINTS to diagnose stroke in the acute vestibular syndrome: Three-step bedside oculomotor examination more sensitive than early MRI diffusion-weighted imaging. *Stroke.* Nov 2009;40(11):3504–3510. doi:10.1161/strokeaha.109.551234

17. Gottesman RF, Sharma P, Robinson KA, et al. Clinical characteristics of symptomatic vertebral artery dissection: A systematic review. *Neurologist.* Sep 2012;18(5):245–254. doi:10.1097/NRL.0b013e31826754e1

18. Chalela JA, Kidwell CS, Nentwich LM, et al. Magnetic resonance imaging and computed tomography in emergency assessment of patients with suspected acute stroke: A prospective comparison. *Lancet.* Jan 27 2007;369(9558):293–298. doi:10.1016/s0140-6736(07)60151-2

19. Ozono Y, Kitahara T, Fukushima M, et al. Differential diagnosis of vertigo and dizziness in the emergency department. *Acta Oto-Laryngologica.* Feb 2014;134(2):140–145. doi:10.3109/00016489.2013.832377

20. Newman-Toker DE, Della Santina CC, Blitz AM. Vertigo and hearing loss. *Handbook of Clinical Neurology*. 2016;136:905–921. doi:10.1016/b978-0-444-53486-6.00046-6

21. Zwergal A, Dieterich M. Vertigo and dizziness in the emergency room. *Current Opinion in Neurology*. Feb 2020;33(1):117–125. doi:10.1097/wco.0000000000000769

22. Stanton M, Freeman AM. *Vertigo*. StatPearls Publishing; Updated 2023. https://www.ncbi.nlm.nih.gov/books/NBK482356/

23. Jain S. Diplopia: Diagnosis and management. *Clinical Medicine (London)*. Mar 2022;22(2):104–106. doi:10.7861/clinmed.2022-0045

24. Low L, Shah W, MacEwen CJ. Double vision. *BMJ*. Nov 18 2015;351:h5385. doi:10.1136/bmj.h5385

25. Ward BK, van de Berg R, van Rompaey V, et al. Superior semicircular canal dehiscence syndrome: Diagnostic criteria consensus document of the committee for the classification of vestibular disorders of the Bárány Society. *Journal of Vestibular Research*. 2021;31(3):131–141. doi:10.3233/ves-200004

26. Cooper CW. Vestibular neuronitis: A review of common causes of vertigo in general practice. *British Journal of General Practice*. 1993;43:164–167.

27. Schubert M, Minor L. Vestibulo-ocular physiology underlying vestibular hypofunction. *Physical Therapy*. 2004;84:373–385.

28. Greene J, Al-Dhahir MA. *Acoustic Neuroma*. StatPearls Publishing; 2023. https://www.ncbi.nlm.nih.gov/books/NBK470177/

29. *Mayo Clinic Contributors*. Acoustic neuroma: Treatment and Quality of Life; 2024. https://www.mayoclinic.org/medical-professionals/neurology-neurosurgery/news/acoustic-neuroma-treatment-and-quality-of-life/mac-20429300#:~:text=Acoustic%20neuromas%2C%20which%20develop%20in%20only%20two%20to,hearing%20loss%2C%20tinnitus%2C%20and%20sometimes%20dizziness%20or%20headache.

30. Sarna B, Abouzari M, Merna C, Jamshidi S, Saber T, Djalilian HR. Perilymphatic fistula: A review of classification, etiology, diagnosis, and treatment. *Frontiers in Neurology*. 2020;11:1046. doi:10.3389/fneur.2020.01046

31. Hidaka H, Miyazaki M, Kawase T, Kobayashi T. Traumatic pneumolabyrinth: air location and hearing outcome. *Otology & Neurotology*. 2012;33:123–131. doi:10.1097/MAO.0b013e318241bc91

32. Reilly JS. Congenital perilymphatic fistula: A prospective study in infants and children. *Laryngoscope*. 1989;99:393–397. doi:10.1288/00005537-198904000-00006

33. Thompson TL, Amedee R. Vertigo: A review of common peripheral and central vestibular disorders. *Oschsner Journal*. 2009;9(1):20–26.

34. Lucieer F, Vonk P, Guinand N, Stokroos R, Kingma H, van de Berg R. Bilateral vestibular hypofunction: insights in etiologies, clinical subtypes, and diagnostics. *Frontiers in Neurology*. 2016;7:26. doi:10.3389/fneur.2016.00026

35. Hall CD HS, Whitney SL, Anson ER, Carender WJ, Hoppes CW, Cass SP, Christy JB, Cohen HS, Fife TD, Furman JM, Shepard NT, Clendaniel RA, Dishman JD, Goebel JA, Meldrum D, Ryan C, Wallace RL, Woodward NJ,. Vestibular rehabilitation for peripheral vestibular hypofunction: an updated clinical practice guideline from the Academy of Neurologic Physical Therapy of the American Physical Therapy Association. *Journal of Neurologic Physical Therapy*. 2022;46(2):118–177. doi:10.1097/NPT.0000000000000382

36. Palmeri R, Kumar A. *Benign Paroxysmal Positional Vertigo*. StatPearls Publishing; Updated 2022. https://www.ncbi.nlm.nih.gov/books/NBK470308/

37. Kalmanson O, Foster CA. Cupulolithiasis: A critical reappraisal. *OTO Open*. 2023;7(1):e38. doi:10.1002/oto2.38

38. von Brevern M, Radtke A, Lezius F, Feldmann M, Ziese T, Lempert T, Neuhauser H,. Epidemiology of benign paroxysmal positional vertigo: A population based study. *Journal of Neurology, Neurosurgery, and Psychiatry*. 2007;78(7):710–715. doi:10.1136/jnnp.2006.100420

39. National Institute of Deafness and Other Communication Disorders. *Ménière's Disease*. NIH Publication No. 10–3404. Updated 2017. 2024.

40. Lopez-Escamez JA, Carey J, Chung WH, et al. Diagnostic criteria for Menière's disease. *Journal of Vestibular Research*. 2015;25(1):1–7. doi:10.3233/VES-150549

41. Staab JP, Eckhardt-Henn A, Horii A, Jacob R, Strupp M, Brandt T, Bronstein A. Diagnostic criteria for persistent postural-perceptual dizziness (PPPD): Consensus document of the committee for the Classification of Vestibular Disorders of the Bárány Society. *Journal of Vestibular Research*. 2017;27(4):191–208. doi:10.3233/VES-170622

42. Knight B, Bermudez F, Shermetaro C. *Persistent Postural-Perceptual Dizziness*. StatPearls Publishing; Updated 2023. Accessed 2024. https://www.ncbi.nlm.nih.gov/books/NBK578198/

43. Smyth D, Britton Z, Murdin L, Arshad Q, Kaski D. Vestibular migraine treatment: A comprehensive practical review. *Brain*. 2022;145(11):3741–3754. doi:10.1093/brain/awac264

44. Lempert T, Olesen J, Furman J, et al. Vestibular migraine: Diagnostic criteria1. *Journal of Vestibular Research*. 2022;32(1):1–6. doi:10.3233/VES-201644

45. Kayan A, Hood JD. Neuro-otological manifestations of migraine. *Brain*. 1984;107:1123–1142.

46. Lempert T, Olesen J, Furman J, et al. Vestibular migraine: Diagnostic criteria (Update) 1. *Journal of Vestibular Research*. 2022;32(1):1–6. doi:10.3233/VES-201644

47. Hac NEF, Gold DR. Advances in diagnosis and treatment of vestibular migraine and the vestibular disorders it mimics. *Neurotherapeutics*. Jul 2024;21(4):e00381. doi:10.1016/j.neurot.2024.e00381

48. Cha YH, Baloh RW, Cho C, et al. Mal de débarquement syndrome diagnostic criteria: Consensus document of the Classification Committee of the Bárány Society. *Journal of Vestibular Research*. 2020;30(5):285–293. doi:10.3233/VES-200714

12

Outcome Measures and Documentation

Chapter Goals

1. Describe recommended outcome measures for vision, neurologic conditions (adults), vestibular, stroke, multiple sclerosis, Parkinson's, and spinal cord injury
2. List parts of the plan of care
3. Discuss the creation of goals
4. List questions to ask while taking a patient history
5. Give examples of documentation
6. Discuss the meaning of *dizziness*

OUTCOME MEASURES

Standardized outcome measures are used to quantify a patient's symptoms, abilities, and progress. They may be used to assist in the creation of plans of care and goals, and may be understood across disciplines. They may take the form of physical measurements, timed/scored objective tests, and subjective questionnaires. Recommended outcome measures are broken into categories: vision, adults with neurologic conditions, vestibular, stroke, multiple sclerosis (MS), Parkinson's disease (PD), and spinal cord injury.

VISION

For vision, there seem to be fewer surveys and standardized tests that are not instrumented when compared to tests for balance and fall risk.

Brain Injury Vision Symptom Survey

A self-administered survey that may be used to test baseline and progress with visual therapy related to vision and traumatic brain injury (TBI) is the Brain Injury Vision Symptom Survey (BIVVS). There is a 28-question (full set) and an 18-item reduced set BIVVS. This survey is designed to "query vision behaviors related to: clarity, comfort, diplopia, depth perception, dry-eye, peripheral vision, & reading with individuals who have suffered mild-to-moderate traumatic brain injury (TBI)."[1] It instructs the patient to rate symptoms (Sx) on a 4-point Likert scale. In a study of 107 TBI subjects, 93.5% were able to answer at least 27 or the 28 questions. Sensitivity and specificity were each found to be 83%.[1]

INTERPRETATION OF THE BIVVS

Cutoff scores indicating a significant vision problem are 31 for the 28-item BIVVS and 18 for the 18-item BIVVS.

DOI: 10.1201/9781003524441-12

Convergence Insufficiency Symptom Survey

The Convergence Insufficiency Symptom Survey (CISS) is a 15-item questionnaire that instructs the patient to rate the frequency of occurrence of Sx on a 0–4 Likert scale. The CISS score was associated with the severity of specific convergence insufficiency (CI) among the young adult subjects. Higher scores predicted a greater likelihood of CI and were associated with all the signs of CI. One study found a greater likelihood of identifying CI for those who were symptomatic versus those who were not. The test has been found to be both valid and reliable in both children and adults.[2,3]

INTERPRETATION OF THE CISS

- A score of ≥21 differentiated adults with symptomatic CI from normal adults.[2]

Ocular Motility Tests

There are several tests of ocular motility beyond the bedside exam, however, they are not free, with some requiring hardware. For example, tracking may be tested using the instrumented Developmental Eye Movement Test and King-Devick Test. The RightEye™ automated sensorimotor testing machine is used to test saccades and pursuits.

ADULTS WITH NEUROLOGIC CONDITIONS

The Academy of Neurologic Physical Therapy (ANPT), part of the American Physical Therapy Association (APTA), created a clinical practice guideline to establish the minimum measures needed to quantify the function of balance, walking speed, walking endurance/distance, and transfer ability. They recommend that these tests/measures should be used across all settings (acute, inpatient, outpatient, home health, skilled nursing) for adults with neurologic conditions.[4] All of these measures are free and may be used over time to assess change.[5] Published results recommend:[5]

- *Static and dynamic sitting and standing balance assessment*: Berg Balance Scale (BBS)
- *Walking balance assessment*: Functional Gait Assessment (FGA)
- *Balance confidence assessment*: Activities-Specific Balance Confidence (ABC) Scale
- *Walking speed assessment*: 10-Meter Walk Test
- *Walking distance assessment*: 6-Minute Walk Test
- *Transfer assessment*: 5 Times Sit-to-Stand Test (5×STS)

VESTIBULAR PATIENTS

The following outcome measures were recommended by the Vestibular Evidence Database to Guide Effectiveness (VEDGE) Task Force of the Academy of Neurologic Physical Therapy (American Physical Therapy Association).[6] The recommendation categories included 4, highly recommended; 3, recommended; 2, reasonable to recommend at this time; and 1, not recommended. They categorized recommendations into clinical, academic, and research settings. The entire recommendations are available at www.neuropt .org. There were many tests/measures rated 2. The definition of this category was that the measure has adequate to good psychometric properties and clinical utility; however, it is not free and may require specialized testing equipment that is beyond the means of many clinicians or clinics; or the measure has been validated in other patient populations but not in persons with vestibular deficits; or the measure has only has adequate clinical utility.[6] Next, the measures rated 3 or 4 are listed.

Acute Acuity Recommendations (Rating 3 or 4)

- *Static postural stability*: None recommended
- *Dynamic postural stability*: 4 Square Step Test, Dynamic Gait Index (DGI) (highly recommended)
- *Function/participation*: Activities-Specific Balance Confidence (ABC) Scale, Dizziness Handicap Inventory (DHI) (highly recommended)

Chronic Acuity Recommendations (Rating 3 or 4)

- *Static postural stability*: None recommended
- *Dynamic postural stability*: 4 Square Step Test, DGI (highly recommended), FGA (highly recommended)
- *Function/participation*: ABC Scale, Dizziness Handicap Inventory (DHI) (highly recommended)

There are many tests for static balance testing listed under category 2, reasonable to recommend at this time. However, according to the authors, the measure "is not free and may require access to specialized testing equipment that is beyond the means of many clinicians or clinics, **OR** this measure has been validated in other patient populations but not in persons with vestibular deficits, **OR** this measure has only adequate clinical utility."[5]

QUESTIONNAIRES

Questionnaires assist the clinician in gathering data regarding fall risk, dizziness, and the ability to perform activities of daily living (ADLs) and instrumental activities of daily living (IADLs). They may be given to the patient while they are in the waiting room or mailed to them prior to their appointments. Many questionnaires are available for specific types of patient reports. For example, there are multiple questionnaires that help quantify a patient's perception of their Sx. All self-rating scales are limited by the fact that they are influenced by the patient's level of skill and literacy; also, not all questions necessarily apply to each patient.[7]

Examples of Questionnaires for Balance, Dizziness, and Vestibular Disorders

DIZZINESS HANDICAP INVENTORY (DHI)

The Dizziness Handicap Inventory (DHI) questionnaire is highly recommended by the Vestibular Evidence Database to Guide Effectiveness (VEDGE). The International Classification of Functioning, Disability and Health (ICF)

components included for this questionnaire include body functions and structures, activities, and participation.

The DHI[8] is a popular questionnaire for the assessment of dizziness handicap.[9] It has been tested in geriatric patients as well as others with vestibular disorders, benign paroxysmal positional vertigo (BPPV), dizziness, MS, and brain injury.[10] There are 25 questions that determine dizziness-dependent changes and are grouped into three domains: functional, emotional, and physical. Example questions from each category include:[11]

- *Functional*: Because of your problem, do you have difficulty getting into or out of bed?
- *Emotional*: Because of your problem, do you feel frustrated?
- *Physical*: Does walking down the aisle of a supermarket increase your problems?

A "yes" response is worth 4 points, "sometimes" is worth 2 points, and "no" is worth 0 points.

Scores range from 0 to 100, with higher scores indicating a worse handicap.[12] In the vestibular population, scores may be interpreted as mild handicap (0–30 points), moderate handicap (31–60), and severe handicap (61–100).[13]

Whitney et al. found that the use of answers from only two questions (rolling over in bed and supine-to-sit) also served as a useful tool for predicting the likelihood of BPPV. By summing the scores for these two items, a score of 4 for this two-item subscale indicated a 2.7 times increased likelihood of BPPV, while a patient who had a score of 8 was approximately 4.3 times more likely to have BPPV than one who scored 0.[14]

Zamyslowska-Szmytke et al. found the DHI total scoring and its vestibular subscale distinguished between patients with compensated and uncompensated vestibular dysfunction, that a low score on the positional subscale may suggest any other reason besides BPPV causing patient symptoms, and the total scoring and subscales were correlated with anxiety and depression.[15]

THE ACTIVITIES-SPECIFIC BALANCE CONFIDENCE (ABC) QUESTIONNAIRE

The Activities-Specific Balance Confidence (ABC) questionnaire is recommended by the VEDGE.

The ICF components included for this questionnaire include activities and participation.

The ABC questionnaire assesses self-perceived balance skill by asking patients to choose how confident they are while performing different functional tasks—feeling that they will not lose their balance or become unsteady. This scale has been recommended to be administered to assess self-reported changes in balance confidence in adults with neurologic conditions.[5] This may be self-administered or administered by another person in 10 or 20 minutes. There is a list of 16 different tasks (ABC-16), for each of which the patient chooses 1 of 11 scores by rating the task from 0% to 100% (e.g., 0%, 10%, 20%, etc.), with higher percentages representing more confidence.[16] There is also a six-question short version of the ABC (ABC-6).

The instructions for the ABC are as follows:[16]

Instruct the patient to indicate their level of confidence in doing the activity without losing your balance or becoming unsteady using percentage points on the scale from 0% to 100%. Instruct them to imagine how confident they would be performing an activity if they do not currently do it. They are to rate the items as if they were using any assistive devices that they currently use.

The total possible score range for the long form is from 0 to 1600, which is then divided by 16 to get the ABC score. Score interpretation depends on the patient population:

- *Parkinson's disease*: 69% is predictive of recurrent falls.[17]
- *Chronic stroke*: 81.1.% indicates relative certainty that the patient does not have a history of falls.[18]
- *Older adults*: <67% indicates risk for falling.[19]
- *Vestibular disorders*: <67% indicates a risk for falling.[19]
- *Multiple sclerosis*: ≤70% (ABC-16) and ≤ 65% (ABC-6) identify fallers.[20]

This questionnaire gives you a structured way to interview a patient about balance problems. It has been tested in the following populations: the elderly and patients with multiple sclerosis, Parkinson's disease, nonspecific patients, vestibular disorders,[21] and lower limb amputees.

STROKE

Core Set of Outcome Measures for Stroke Patients

According to Pohl et al., outcome measures regarding stroke operate on a national level and lack international consensus.[22] Because of this, they set out to gain consensus from 33 experts from 18 countries and published the results, summarized next.[22] These experts recommended measurement time points of days 2±1 and 7; weeks 2, 4, and 12; and 6 months poststroke and every following sixth month.

- Fugl-Meyer Assessment (FMA)
- 10-Meter Walk Test
- Timed Up-and-Go (TUG)
- Berg Balance Scale (BBS)
- Barthel Index (BI)
- Functional Independence Measure (FIM) for the ADL/stroke-specific section
- Stroke Impact Scale (SIS)

Outcome Measures for the Upper Extremity after Stroke

- Fugl-Meyer Assessment of Upper Extremity (FMA-UE)
- Action Research Arm Test (ARAT)

Outcome Measures for the Lower Extremity after Stroke

- Fugl-Meyer Assessment of the Lower Extremity (FMA-LE)
- 10-Meter Walk Test

Outcome Measures for the Active Domains

- TUG
- BBS

Outcome Measures for ADL/Stroke-Specific

- National Institutes of Health (NIH) Stroke Scale
- BI or FIM

Outcome Measures—All International Classification of Functioning (ICF), Disability and Health Domains

- SIS

MULTIPLE SCLEROSIS (MS)

The ANPT's Multiple Sclerosis Task Force reviewed 63 outcome measures for MS, and recommended measures for acute care, in-patient rehab, home health, skilled nursing facilities, and outpatient clinic settings. The full list is available at ANPT's website (www.neuropt.org); here we will only review the highly recommended measures. Results have been published.[23]

Highly Recommended Measures

- 12-Item MS Walking Scale
- 6-Minute Walk Test
- 9-Hole Peg Test
- BBS
- Dizziness Handicap Inventory (outpatient settings only)
- MS Functional Composite (outpatient settings only)
- MS Impact Scale (MSIS-29)
- MS Quality of Lift (MS Qol-54)
- Timed 25-Foot Walk
- TUG (Cognitive and Manual)

PARKINSON'S DISEASE

The ANPT's Parkinson's Disease Task Force reviewed 60 outcome measures and formulated and published recommended outcome measures.[24] The complete materials are available via the ANPT's website (www.neuropt.org), with highly recommended measures listed next, divided into ICF classifications. Next to each measure is the recommended Hoehn and Yahr (H&Y) disease stage appropriate for the test.

Body Structure and Function

- Movement Disorder Society-Sponsored Revision of the Unified Parkinson's Disease Rating Scale (MDS-UPDRS)—Part 3 (H&Y I, II, III, IV, V)
- MDS-UPDRS—Part 1
- Montreal Cognitive Assessment (MoCA) (H&Y I, II, III, IV)

Activity

- 6-Minute Walk Test (H&Y I, II, III, IV)
- 10-Meter Walk Test (H&Y I, II, III, IV)
- Mini-Balance Evaluation Systems Test (Mini-BESTest) (H&Y I, II, III, IV)
- MDS-UPDRS—Part 2
- FGA (H&Y I, II, III, IV)
- 5xSTS (H&Y I, II, III, IV)
- 9-Hole Peg Test (H&Y I, II, III, IV)

Participation

- Parkinson's Disease Questionnaire, short version (PDQ-8) (H&Y I, II, III, IV, V)
- PDQ-39 (H&Y I, II, III, IV, V)

Specific Constructs

- Freezing of Gait Questionnaire (H&Y II, III, IV)
- Parkinson's Fatigue Scale (H&Y I, II, III, IV, V)
- ABC Scale (for fear of falling) (H&Y I, II, III, IV)
- TUG-Cognitive (to test dual task) (H&Y I, II, III)

3-Meter Backward Walk Test (3MBWT)

The 3MBWT tests the patient's ability to ambulate backward. It has demonstrated excellent test–retest reliability (ICC = 0.965), a minimal detectable change (MDC) of 2.13 seconds, and has high correlations with other outcome measures.[25] The cutoff time that best discriminates fallers from non-fallers with PD was 10.31 seconds.[25]

SPINAL CORD INJURY (SCI)

The SCI Taskforce of the ANPT reviewed 63 outcome measures for individuals with SCI, recommended and published those that entry-level students should be made aware and learn to administer.[26] The full list of recommendations is available via the ANPT website (www.neuropt.org).

Students Should Learn

- 6-Minute Walk Test
- 10-Meter Walk Test
- ASIA Impairment Scale
- BBS
- FIM
- Handheld Myometer
- Manual Muscle Test
- Numeric Pain Rating Scale
- TUG

TAKING A PATIENT HISTORY

Before you begin taking a patient's history, it is important to introduce yourself and anyone who accompanies you into the patient's room. Confirm you are speaking with the patient by using a patient identifier (such as name and date of birth). Ask permission to ask questions. When possible, sit in a chair a few feet away and at the same eye level while taking a history. If the patient is a minor, make sure there is another adult present in the room, even if it is a coworker or employee, if a family member is not available, and document their presence.

According to the APTA, the following elements may be included in a history: general demographics, social history, employment/work/school/play, growth and development, living environment, general health status, social/health habits, family history, medical/surgical history, current condition/chief clinical report, functional status and activity level, medications, and other clinical tests.[27]

According to the American Occupational Therapy Association (AOTA), the essential components of an occupational therapy evaluation include (1) an "occupational profile" consisting of

a summary of the patient's occupational history and experiences, patterns of daily living, interests, values, needs, and relevant contexts; and (2) an analysis of occupational performance.[28] There are several AOTA Evaluation & Quality Measures Checklists available on the AOTA website (www.aota.org).

What makes a patient's history important? About 75% of the time, a diagnosis can be determined on the basis of a history alone.[29] You can get much if not most of the information you need to begin your investigation by carefully questioning and listening to the patient during the history-taking process. The way you ask questions is critical if you want to get information that is helpful. Patients do not always make this process easy. Often, they tell you things that have no bearing on their current clinical report, or the family members want to interject and discuss their own past medical history (PMH) or symptoms. At times this may require you to interrupt a patient and gently redirect the conversation to more quickly get to the relevant information. You can use phrases such as:

- "I'll answer all of your questions when we are through with the examination, but right now we have a lot of things to look at. Is that OK?"
- "Because we have such little time together, for now let's focus on (state the reason the patient came to see you). Is that OK?"

Questions to Ask Regarding Dizziness

It can be difficult to get a clear description of dizziness. You may ask, "What do you mean when you say you feel dizzy?" Often, the patient may provide other nonhelpful descriptors, such as woozy, or worse, the patient may reply with nonessential information offering a statement such as, "In 1964, when my husband had his hip replaced..." In these circumstances, it may be helpful to limit the patient's choices in discussing dizziness by providing descriptors from which to choose. Phrase your question in a similar way to the following: "When you say you are dizzy, do you mean you feel lightheaded, that you see or feel the room spin, that you are off balance, or something else, like floating?"

If a fall is part of the patient's history, make sure you find out the circumstances surrounding it. What activity was the patient doing when they fell? Describe the environment (light, dark, firm or unstable standing surface, inside/outside, etc.). Was the patient standing still or moving when they fell? Has the patient fallen before, and if so, how often and when? What type of shoe was the patient wearing during the fall? Was the patient ascending/descending stairs or stepping over anything? Was the patient using an assistive device (walker, cane)? Do they own an assistive device and who gave it to them?

While there are a few questions that are unique to the dizzy patient, most questions for the patient report of dizziness/balance problems are the same as those you already use when questioning any patient. They include but may not be limited to:

- A description of the current clinical report.
  - Make sure not to interrupt the patient's first few sentences. Prompt the patient to give information regarding their Sx.
    - Timing (onset, duration of Sx when present, time of day Sx are present).
    - Triggers: Alleviating/Exacerbating factors.
    - Severity.
    - Character of symptoms (description).
  - "Associated symptoms that would suggest a central (neurologic) etiology, such as dysarthria, dysphagia, diplopia, truncal ataxia, or cerebellar signs."[30]
  - "Associated signs and symptoms may suggest a cardiovascular etiology, such as chest pain, arrhythmia, dyspnea, or orthostatic blood pressure changes."[30]
  - Any reports of dizziness (vertigo vs. non-vertigo).
- Drugs/Medications
  - PMH including any chronic medications (and when last taken).
  - Any recent changes to medications.
  - When did you last take any sedating medications, such as antihistamines, benzodiazepines, or anticholinergics? (These drugs may skew test results by suppressing eye motions.)

- Do they take antidepressants and antipsychotic agents? (They may impair oculomotor function and cause loss of balance.)
- Any other drugs taken: Over the counter, illicit/recreational (and when last taken/used).
- Any recent head trauma, falls, near-falls, or car accidents within the last year.
- Describe the living situation, including a description of their living accommodations.
  - Stairs/steps.
  - Durable medical equipment (DME), and when they use it.
  - Do they live alone?
  - Have prescription spectacles (eyeglasses)?
- Any recent changes to vision/eyeglasses prescription/hearing?

While these questions gather most of the information regarding symptoms, there are some additional questions you should ask that are unique to dizziness. These questions include the following:

- Worse in a specific body/head position or motion?
- Worse in light or darkness? (This question helps to differentiate between central causes that may be worse in the light and peripheral vestibulopathy, which may be worse in the dark.)
- Provoked by visually stimulating environments? (Points to vestibular or vision issues.)
  - While watching TV.
  - Walking in grocery stores or shopping malls.
  - When watching cross traffic while in a car.
  - When seeing moving ceiling fans.
- Any dizziness reports?
  - If dizzy, what does *dizzy* mean?
    - Vertigo (seeing or feeling the room move).
    - Disequilibrium (being off balance).
    - Lightheadedness (presyncope).
    - Floating sensations.
  - Any previous history of dizziness? (This helps to differentiate various conditions, like BPPV or Ménière's syndrome.)
  - Any previous treatment or tests for dizziness?

- Patient's goal (typically the resolution of symptoms, but sometimes they give examples of ADL performance or activities they have been having difficulty with).

Ask about the patient's ability to perform functional movements. Is the patient having trouble ambulating or performing ADLs? It is very common for elderly patients who have balance problems to deny any issues. When asked if they have any difficulties ambulating or performing ADLs, they report that they are doing just fine. When you ask the patient if they touch furniture when they walk around the house or perform ADLs, they tend to think that *if* they can function by holding onto furniture or walls while walking, they *can* function and must be OK. However, a positive answer to this question reveals an underlying balance problem. During your history taking, you want to be able to create a list of physical deficits as well as a list of functional ones.

A Discussion about Dizziness

WHAT DOES *DIZZY* MEAN?

Often clinicians fail to ask the right questions to figure out what the patient means when saying, "I'm dizzy." As you know, there are many different causes of dizziness. When a patient says they feel dizzy, this may mean a variety of things because the word *dizzy* is an umbrella term that may include a sensation of movement (vertigo), lightheadedness (presyncope), lack of balance (disequilibrium), or a "floating out of the body" feeling. Each of these descriptors is very different from the others, yet they may all fall into the category of dizziness. The problem with using only patient descriptions to diagnose conditions is that "descriptions of the quality of dizziness are unclear, inconsistent, and unreliable, casting doubt on the validity of the traditional approach to the patient with dizziness."[31] Patients also use the term *vertigo* synonymously with *dizziness* not understanding the true meaning of the word.

Patients may have multiple "dizziness" sensations occurring at the same time. If you wish to have the patients describe their reports of dizziness, give this list to patients and ask them to choose the descriptors that best fit their reports by asking them to choose one or more of the following:

When you say you are dizzy (or vertigo), do you mean that you:

- See or feel the room spin?
- Feel lightheaded?
- Feel off balance?
- Or something else (floating)?

An impaired vestibular system, or even a central deficit affecting the vestibular system from a stroke or even MS may produce a sensation of vertigo (movement, usually spinning for vestibulopathy but may also be a room shift for MS). Knowing this, if the patient reports true vertigo, you may suspect that the vestibular system is somehow involved.

Feelings of lightheadedness have multiple etiologies but are commonly caused by things like orthostatic hypotension, hypoglycemia, cardiac arrhythmias, medication side effects, anxiety, and even vestibular dysfunction. When a patient reports feeling off balance, the descriptor is not by itself enough to give you a hint of where to look for a problem.

The last descriptor is "something else." Some patients report a feeling of floating out of their bodies. These sensations are usually caused by either psychiatric issues or central nervous system problems. However, floating sensations have also been reported by patients who are experiencing early symptoms of brain tumors.

It has been suggested that by inquiring about dizziness, *timing and triggers* may be a better way to question patients.[32] In some cases, the time of symptom occurrence is itself a clue. For example, when a patient reports being dizzy upon getting up in the morning, it is helpful to ask what happens when they lie down or rolls in bed. This will help you differentiate between BPPV (occurs when pitching the head when getting up and lying down), orthostatic hypotension (occurs when getting up only), and hypoglycemia (in which the Sx is constant). If the patient is diabetic, you may consider assessing blood sugar at different times of the day. If the patient has a history of cardiac problems, you may wish to have their blood pressure recorded at different times of the day.

The patient history can reveal very important data but may require skilled questioning to uncover the needed information. Open-ended questions asking someone to describe their Sx can be very imprecise and of limited value with regard to dizziness. A study of 300 acutely dizzy patients presenting to the emergency room showed the type of dizziness to be an imprecise metric, with more than half of the patients unable to reliably report which symptom type most accurately reflected their clinical reports.[20]

TIMING AND TRIGGERS

A newer approach to patient inquiry when it comes to dizziness divides patients into three categories using timing and triggers:[32]

1. *Acute vestibular syndrome*: Exam differentiates vestibular neuritis from stroke.
2. *Spontaneous episodic vestibular syndrome*: Exam differentiates vestibular migraine from a transient ischemic attack (TIA).
3. *Triggered episodic vestibular syndrome*: Exam differentiates BPPV from posterior fossa structural lesions.

Edlow et al. point out that dizziness is frequently misdiagnosed, in part due to the traditional approach of relying on dizziness Sx quality or type to guide inquiry that does not distinguish between dangerous causes and is inconsistent with current best evidence.[32] Almost 10% of strokes are misdiagnosed, and these patients are more likely to be under the age of 50, women, and minorities.[33] In a 2007 study of emergency room patients, the subjects were asked questions to determine the reliability and consistency of eliciting symptom quality (i.e., describe your dizziness). When the question was asked again, an average of 6 minutes later, half of the patients changed their primary dizziness type, and more than 60% endorsed more than one type of dizziness.[31,32,34] Does this mean that you should never ask a patient to describe their dizziness? No. It does mean that you should not base your diagnosis solely on the description they give and to include timing and trigger questions. According to Gurley and Edlow, patients are far more consistent in their responses to timing and triggers than they are for dizziness type.[33]

Example Cases Where Careful Questioning Assisted the Examination

Discussed next are four true-life examples of how careful questioning as well as a thorough examination assisted in determining the cause of dizziness.

Example 1 involves a male patient whose primary clinical report was dizziness. The patient was given sedating medication to treat the dizziness and was referred to a physical therapist. At the therapy office, he was asked to choose a descriptor from a list (lightheaded, off balance, room spinning, or other) and chose lightheadedness. Next, the patient was asked to explain when (timing) he became lightheaded or dizzy. Was he lightheaded at certain times of day or in certain circumstances (triggers)? The response was that he typically woke up dizzy but felt better after eating breakfast. Then he became dizzy again around lunchtime and again in the early evening. Eating seemed to resolve each episode. Further questioning revealed that this patient was diabetic, even though this fact was not reflected in his medication list. After reviewing this interaction, what type of issue do you suspect this patient may be having? What tests should be performed? Which members of the health care team would best assess the suspected issues? These symptoms are common for patients who have blood sugar irregularities. Even though the patient history was not suggestive of a vestibular issue, a thorough assessment was performed, and it was negative for vestibular or central deficits. The patient was referred back to the physician with the suggestion to investigate blood sugars.

Example 2 involves an elderly woman who told her doctor that she was dizzy. This patient was given a benzodiazepine to control the dizziness and sent to a physical therapist. When asked what *dizzy* meant, the patient said that she felt off balance and unable to walk a straight line when ambulating (timing and trigger). She denied any lightheadedness or vertigo. While a therapy evaluation was indicated, the choice of medication for this patient may not have been the best option, as classes of medications used to treat dizziness, such as benzodiazepines, antiarrhythmics, digoxin, diuretics, sedatives, psychotropics, and other medications that patients may be on, such as antidepressants, have been associated with increased falls.[35,36] This patient, who had a balance problem, was given a medication known to be statistically associated with falls because she used the word *dizzy* to describe her problem of disequilibrium. Obviously, there are times when these medications are not only indicated but also very helpful. Good history-taking questions will guide the clinician toward the best treatment and intervention.

Example 3 is that of a young woman in her late 20s who reported dizziness and had sensations of movement (vertigo). These sensations did not seem to be provoked by motion or position. She was not taking any prescribed medications. The examination ruled out vestibular issues, but the patient had an abnormal oculomotor examination (vertical skew with alternate cover test). Are there any red flags for this patient? The patient was young, female, and dizzy, with a central sign (vertical skew deviation). This patient was referred to neurology, and a magnetic resonance imaging revealed neural plaque consistent with multiple sclerosis. Her age, gender, and positive central sign were initial clues that multiple sclerosis could be causing her dizziness.

Example 4 is a middle-aged male reporting dizziness when getting out of bed. Careful questioning revealed he became vertiginous also when lying down, but not when sitting or lying still. The timing and triggers led the examiner to perform tests of BPPV, which were positive. The patient was treated for BPPV and released on the same visit.

To summarize, the patient history adds immense value to the clinical examination in the following ways:

- Providing clues based on the patient's subjective symptom, timing, and triggers to help guide the examination
- Helping the examiner to form a hypothesis as to the etiology of the patient's clinical report and arrive at a diagnosis
- Identifying previously performed tests

- Identifying any medications that may be additive to the patients' current reports
- Identifying medications that may impede the examination or impair progress
- Alerting the clinician to patient conditions that require the expertise of other health professionals
- Uncovering the patient's goals for seeking treatment

DOCUMENTATION

In 2001, the World Health Organization (WHO) implemented the International Classification of Functioning, Disability and Health (ICF) to measure health and disability at both individual and population levels, focusing on three domains:

1. Body functions (physiological functions of body systems) and structures (anatomical body parts).
2. Activities (individual and societal levels) are the execution of a task or action by an individual.
3. Participation is involvement in a life situation.

These three domains are used to describe functioning and disability in relation to health conditions, as well as the environmental and personal factors that impact them. A detailed description of the ICF as well as learning tools are available on the WHO website.[37] According to the WHO, the ICF provides a scientific basis for understanding health, a common language for describing health and health-related states, allows comparison of data across countries and health care disciplines, and provides a systematic coding scheme. Qualifiers are used to describe the "magnitude of the level of health or severity of the problem."[38]

Most documentation contains these four components: subjective, objective, assessment, and plan. They may have different labels, but the information is the same.

The subjective section allows the practitioner to record the patient's subjective experiences and personal views of the patient or caregiver.[39] Here you will record the patient's chief clinical report(s), current medications/allergies, history (medical, surgical, family, social), and questions regarding a "review of systems" that may help uncover Sx not otherwise mentioned.[39] The objective section contains things you observe, measure, or record, such as vital signs, physical examination findings, laboratory data, imaging results, other diagnostic data, and recognition and review of the documentation of other clinicians.[39] The assessment section synthesizes the subjective and objective evidence to arrive at a diagnosis (Dx).[39] It includes a list of problems in order of importance, and a list of different possible Dx from most to least likely.[39] Finally, the plan section includes steps to be taken to treat the patient, including the need for additional testing and consultation with other clinicians.[39]

PLAN OF CARE (POC)

The plan of care (POC) is your roadmap to treating your patient. According to the Centers for Disease Control and Prevention (CDC), medical practitioners should include the following in their POC:[40]

1. Patient name, date of birth, and contact information
2. Health condition(s)
3. Medicines, dosages, and when/how they are given
4. Health care providers with contact information
5. Health insurance information
6. Emergency contacts

The APTA guidelines call for the POC to include:[27]

- Overall goals stated in measurable terms that indicate the predicted level of improvement in functioning
- A general statement of interventions to be used
- Proposed duration and frequency of service required to reach the goals
- Anticipated discharge plans

GOALS

When writing goals, a good way to remember the components is using the acronym *SMART*. A SMART goal is specific, measurable, achievable, relevant, and time-bound. If you are a physical or occupational therapist, the goal should include a function (e.g., walking, transferring, performing an ADL).

- *Specific*: Clearly articulate what will be accomplished.
- *Measurable*: Quantify the goal in order to track progress.
- *Achievable*: The goals should be realistic, which will keep the patient engaged in trying to achieve them. You can always update patient goals! When the patient achieves a goal, increase its difficulty, distance, time, or write a new goal.
- *Relevant*: The goal should be in line with the plan of care.
- *Time-bound*: Give a deadline for the achievement of the goal (both short- and long-term goals).

An example of a SMART goal from a physical therapist:

> The patient will improve ambulation distance from 60′ to 100′, independently using a straight cane with a step-through gait pattern within 2 weeks in order to allow access to her mailbox.

An example of a SMART goal from a physical therapist:

> The patient will perform upper extremity dressing with an improvement from mod verbal cues to minimal verbal cues within 2 weeks to increase independence in the home.

You will notice that we did not make an outcome measure a goal. For example, a goal should not be: "The patient will score 41/56 on the Berg Balance Scale in 2 weeks." You may, however, use an outcome measure as evidence of improvement. *For example*: "The patient will improve dynamic standing balance (Specific) in 2 weeks (Time-bound), as evidenced by a Berg Balance Scale score increase from 30 to >40 (Measurable and Achievable), to decrease risk of falls in the home." In the second example, the goal is not to score a certain number, but instead to reduce fall risk (relevant).

A POC that includes *vestibular rehabilitation therapy*, or *vestibular rehab (VR)* for short, encompasses more than just interventions for an impaired vestibular system. It includes interventions that address *any system* that contributes to balance and functional movement. The patient in VR may have interventions for any of the systems of balance (oculomotor, vestibular, somatosensory, cerebellar, and musculoskeletal). They may have interventions that address specific functional limitations or activities (e.g., gait, ADLs). The goal of these interventions is ultimately to return the patient to improved function or to reduce Sx that may impair function. Sometimes these interventions induce changes in the system that is targeted by the exercise, while at other times they act as a stimulus forcing the patient to find different ways to collect/process information or perform a given task when a particular system is deficient.

There are various methods to document a patient encounter. The basic *SOAP* note method involves recording the patient's *s*ubjective report, *o*bjective measures that are observed or taken, the clinician's *a*ssessment of the patient's condition, and the *p*lan. Another method to remember these parts of the clinical note is to separate information gained from a patient encounter using *P-ABC-P*.

- **P**: Prior List the previous medical history (including medications), any previous episode of the patient's current medical issue, any prior tests or treatments, and outcomes. The patient's subjective story also falls under the prior category. It answers the question, "What has already happened?"
- **A**: Actions Any recorded measures taken or intervention actions by the clinician, any activity or exercise the patient performs (that is to say, the patient's treatment), how they perform, and their tolerance/disposition after the treatment/exercise.
- **B**: Behaviors Any observations of the patient made by the clinician (e.g., gait patterns, posture, observed avoidance behaviors).
- **C**: Conclusion The clinician's assessment of the patient's condition.
- **P**: Plan The clinician's plan of care.

EXAMPLES OF DOCUMENTATION

Balance and Gait Documentation

Observations made during interventions or evaluations should lead to the documentation of any deficiencies, limitations, or substitutions. Descriptions of gait should describe any problems observed during the gait cycle, such as a short step length, the lack of heel strike or toe off, asymmetrical stance time between the limbs, circumduction in swing phase, hip hiking, and loss of balance. For therapists documenting balance and gait interventions, remember to show the skill involved. Simply describing the exercise, activity, or distance a patient ambulated is not enough to justify reimbursement. Describing the gait shows why the clinician was needed, as a layman would likely not be able to observe these signs and know how to address them.

After noting your intervention, exercise, or activity, ask yourself if it is something your nonclinical neighbor could have done. If it is, you probably need to add phrases to show the skill you provided to instruct or improve the patient's ability to ambulate or perform an exercise. Some examples include the following.

Verbal cues were needed to:

- Improve step length
- Increase heel strike
- Narrow stance width

Tactile cues were needed to:

- Recover loss of balance
- Correct placement of walker
- Initiate hip abductor activation

An example of documentation reflecting gait training:

> *Therapist's note*: "Ambulated 150 feet × 2, min assist with rolling walker."

Looking at this example, we need to ask ourselves if the neighbor could ambulate with the patient for 150 feet. they probably could. The phrase "min assist" does not by itself show skill. Could the neighbor offer min assist to the patient? No skill is evident in this example. Next, is 150 feet significant in some way? Does the patient need to walk 150 to be functional within their environment, such as to reach his mailbox, or is this an improvement in distance to reach the goal of ambulating to the mailbox? Finally, a description of the gait mechanics is missing, as well as any instruction that improved it. To improve this note, first, indicate how the skill of a therapist can improve the patient's gait and thereby make patient more functional in their environment or reduce fall risk. How do you show skill during gait training? Helpful phrases such as "Verbal cues needed for …" and "Tactile cues needed to …" help you show that you have provided professional skill that will improve the patient's condition.

Improved example:

Ambulated 150 feet × 2 (distance from bedroom to kitchen) with min assistance using a rolling walker. Verbal cues were needed to increase knee extension in terminal swing phase and to increase heel strike to reduce fall risk. Tactile cues were needed to instruct proper advancement and placement of the walker for gait stability.

Now let's look at an example of a balance exercise. Like the first example, it will not be ideal, and we will use this as a way to highlight ways to document meaningful exercises.

Therapist's balance exercise note:

Performed balance exercises × 15.

Can you identify what is missing in this example? Which balance exercise? What were the deficiencies during patient performance that required the skill of a therapist? What skilled interventions were provided during the exercise? What does 15 represent: time or repetitions? Remember, the exercise should address a deficit you record in your evaluation or add to the plan of care later. If the exercise or activity does not reflect the evaluation findings or plan of care, a reviewer may question its need.

Example of an improved balance note:

Diagonal weight shifting × 15 reps (holding the final stance position 3 seconds) to an advanced right foot. Tactile cues were needed for instructing positioning of the center of gravity over the base of support and for proprioceptive cues to maintain balance while in asymmetrical stance. Loss of balance × 3 was corrected with minimal tactile cues during the exercise.

Documentation of Vestibular Rehab

In documenting a vestibular test, document the name of the test, which ear was tested, any modifications you made, and findings. For cases of BPPV, describe:

- The test used
- The involved ear
- The involved canal (describe nystagmus)
- Classification of canalithiasis vs cupulolithiasis
- Which canalith repositioning maneuvers were performed, and outcome/disposition post-maneuver

The plan of care should list "canalith repositioning" as the intervention when you plan to use repositioning maneuvers. Avoid naming maneuvers, such as "the Epley maneuver," in your plan of care, as this will limit your choice of interventions. By using the broad category of canalith repositioning, you may use any number of maneuvers that you will describe in your treatment documentation.

TESTS FOR BENIGN PAROXYSMAL POSITIONAL VERTIGO

Example of a Canalithiasis Evaluation

Positive Dix–Hallpike for right posterior canal canalithiasis. (Latency ~5 seconds. Right torsional and upbeating nystagmus observed <1 min.)

The use of the word "positive" indicates the presence of BPPV. Next, the name of the test that was employed is documented: "Dix-Hallpike." The words "right posterior canal" indicate that the involved canal and the ear that was tested. The use of "canalithiasis" indicates loose crystals, that observed nystagmus lasted less than 1 minute, and that it had a latency prior to onset. This description of nystagmus justifies the diagnosis of right posterior canalithiasis. If you are sending a report to another clinician who may not have a lot of vestibular patients or experience reading reports regarding vestibular tests, it is often helpful to include the description of nystagmus.

Example BPPV of an Intervention

Performed canalith repositioning maneuvers for the treatment of BPPV, including the modified Epley × 2, Semont-liberatory × 1. Minimal nausea reported. Negative Dix–Hallpike following repositioning.

Your plan for this patient would include retesting for BPPV at the next clinical visit.

Example of a Cupulolithiasis Evaluation

Positive Dix–Hallpike for right posterior canal cupulolithiasis.

This note indicates that:

- The test used was the Dix–Hallpike.
- The right ear was tested.
- BPPV was found (i.e., the test was positive).
- The involved canal was the posterior.

"Cupulolithiasis" implies an immediate onset of nystagmus that lasted longer than a minute and that crystals were either stuck to the cupula or trapped in the short arm of the canal.

While not required, you could write a more descriptive note describing the latency and duration of nystagmus. The term "cupulolithiasis" already implies this information, but sometimes it is good to describe, depending on the intended audience of the note.

A more descriptive example:

Positive Dix–Hallpike for right posterior canal cupulolithiasis with right-torsional and upbeating nystagmus. Latency: none; duration >60 seconds. The patient was taken out of the test position after 60 seconds.

TESTS OF VESTIBULAR FUNCTION

These examples review how to describe positive bedside tests of the VOR and oculomotor observations and tests. Descriptions reflect positive test results. Negative tests indicate normal function.

We will use a patient who has a left unilateral vestibular loss for our example.

- *Example*: Positive left head thrust test indicating possible left unilateral vestibular weakness.
- *Example*: Positive head shake test with right-beating post-head shake nystagmus, indicating a possible left unilateral vestibular weakness.

Remember, if you find positive tests of VOR function, recommend further testing, such as an electronystagmography/audiography to help confirm vestibular loss and rule out central pathologies.

VESTIBULAR REHAB TREATMENT EXAMPLES

In general, describe or name the exercise/activity, time or repetition performed, patient tolerance, and the skill involved.

- *Example*: Performed VOR × 1, 2 × 1 min with verbal cues needed to keep frequency of head motion >0.5 Hz. The patient became slightly nauseous and required 2 minutes to recover after exercise.
- *Example*: Performed motion habituation exercise of seated left-ear to left knee × 15 reps with verbal cues for timing and head position. Positions were held until dizziness symptoms lessened (less than 40 seconds were required for each repetition).

For therapists, when documenting exercises and interventions, it is extremely important to include the skill that was used. This is easy to do if you get used to including phrases like, "Verbal cues needed for …" and "Tactile cues needed to …" Without an explanation of the clinician's skill, many insurance companies refuse to pay for the service. Read your clinical note and ask yourself if the described intervention could be performed by the patient's neighbor.

Oculomotor Function Test Examples

FIXATION

Document any inability to maintain fixation.

- *Example*: Ms. Smith is unable to maintain fixation for longer than 5 seconds.

GAZE NYSTAGMUS

You should recall that there should be no observed nystagmus prior to near end-ranges. If noted, you should document how many beats of nystagmus you see and in which direction they are beating. Vertical gaze nystagmus typically represents a central finding.

- *Example*: Positive right-gaze nystagmus at 45 degrees, >3 beats, with increased quick phases with rightward gaze, indicating a possible vestibular asymmetry (e.g., left unilateral vestibular loss).
- *Example*: Positive right-gaze nystagmus at end-range, >3 beats observed, indicating a possible vestibular asymmetry (e.g., left unilateral vestibular loss). No other gaze nystagmus noted.
- *Example*: Positive up-gaze nystagmus representing a possible central finding.
- *Example*: Positive left-gaze nystagmus of 3 beats (likely physiological).

Remember, if you find positive gaze nystagmus, recommend further testing, such as an electronystagmography/audiography, to help confirm vestibular loss and rule out central pathologies.

SMOOTH PURSUIT

When patients lack smooth pursuit, they will use saccades (if available) to substitute. In a positive test, the patient is unable to generate smooth tracking motions, and you will see a series of saccades.

Document this as positive saccadic smooth pursuit. If the patient is near or over the age of 60, this may be an age-related change and may be documented as such.

- *Example*: There is a lack of smooth pursuit, with the patient substituting saccades. As she is <60 years of age, further assessment may be warranted.
- *Example*: There is a lack of smooth pursuit, with the patient substituting saccades. As she is >60 years of age this is likely an age-related change.

SACCADES

Deficiencies you will record are:

- *Hypometric saccades*, which are undershooting saccades with >2 required to reach targets held within the patient's visual field.
- *Hypermetric saccades*, which are overshooting saccades with a corrective saccade in the reverse direction required after the eyes pass the target. This was repeatable.

OCULAR RANGE OF MOTION

Document any loss of range, such as:

- Limited upward gaze
- Inability to perform upward gaze
- Limited left gaze to the left eye—does not move left past primary gaze position

VERGENCE

Vergence limitations are noted at bedside, usually by a limitation of binocular fusion during convergence. Measure the distance from the tip of the patient's nose to the point where they lose fusion.

- *Example*: Vergence to 25 cm prior to loss of fusion and reports of diplopia.
- *Example*: Convergence insufficiency with diplopia reported at 25 cm.

COVER TESTS

The terminology of eye motions and positions can be intimidating, especially when not used routinely. Recall that the unilateral cover test checks for heterotropia (also known as *manifest strabismus*), which is an abnormal eye deviation. Document the following abnormalities:

- Any corrective eye motion during testing of the uncovered eye
- The eye position noted during the unilateral cover test: Exotropia, esotropia, hypertropia, hypotropia
- The eye position noted during the alternate cover test: Exophoria, esophoria, hyperphoria, hypophoria
- Which eye is involved or if both are positive
  - *Example*: Positive right eye esotropia during unilateral cover test.
  - *Example*: Positive left eye hypophoria during the alternate cover test.

If you cannot recall these terms, use the word *strabismus*, which is a general term describing improper alignment of the eyes, and include if the eyes were moving laterally or vertically. Recall that vertical skews are significant central findings.

- *Example*: Positive unilateral cover test with a left eye lateral strabismus.
- *Example*: Positive alternating cover test with vertical strabismus bilaterally, recommend further investigation.

This general description is enough for an oculomotor specialist, such as a neurologist; neurotologist; or ear, nose, and throat doctor to understand what you observed in the patient's eye motions. Vertical corrective eye motion requires further examination by one of these specialists.

REFERENCES

1. Laukkanen H. Research Summary for Brain Injury Vision Symptom Survey: (BIVSS) comparison data and Rasch analysis. Presented at: *7th International Congress of Behavioral Optometry*; 2014; Birmingham, UK. https://ovpjournal.org/uploads/2/3/8/9/23898265/f.pdf

2. Rouse MW, Borsting EJ, Mitchell GL, et al. Validity and reliability of the revised convergence insufficiency symptom survey in adults. *Ophthalmic Physiol Opt*. Sep 2004;24(5):384–90. doi:10.1111/j.1475-1313.2004.00202.x

3. Borsting EJ, Rouse MW, Mitchell GL, et al. Validity and reliability of the revised convergence insufficiency symptom survey in children aged 9 to 18 years. *Optom Vis Sci*. Dec 2003;80(12):832–838. doi:10.1097/00006324-200312000-00014

4. *Academy of Neurologic Physical Therapy Contributors*. Core Set of Outcome Measures for Adults with Neurologic Conditions; 2024. https://www.neuropt.org/practice-resources/anpt-clinical-practice-guidelines/core-outcome-measures-cpg

5. Moore JL, Potter K, Blankshain K, Kaplan SL, O'Dwyer LC, Sullivan JE. A core set of outcome measures for adults with neurologic conditions undergoing rehabilitation: A clinical practice guideline. *J Neurol Phys Ther*. Jul 2018;42(3):174–220. doi:10.1097/npt.0000000000000229

6. Scherer MR HL, Dannenbaum E, Fay JL, Lambert KH, Rice TA, Stoskus JL, Wrisley DM. *The Vestibular Evidence Database to Guide Effectiveness (VEDGE)*; 2024. https://www.neuropt.org/practice-resources/neurology-section-outcome-measures-recommendations/vestibular-disorders

7. Cohen HS. Assessment of functional outcomes in patients with vestibular disorders after rehabilitation. *NeuroRehabilitation*. 2011;29(2):173–178.

8. Jacobson GP, Newman CW. The development of the dizziness handicap inventory. *Arch Otolaryngol*. 1990;116(4):424–427. doi:10.1001/archotol.1990.01870040046011

9. Mutlu B., Serbetcioglu B. Discussion of the dizziness handicap inventory. *J Vestibular Res*. 2013;23:271–277. doi:10.3233/VES-130488

10. Shirley Ryan Ability Lab Contributors. *Dizziness Handicap Inventory*. AbilityLab; 2024. https://www.sralab.org/rehabilitation-measures/dizziness-handicap-inventory

11. Jacobson GP, Newman CW. The development of the Dizziness Handicap Inventory. *Arch Otolaryngol Head Neck Surg.* Apr 1990;116(4):424–427. doi:10.1001/archotol.1990.01870040046011

12. Tamber AL, Wilhelmsen KT, Strand LI. Measurement properties of the Dizziness Handicap Inventory by cross-sectional and longitudinal designs. *Health Qual Life Outcomes.* 2009;7:101. doi:10.1186/1477-7525-7-101

13. Whitney SL, Wrisley DM, Brown KE, Furman JM. Is perception of handicap related to functional performance in persons with vestibular dysfunction? *Otol Neurotol.* 2004;25(2):139–143. doi:10.1097/00129492-200403000-00010

14. Whitney S, Marchetti G, Morri L. Usefulness of the dizziness handicap inventory in the screening for benign paroxysmal positional vertigo. *Otol Neurotol.* 2005;26(5):1027–1033. doi:10.1097/01.mao.0000185066.04834.4e

15. Zamyslowska-Szmytke E, Politanski P, Jozefowicz-Korczynska M. Dizziness handicap inventory in clinical evaluation of dizzy patients. *Int J Environ Res Public Health.* 2021;18(5):2210. doi:10.3390/ijerph18052210

16. Powell LE, Myers AM. The Activities-specific Balance Confidence (ABC) scale. *J Gerontol A Biol Sci Med Sci.* Jan 1995;50a(1):M28–M34. doi:10.1093/gerona/50a.1.m28

17. Mak MK, Pang MY. Fear of falling is independently associated with recurrent falls in patients with Parkinson's disease: a 1-year prospective study. *J Neurol.* 2009;256(10):1689–1695. doi:10.1007/s00415-009-5184-5

18. Beninato M, Portney LG, Sullivan PE. Using the international classification of functioning, disability and health as a framework to examine the association between falls and clinical assessment tools in people with stroke. *Phy Therapy.* 2009;89(8):816–825. doi:10.2522/ptj.20080160

19. Lajoie Y, Gallagher SP. Predicting falls within the elderly community: comparison of postural sway, reaction time, the Berg balance scale and the Activities-specific Balance Confidence (ABC) scale for comparing fallers and non-fallers. *Arch Gerontol Geriatri.* 2004;38(1):11–26. doi:10.1016/s0167-4943(03)00082-7

20. Abasıyanık Z, Kahraman T, Baba C, Sağ ıcı Ö, Ertekin Ö, Özakbaş S. Multiple Sclerosis Research Group. Discriminative ability of the original and short form of the Activities-specific Balance Confidence scale and its individual items for falls in people with multiple sclerosis. *Acta Neurol Belgica.* 2024;124(3):957–964. doi:10.1007/s13760-024-02515-y

21. Shirley Ryan Ability Lab Contributors. *Activities-Specific Balance Confidence Scale.* AbilityLab; 2024. https://www.sralab.org/rehabilitation-measures/activities-specific-balance-confidence-scale#non-specific-patient-population

22. Pohl J, Held JPO, Verheyden G, et al. Consensus-based core set of outcome measures for clinical motor rehabilitation after stroke-A Delphi study. *Front Neurol.* 2020;11:875. doi:10.3389/fneur.2020.00875

23. Cohen ET, Potter K, Allen DD, et al. Selecting rehabilitation outcome measures for people with multiple sclerosis. *Int J MS Care.* Jul–Aug 2015;17(4):181–189. doi:10.7224/1537-2073.2014-067

24. Osborne JA, Botkin R, Colon-Semenza C, et al. Physical therapist management of Parkinson disease: a clinical practice guideline from the American Physical Therapy Association. *Phys Ther.* Apr 1 2022;102(4) doi:10.1093/ptj/pzab302

25. Kocer B, Soke F, Ataoglu NEE, et al. The reliability and validity of the 3-m backward walk test in people with Parkinson's disease. *Ir J Med Sci.* Dec 2023;192(6):3063–3071. doi:10.1007/s11845-023-03384-9

26. Kahn JH, Tappan R, Newman CP, et al. Outcome measure recommendations from the spinal cord injury EDGE task force. *Phys Ther.* Nov 2016;96(11):1832–1842. doi:10.2522/ptj.20150453

27. American Physical Therapy Association Contributors. *Guidelines: Physical Therapy Documentation of Patient/Client Management.* American Physical Therapy

Association; 2024. https://www.apta.org/siteassets/pdfs/policies/guidelines-documentation-patient-client-management.pdf

28. American Occupational Therapy Association. Occupational therapy practice framework: domain and process: Fourth edition. *Am J Occupat Therapy.* 2020;74(Suppl. 2):7412410010p1–7412410010p87. doi:10.5014/ajot.2020.74S2001

29. Erickson M, McKnight R, Utzman R. *Physical Therapy Documentation: From Examination to Outcome.* SLACK, Inc.; 2008.

30. Davis AJ, Pozun A. *Evaluation of the Dizzy and Unbalanced Patient.* StatPearls Publishing; Updated 2023. Accessed 2024. https://www.ncbi.nlm.nih.gov/books/NBK589645/

31. Newman-Toker DE, Cannon LM, Stofferahn ME, Rothman RE, Hsieh YH, Zee DS. Imprecision in patient reports of dizziness symptom quality: a cross-sectional study conducted in an acute care setting. *Mayo Clin Proc.* 2007;82:1329–1340. doi:10.4065/82.11.1329

32. Edlow J, Gurley K, Newman-Toker D. A new diagnostic approach to the adult patient with acute dizziness. *J Emer Med.* 2018;54(4):469–483. doi:10.1016/j.jemermed.2017.12.024

33. Gurley KL, Edlow JA. Acute dizziness. *Semi Neurol.* 2019;39(1):27–40. doi:10.1055/s-0038-1676857

34. Newman-Toker DE. Charted records of dizzy patients suggest emergency physicians emphasize symptom quality in diagnostic assessment. *Annal Emerg Med.* 2007;50(2):204–205. doi:10.1016/j.annemergmed.2007.03.037

35. Appeadu MK, Bordoni B. *Falls and Fall Prevention in Older Adults.* StatPearls Publishing; Updated 2023. https://www.ncbi.nlm.nih.gov/books/NBK560761/

36. Bronstein A, Lempert T. *A Practical Approach to Diagnosis and Management.* Cambridge University Press; 2007.

37. World Health Organization Contributors. *International Classification of Functioning, Disability and Health (ICF).* World Health Organization; 2024. https://www.who.int/standards/classifications/international-classification-of-functioning-disability-and-health

38. World Health Organization Contributors. *ICF 3-Learning.* World Health Organization; 2024. https://www.icf-elearning.com/

39. Podder V, Lew V, Ghassemzadeh S. *SOAP Notes.* StatPearls Publishing; Updated 2023. https://www.ncbi.nlm.nih.gov/books/NBK482263/

40. *Centers for Disease Control and Prevention Contributors.* Steps for Creating and Maintaining a Care Plan; 2024. https://www.cdc.gov/caregiving/guidelines/index.html

13

Vision Interventions

This chapter reviews suggestions for interventions for vision deficits. There are also websites and apps for smartphones, tablets, and computers that have various exercises for vision, such as pursuits and saccades, that may be downloaded or watched on a computer. Search for "saccade exercise," "pursuit exercise," etc.

OCULOMOTOR NERVE PALSY

Treatment of ocular nerve palsy depends on the underlying condition/cause of the palsy. Treatments, therefore, vary. For palsy of cranial nerves III, IV, and VI, the following are treatment options:

1. Often, spontaneous recovery occurs within 6–8 months.

2. Antibiotics for bacterial infections.
3. Corticosteroids.
4. Surgery.
5. Eye patch. The eye patch should be semi-clear and switched from one eye to the other so that one eye doesn't get weak or lazy. Prolonged patching of an eye encourages vision suppression.
6. Partial visual field occlusion (for diplopia).
7. Neuro-optometric rehabilitation/vision therapy.
8. Spontaneous recovery often occurs within 6–8 months.
9. Prism glasses to reduce diplopia.
10. Botox.
11. Treatment of underlying disorders.

VISUAL FIELD LOSS

Visual field loss includes a central field loss, hemianopia, homonymous hemianopia, quadrantanopia, and scotoma.

CENTRAL FIELD LOSS

ECCENTRIC READING/VIEWING

Eccentric viewing is a technique used for people with ventral field loss (such as macular degeneration or scotomas) to read and perform activities of

DOI: 10.1201/9781003524441-13

daily living (ADLs). The patient is taught to use the intact visual field to view an object of interest or read. While the object or word will not be sharply seen, people can learn to read using the parts of the visual field that are intact.

SCANNING/SACCADES

Using the intact visual field, the patient is taught to scan the environment to avoid obstacles or find and interact with objects they need.

VISUAL FIELD INATTENTION (NEGLECT)

Patients typically deny having a visual deficit. The patient does not pay attention to the side opposite of the side of the brain lesion. However, this is not a visual field cut. This is often secondary to a right middle cerebral artery (MCA) stroke causing left inattention. They may or may not have intact vision on the side of inattention. A visual field test will indicate which of these is the situation. While treating a patient with visual inattention, if you need to show them something important, do it on the side of attention (strong side). During treatment, however, you want to promote the use of the side of inattention.

TREATMENTS FOR PERIPHERAL VISUAL FIELD LOSS AND HEMI-INATTENTION

The examples described next are assuming a left inattention. If you have a patient with a right inattention, you may use the same techniques, but swapping "left" for "right" in the instructions.

OPTOKINETIC STIMULATION

Optokinetic stimulation (OKS) is a large visual-field motion stimulus that the patient watches. This stimulus should induce optokinetic nystagmus (OKN). OKS can be generated by apps for smartphones and tablets, by using a disco ball, or simply moving a piece of paper with lines drawn on it across the visual field.

PRISM THERAPY

How many prism diopters (PD) are needed? To convert prism diopters to degrees:[1]

> Prism diopter = 100 × tan Angle (Angle is the angle of deviation in degrees.)
> Angle = Arctan (Prism diopter/100)

For small angles: 1 prism diopter for every 0.57 degrees and 1 degree for every 1.75 prism diopters.

Prisms for Hemifield Loss

Under the guidance of an optometrist, use base-left yoked prisms to shift the visual field at least 10 degrees, using prisms that are up to 40 PD. Use this rule of thumb for prism diopters and degrees: When the prisms are base left, they will shift images from the left visual field closer to the right. While wearing the prisms, have the patient reach for objects in the blind field 50–100 times in a row daily while in therapy.

Prisms for Hemi-Spatial Inattention (aka Neglect)

Under the guidance of an optometrist, the patient wears prisms with the base toward the side of field loss, from 10 to 40 PD. While wearing prisms, the patient is instructed to point toward objects or sounds and perform tasks toward the side of inattention.

MARGOLIS EYE-THROWING

Mobility and Orientation Strategies

Use the Margolis eye-throwing technique instead of asking the patient to turn their head. The goal is to get the eye moving past the primary eye position (midline) while scanning. If you only ask them to turn their head, they will keep the eye in the primary position, and this will embed the hemi-inattention.

MARGOLIS EYE-THROWING TECHNIQUE (FOR LEFT INATTENTION)

1. Instruct patients to close their eyes and then move their eyes as far to their left as they can. This encourages them to use non-visual cues for eye movements.
2. Once the patient moves their eyes to the farthest point left as the ocular muscles allow, instruct them to open their eyes and describe objects they can see. No sclera should be visible on the temporal side in the direction of eye turn. If they do not move the eyes far enough, use verbal cues.
3. Teach them to "throw" their eyes left and scan right.

BODY IMAGE AWARENESS

Angels in the Snow

If you live in an area that snows, you will understand this one immediately. The patient begins in supine with eyes open. The patient is instructed to move limbs outward into abduction when the clinician taps them. Begin with one limb at a time, progressing the tapping limbs on both sides simultaneously. Next, repeat with the patient's eyes closed. You may again progress the patient to moving a limb that the therapist points to (obviously with the patient's eyes open).

Mannequin Projections

The patient stands behind another person who will be the mannequin (best if they are of similar sizes). The therapist touches the mannequin and instructs the patient to touch them in the same spot. Begin by touching points of the mannequin that are farther away from the mannequin's midline.

Mirrors

Place a thin strip of colored tape vertically down the length of a full-length mirror. Patients are instructed to walk (from a distance) toward the mirror, keeping the tape in the center of their reflection.

USE OF ANCHORS FOR READING

A visual anchor is a visual target used as a starting point when reading. It is usually brightly colored.

1. Place a strip of brightly colored Velcro along the left margin of the text. Instruct the patient to rub a finger on the Velcro as a reminder to move their eyes all the way to the left when beginning to read a new line of text.
2. Use a T-square with a brightly colored vertical arm. The horizontal arm prevents the patient from skipping lines, while the vertical arm is used as an anchor to remind them to move their eyes all the way to the beginning of the sentence.
3. Use a highlighter or brightly colored marker to mark the left edge of the page to use as an anchor.
4. Number sentences along the left margin to assist in keeping track of lines of text.

OTHER TECHNIQUES TO ASSIST READING WITH FIELD LOSS

Have patients draw a pen line below sentences they are reading.

1. Tracking printed words while listening to a book on tape.
2. Have patients call out the first and last letter on each printed line of text. Begin with large print, and progress to standard print sizes.
3. Count specified words in paragraphs.
4. Cancellation tasks: Use printed letters, numbers and symbols. Instruct the patient to find and cross out (cancel) a specific stimulus when it appears.
5. For right visual field cuts, you can train the patient to read by turning the text sideways or at an angle to which they are not trying to find the next word in their blind spot.

BALLOON BUNT

The patient is instructed to bunt a balloon with the limb to which it is thrown. If the patient has left inattention, most balloon tosses should be toward the patient's right.

OBSTACLE COURSE

Patients are instructed to negotiate obstacle courses by staying in the middle of the path and not touching any obstacles on either side. Begin with large spaces such as hallways and doorways.

LIGHTLY WEIGHTED DOWEL ROD

Instruct the patient to pick up dowel rods of various sizes by their middle. The dowel rod weight as well as verbal cues will assist the patient in realizing how accurate they are with the task.

MEALTIME ACTIVITIES

- Sit on the patient's affected side asking for eye contact when speaking.
- Put brightly colored tape on the affected side of the table/tray as an anchor.
- Place utensils on the neglected side to encourage visual scanning.
- Cooking: Have the patient find safety hazards, ingredients needed, pots/pans, and utensils they will need while cooking.

VISUAL SCANNING SEARCH TASKS

- Place common and familiar objects in front of the person and on their affected side, asking them to find a specific item. Use verbal cues to look farther left.
- Place sticky notes with numbers or letters on the walls of the hallway and have the patient find them in order.
- Have the patient complete paper/pen mazes.
- During ambulation, instruct the patient to scan into the blind field every five or six steps. This should become a habit.

DIPLOPIA

BINOCULAR DIPLOPIA

In most cases double vision, called diplopia, is due to a misalignment of the eyes. Think of the eyes as cameras. If both cameras are pointed at the same object, the brain can make one picture out of the images coming from each eye. However, if the eyes (cameras) are not pointing closely enough at the same object, the brain can no longer fuse the images, and the patient will see two images. This vision deficit may be addressed using a monocular prism to shift images into view (called a corrective prism) or used to strengthen the eye muscle involved by using a prism that is 1 PD less than needed to correct the issue, forcing the patient to use the offending muscle and thereby strengthening it (called a therapeutic prism). Once diplopia is resolved using the prism this way, it is no longer needed.

Another way to treat diplopia from an eye that is either exo- or esotropic is to use partial occlusion. This is a good option for therapists, as they do not need to consult with an optometrist to implement but should refer the patient to an optometrist at some point. As an example, let's use a real-life example. A 23-year-old woman drove her car into a house and ended up in the hospital. Among the many medical problems that resulted, she had a left exotropia result secondary to a head injury. She normally wore prescription spectacles, so a piece of semiclear tape was placed on the lateral boarder of the spectacles, just immediately adjacent to but not covering her pupil. As the eye eventually came back to the primary position, the tape was adjusted to always be adjacent to the pupil, until she no longer needed the tape. Many patients with mild traumatic brain injury (TBI) complain of diplopia as a result. Partially occluding the eye that is abnormally turned not only relives the patient of diplopia (at least in the primary position) but also encourages the eye to move back to its correct position.

MONOCULAR DIPLOPIA

Sometimes the patient has double vision out of only one eye (monocular diplopia), and corrective lenses are used to alleviate the diplopia.

SACCADE TRAINING

When training saccades, it is important to begin training the intact visual field first with large

Table 13.1 Saccade Training Techniques

Large Saccades Training	Small Saccades Training	Saccadic Speed Training
• Dynavision D2™ • Eye–head shifts • Descriptive walking • Post-it notes in hallway	• Word puzzles • Double Hart chart • Newspaper cancellation tasks • Boundary marking • Michigan saccades workbook	• Dynavision D2™ • Table tennis

Source: From S Whittaker, M Scheiman, D Sokol-McKay, *Low Vision Rehabilitation–A Practical Guide for Occupational Therapists*, 2nd ed., Thorofare, NJ: Slack Inc., 2016.

saccades, and progress to small and the quick saccades. Then progress to moving into the affected visual field. Table 13.1 lists various techniques for each of these categories.

HOMEMADE SACCADE CHARTS

You may make a simple saccades chart by drawing a circle on a piece of paper, marking the middle with an *X*, and placing two letters each (*A*, *B*, *C*, *D*) around the circle, with each letter across from its pair (e.g., *A* is across from *A*). Instruct the patient to sit in front of the chart and look at one target, then to the *X* in the middle, then to the corresponding target on the other side of the circle, and then back to the *X*, and finally the starting point again. Using the letter *A* as an example, the patient would look in this order at *A* (left)–*X*–*A* (right) (counts as one repetition), then back to *X*, then *A* (left) again (counts as another repetition). Repeat for the prescribed number of repetitions (commonly 20 to 40 repetitions, or timed), then move to the next letter. An example of an entire round of exercises would be (Figure 13.1): *A–X–A–X–A* (*X*10), *B–X–B–X–B* (*X*10), *C–X–C–X–C* (*X*10), *D–X–D–X–D* (*X*10), etc.

You may also use different types of lines marked at either even or varied intervals. Refer to the charts

in Figures 13.2 to 13.4. The lines do not all have to be straight. By varying the lines to use waves or zigzags, you increase the variety of angles the patient must use during the exercise. You may also turn the charts 90 degrees and use them to practice vertical saccades.

Just draw or print a line and put hash marks along it. The hash marks may have even or varying spaces between them. If you are trying to train saccades of a certain size to use as a substitute for the loss of other motions (like a VOR), you would want evenly spaced hash marks. If you are trying to challenge the brain to improve the saccades themselves, you may wish to use a mix of evenly spaced and variably spaced hash marks. Using the lines with hash marks, have the patient scan each line L → R and R → L. Then turn the chart and have the patient scan the lines vertically, top → bottom, and then bottom → top.

A great exercise to teach scanning of the environment, which is an intervention often used in treating visuospatial neglect in stroke patients, involves hiding easily identified objects (like tennis balls) in a room and then having the patient visually scan the room using saccades until they find the objects. Make sure you incorporate vertical eye motions, not just left and right scanning. Prompt the patient to scan the environment using saccades and a still head. Make sure that all targets are within the patient's visual field.

DYNAVISION D2

The Dynavision D2™ is a light board with 64 light switches that are arranged in five concentric rings. The patient stands in front of the light board and

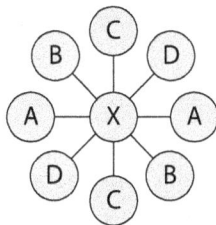

Figure 13.1 Simple Saccade Chart

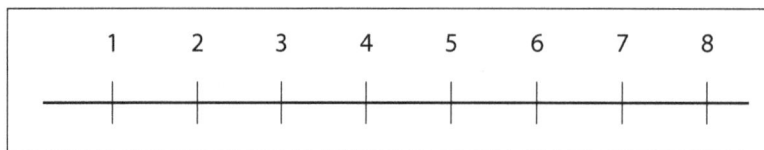

Figure 13.2 Example of a Saccades Chart

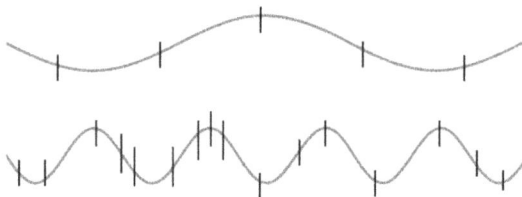

Figure 13.3 Example of a Saccades Chart

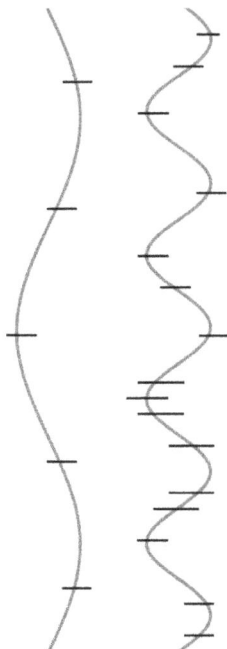

Figure 13.4 Vertical Saccades

taps each light that illuminates. Patients must focus on the middle of the board, using their peripheral vision.

EYE–HEAD SHIFTS

Patients are instructed to shift their eyes as far to one side as possible. Once their eyes are shifted, the patient moves their head in the same direction.

DESCRIPTIVE WALKING (SACCADES)

Place items on the wall (pictures, sticky notes, etc.). As the patient ambulates slowly down the hall, instruct them to use the eye/head shift technique and call out what they see on the walls. Begin on the intact visual field side, progressing to the affected side. Finally, have them call out items on both sides of the hall.

HART CHARTS

Hart charts are blocks of letters in rows and columns. They come in a variety of font sizes and colors, and there are many activities you can do to promote saccades using them. A few examples are as follows:

1. In this example we will use a ten-column Hart chart. Number the columns and rows. Instruct the patient to alternately read the letters from columns 1 and 10 of each row. Next instruct the patient to read from columns 2 and 9. Continue until they have read every letter on the chart.
2. Have a phrase the patient needs to decode, e.g., "My saccades are improving." On a piece of paper next to the Hart chart, have each letter of the phrase indicated by an underscore, with the location of the letter (column, row number) underneath. The patient must find the letter using the locator and then fill the letter in for each underscore until they can read the phrase.
3. Double Hart charts: Use two Hart charts side by side. Instruct the patient to read each letter in the first column of each chart, and then the second letter from each first column. Continue until each letter of each column has been read aloud.

4. Michigan saccade workbooks: These are available for purchase online. The workbooks have pages of groups of letters that look as if they form paragraphs; however, the letters do not form words. One example instructs the patient to read each letter/line and circle letters in succession. For example, "As you read the letters, circle the first letter *a* that you come to, next circle *b*, then *c*, and so on."

PURSUIT TRAINING

PIE PAN

Place a large marble in a pie pan. Instruct the patient to roll the marble around the edge of the pie pan while pursuing. Do this both clockwise and counterclockwise.

MIRROR

Instruct the patient to look at themselves in a handheld mirror as they move the mirror in different directions (horizontally, vertically, circles). Repeat using the other eye.

MARSDEN BALL

- Cover one of the patient's eyes and ask them to read the letters on the ball as it swings by. Swing the ball around the patient and instruct them to pursue it as it passes. Do this both clockwise and counterclockwise.

FLASHLIGHTS

The clinician shows a red light on the wall. The patient is given a green light and instructed to shine their light on the of the clinician's red light. Now, move the red light and instruct the patient to keep their greenlight on top of the red light.

VISUAL ACCOMMODATION

Accommodative Rock Cards and lens flippers (2+/2– lenses) are used to improve accommodation.

The patient focuses on a card with letters, numbers, or images printed in rows while holding the plus lenses over their eyes. Once the image is in focus, they "flip" the lenses such that the minus lenses are over their eyes. They will do 20 cycles in 60 to 90 seconds.

CONVERGENCE/DIVERGENCE

Before beginning convergence/divergence training, make sure the patient is pursuing well and can perform saccades. If they cannot do those things, work on them prior to beginning convergence/divergence. There are multiple ways to work on convergence/divergence such as barrel cards, Brock string, reaching tasks, Marsden ball, tranaglyphs, and vectograms.

BARREL CARDS

These are small cards (called barrels) at the same distances. The patient is instructed to focus on each barrel, one at a time, until they can form a single image for each one.

BROCK STRING

Brock strings may be used for close convergence/divergence (~40–50 cm) or for distance (~3 feet/1 m). The rope or string typically has at least three different colored beads on it. For near saccades, the patient holds one end of the string (or yarn) to the end of their nose, while they hold the other end with their outstretched arm/hand (Figure 13.5). They next focus on the closest bead until they can form only one image (i.e., see only one bead). If they cannot fuse the image and only see one bead, it is moved farther away until they can see one bead. Next, they look at the next distant bead and do the same. They progress down the string, focusing on each bead until they see one bead. Keep in mind that when patients are using both eyes and focusing on one bead, the parts of the string that are closer and farther from the point on which they are focusing will be doubled. The point of focus looks like the center of an *X*. If the patient is only seeing one string, then they are visually suppressing images of one eye and need the attention

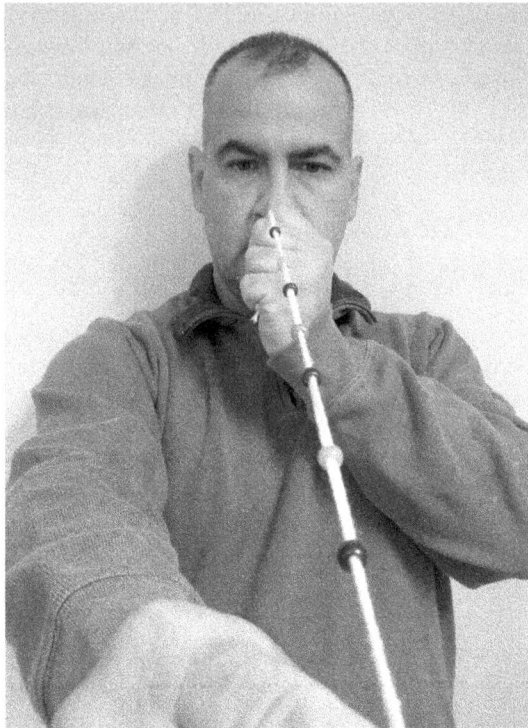

Figure 13.5 Brock String Near-Vergence

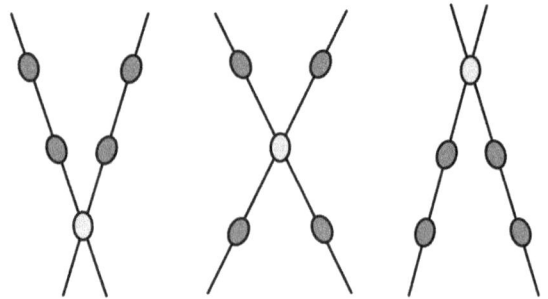

Figure 13.6 Brock String Diagram: Lighter-Colored Beads Indicate the Point of Visual Fixation

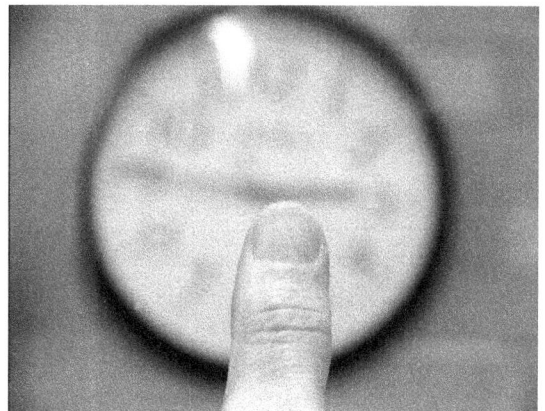

Figure 13.7 Thumb in Focus

of an optometrist. You can purchase Brock strings online or make your own by doubling a stretch of yarn, placing three different colored beads on it, and tying the ends. Brock strings used for distance vergences are used in the same way, only the distant end of the rope/string is tied to something to anchor it (e.g., a doorknob or shut in a door).

When the patient is able to see only one image for each bead on which they are fixating, the beads are spread farther apart, moving the closest bead a little bit closer and the farthest bead more distant. Keep in mind that beads that are closer and farther than the bead that is the fixation point will seem to be doubled (Figure 13.6). (Try it yourself.)

If you do not have a Brock string, you may have the patients hold their thumb with arm extended in front of themselves, focus on the thumbnail, and then focus on an object (e.g., a clock) behind the thumb that is on the wall (Figures 13.7 and 13.8).

REACHING TASKS

Reaching tasks are only limited by your imagination. An example of a reaching task is to instruct

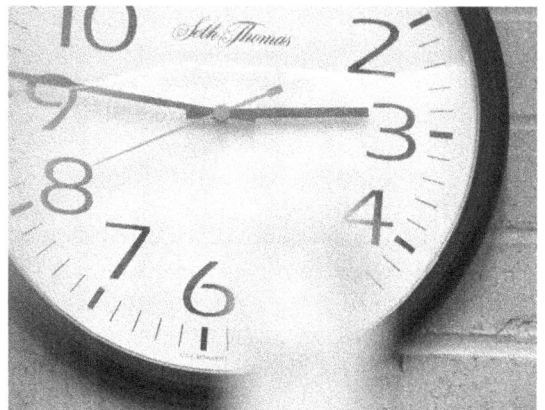

Figure 13.8 Clock in Focus

the patient to place toothpicks in a row along a foam tube (like a pool noodle). You can then ask them to place beads on each toothpick.

TRANAGLYPHS

The patient is instructed to wear a pair of red/green glasses (one eye red, one green). When looking at the image (tranaglyph) printed on the card, the patient will need to fuse the red and green images into one 3D image. You must purchase tranaglyphs.

VECTOGRAMS

The patient places two transparent cards, each with part of an image printed on it, into the vectogram machine. They then wear polarizing glasses to create depth. The patient is then instructed to either converge or diverge to fuse the partial images into one 3D image. You must purchase vectograms.

HAND–EYE COORDINATION

Examples of hand–eye coordination activities are discussed in the following sections.

MARBLE ROLL

The clinician rolls a marble across a table toward the patient, who is instructed to stop the marble by placing an upside-down cup over it.

BUNTING ACTIVITIES

The patient is instructed to bunt an object that is moving toward them, such as a balloon tossed by the clinician or a Marsden ball.

HECOstix

A HECOstix is a three-handled stick (think of the letter Y with equal angles between the lines). Each end is colored differently. The HECOstix is tossed between the clinician and patient, with the clinician calling out what color the patient should catch. This is a good activity for athletes. You can have the patient perform a walking or balance activity to increase difficulty.

SPATIAL ORIENTATION

SPATIAL ORIENTATION ACTIVITIES FOR CHILDREN

There are a number of activities used for children to learn spatial orientation, depending on their age. Examples include jigsaw puzzles, obstacle courses, and follow-the-leader that includes jumping, crawling, walking on tip toes, and placing hands on hips or shoulders. For older children you may include sports (e.g., basketball, baseball, soccer [football]), jigsaw puzzles, or using a map to navigate.

SPATIAL ORIENTATION ACTIVITIES FOR ADULTS

On their own, patients may use hobbies to improve spatial awareness through activities such as drawing/painting or photography, solving jigsaw puzzles, mental mapping (sketching maps of familiar spaces such as the layout of a patient's home), and games such as checkers or chess. In therapy, you may have the patient perform a quick scan of the room using saccades and then describe what they see and point to each object. Next, you may have the patient use their memory to walk through the room or a simple obstacle course. You may use colored tape (one color for the left and a different one for the right) to mark the sides of a door or room.

LOW-VISION TREATMENTS/ ACTIVITIES

Patients with low vision first need to be evaluated by an optometrist and have the correct prescriptions for their spectacles. While wearing their spectacles, have them work on visual scanning, saccades, and fixation. Optimize vision using high contrast materials/tape, lighting, and magnification. Increase font sizes for reading. Treatment of low vision is a combination of adapting the patient's environment (e.g., high contrast) and visual therapy exercises.

FOCAL BINDING

For those suffering from cerebrovascular accident (CVA), TBI, mild TBI, convergence excess, esotropia, visual overstimulation, or divergence insufficiency, use binasal visual field occlusion. If the patient wears spectacles, tape the medial (i.e., nasal) aspects of the lenses with semiclear tape. This will reduce the images the brain needs to process, and typically gives the patient relief. Instruct the patient to wear the tape on the lenses for 3 to 4 weeks. If the patient does not wear spectacles, purchase clear nonprescription spectacles online, and tape them (search online for "vintage sunglasses with clear lens many colors frame").

REFERENCE

1. Childrenseye.org contributors. *Converting Prism Diopters to Degrees*. Childrenseye.org. 2024. https://childrenseye.org/wiki/doku.php?id=converting_prism_diopters_to_degrees

14

Vestibular and Balance Interventions

Chapter Goals

1. List the goals of vestibular rehab therapy
2. Discuss pharmacological and non-pharmacological treatment strategies for vestibular deficits
3. Discuss the vestibular clinical practice guideline
4. Explain traditional vestibular hypofunction interventions
5. Explain new vestibular interventions for vestibular hypofunction
6. Explain the use of optokinetic stimulation for vestibular hypofunction
7. List interventions for benign paroxysmal positional vertigo
8. Explain the use of motion habituation for dizziness
9. Discuss research that impacts ankle proprioception
10. List and explain balance exercises

The goals of vestibular rehab therapy (VRT) include:[1,2]

1. Decrease anxiety
2. Enhance gaze stability/improve VOR function
3. Enhance postural stability/balance
4. Improve vertigo/dizziness
5. Decrease fall risk

6. Improve gait, especially with head movements
7. Improve activities of daily living (ADLs)
8. Improve endurance

Underlying physical deficits may impact a patient's ability to perform functional movements with precision and skill. As no one exercise program or protocol is effective for all patients, it is critical that you customize each patient's interventions based on their underlying physical and functional impairments, tolerance to treatment and interventions, and functional needs and personal goals. This chapter will review evidence-based vestibular treatments for various conditions, VRT, vestibular rehab clinical practice guidelines, and specific intervention examples. Vestibular treatments fall into one of two categories: pharmacologic and non-pharmacologic.

PHARMACOLOGIC TREATMENTS OF VESTIBULAR DYSFUNCTION

Pharmacologic treatments of symptoms are listed in Table 14.1.[3,4]

The safety and efficacy of VRT combined with anti-vertigo drugs in patients with vestibular neuritis have been established.[4] The benefit of anti-vertigo drugs in combination with VRT is the patient's reduced symptoms, which may increase compliance with VRT exercises. However, recovery may

Table 14.1 Pharmacologic Treatments of Vestibular Dysfunction (Symptomatic Management)

Medication Type	Examples
Antiemetics	Metoclopramide, ondansetron, prochlorperazine, promethazine
Vestibular suppressants	Diphenhydramine, dimenhydrinate, meclizine, promethazine, betahistine
Benzodiazepines	Alprazolam, clonazepam, diazepam, and lorazepam
Steroids	Methylprednisolone, prednisolone, dexamethasone
Endogenous coenzyme B12	Mecobalamin
Alkaline	Sodium bicarbonate

be longer while taking them. The management of peripheral recovery of function after vestibular neuritis has not yet been established, with the therapeutic choices being corticosteroids, antiviral therapy (acyclovir), a combination of corticosteroids and an antiviral agent, and finally VRT.[5]

One systematic review and meta-analysis of randomized controlled trials comparing VRT to corticosteroid treatment for vestibular neuritis concluded that corticosteroids enhanced earlier canal paresis improvement, but that their long-term efficacy does not appear to be different than VRT.[6] VRT showed an earlier Dizziness Handicap Inventory (DHI) score improvement compared to steroid treatment alone.[6] The study stated VRT has to be offered as the primary option, and corticosteroids can be added to provide better recovery in the absence of its contraindication, and that treatments of VRT, corticosteroids, or their combination should be tailored to the patient's condition and health status.[6]

It is a rare occurrence to evaluate an adult patient who is not taking medications. The increasing understanding of pharmaceuticals has dramatically improved and extended lives. While medications are useful to address problems, they may also have unintended side effects involving other systems or functions. We do not all need to be pharmacists, but we should be familiar with the more common medications that affect the balance/dizziness patient for good or ill.

MEDICATIONS USED TO TREAT SYMPTOMS OF DIZZINESS

Three classes of medications are commonly used to suppress symptoms of dizziness: antihistamines,

benzodiazepines, and anticholinergic agents. Physicians prescribe these agents to reduce symptoms because they are sedating to the vestibular system and CNS or increase tolerance to motion. Often, however, one or more of these medications are prescribed for chronic use. As people take medications for different reasons, it is important to identify the reason for their use and assess the impact they have on the patient's function. Do not assume that a patient is taking a medication for its primary indication.

Sometimes it is helpful for the patient to take medications for their symptoms of dizziness if their symptoms interfere with vestibular therapy. A good example of this is when we are teaching vestibular exercises to those with inner ear deficits or habituation exercises for central dizziness. If the dizziness and nausea are too bothersome during the intervention, the patient's unwillingness to participate may reduce compliance with home exercises. When this is the case, it may be beneficial for the patient to take a medication that will reduce symptoms to a level where the intervention is tolerable.

Sedating medications may prolong the adaptation or habituation process, which means that the patient may need therapy for a longer period of care than if they were not taking the medication. However, this is a small price to pay to resolve symptoms if the alternative is to be chronically sedated. For these patients, medications may reduce symptoms, anxiety, or fear and thereby allow greater participation, which in turn will lead to improved compensation and function. Later in the treatment period when the brain has begun its adaptation/habituation, the medications may be weaned or eliminated under the care of the referring clinician.

When you evaluate a patient who is complaining of balance or dizziness problems, it is helpful to get hold orders for medications that are sedating, as they may hide symptoms. If you cannot get these medications held for medical reasons or physician choice, then clearly document which medications the patient was taking when they were evaluated (or if they are being taken during interventions) along with an explanation indicating that these medications may have altered your findings.

MEDICATIONS THAT MAY CAUSE DIZZINESS

Now let's look at medications that commonly *cause* dizziness. When we hear patients complain of dizziness, medications that can change blood pressure, heart rate, and blood sugar come to mind. This is especially true when these types of medications have recently been added or adjusted. However, there are other types of medications that frequently cause patients to feel dizzy.[7,8] The following list from Rogers et al.[9] was adapted by the authors from the original article from Muncie et al.[10] and Roscol et al.[11] These lists provide the class of medications and the causal mechanisms of dizziness:

MEDICATIONS AND SUBSTANCES ASSOCIATED WITH DIZZINESS

Realize that taking these medications does necessarily cause dizziness. However, if such medications were recently added or adjusted and symptoms seem to coincide with their use, then they move up the list of possible or likely causes. If other tests fail to find a cause, review current medications closely. You should clearly list in your report any medications that are being used to treat symptoms of dizziness or that may cause dizziness/imbalance when evaluating patients report dizziness and/or disequilibrium.

A real-life example will help to highlight this point. A female patient was referred to a balance clinic by a neurologist to address falls and balance problems. The patient was dependent on her husband for walking and static sitting balance. She needed 24-hour supervision and even needed help to remain seated on a commode. She was being treated by other medical professionals for clinical depression and anxiety as well as hypertension. As a result, she was taking mood-altering medications and anxiety medications as well as a medication to control her blood pressure. The patient failed every balance test given; she had abnormal smooth pursuit, gaze nystagmus, and saccades as well as post–head-shake nystagmus and orthostatic hypotension. She could not sit on the exam table without verbal cues to keep her from falling over. Electronystagmography/audiography was ordered to help in the differential diagnosis. It took a couple of weeks, with the assistance of the physician, to wean the patient from all medications that might have impaired the test results. The results of the audiology test were that vestibular function was normal and there were only minor oculomotor findings. However, given the patient's history, the audiologist recommended a head scan based on the abnormal oculomotor findings. The head scan was ordered, and results were all within normal limits. It was concluded that the medications

Table 14.2 Medications Causing Dizziness: Cardiac Effects or Sedation

• Antiarrhythmic, class 1a	• Attention-deficit agents
• Antidementia agents	• Hyperactivity disorder agents
• Antihistamines	• Digitalis glycosides
• Antihypertensives	• Dipyridamole
• Antidepressants	• Narcotics
• Anti-infectives	• Nitrates
• Anti-influenza agents	• Phosphodiesterase type 5 inhibitors
• Antifungals	• Skeletal muscle relaxants
• Quinolones	• Sodium-glucose cotransporter-2 inhibitors
• Antiparkinsonian agents	• Urinary anticholinergics

Table 14.3 Medications Causing Dizziness: Central Anticholinergic Effects

- Skeletal muscle relaxants
- Urinary anticholinergic and gastrointestinal antispasmodics

Table 14.4 Medications Causing Dizziness: Cerebellar Toxicity

- Alcohol
- Antiseizure medications
- Benzodiazepines
- Lithium

Table 14.5 Medications Causing Dizziness: Hypoglycemia

- Antidiabetic agents
- Beta adrenergic blockers

Table 14.6 Medications Causing Dizziness: Ototoxicity

- Aminoglycosides
- Antirheumatic agents

Table 14.7 Medications Causing Dizziness: Bleeding Complications

- Anticoagulants

Table 14.8 Medications Causing Dizziness: Bone Marrow Suppression

- Antithyroid agents

were the primary cause of the patient's complaints of disequilibrium and dizziness. The patient still needed the psychiatric medications to keep a stable mood, allowing for normal social function, and she still needed medication to control her hypertension. With a combination of the physician adjusting medication dosages and continued therapy to retrain balance, the patient was ultimately discharged with a good outcome and normal balance test scores. She no longer was a fall risk according to multiple standardized tests and could ambulate independently. The moral of the story is that one should not discount the possibility that a patient's medications might be involved in their symptomology. Also, a team approach helped not only to discover the cause of the problem, but also to recover the patient's motor function.

MEDICATION EFFECTS ON RECOVERY OF VESTIBULAR LOSS

There is evidence that medications that are sedating to the CNS and vestibular system slow the progress of recovery during adaptation. Shepard et al. examined the extent of this interference and found that patients taking vestibular suppressants, antidepressants, tranquilizers, and anticonvulsants ultimately achieve the same level of compensation as those who are not taking such medications, but that the length of therapy is significantly longer.[12-14]

RESEARCH OF MEDICATIONS VERSUS VESTIBULAR REHABILITATION

It is not at all uncommon for physicians to prescribe sedating medications for patients who have vestibular deficits to help control their symptoms of dizziness. Often, they do not refer these patients to therapy. According to research, compared with medications, vestibular rehabilitation was superior to medication in improving subjective reports of dizziness in people with unilateral peripheral vestibular dysfunction.[15,16]

One study found exercise to be a better treatment choice than medication and may be preferable for patients with persistent or chronic vertigo stemming from BPPV. This makes sense as BPPV is a condition where otoconia are in the canals and not in the utricle. Medications cannot correct this problem, and the best option to relieve symptoms from this condition is to reposition the offending otoconia back to the utricle.

Comparing vestibular rehab to medications (diazepam and meclizine) and "general exercise" in patients with chronic vestibular symptoms, a study by Horak et al. found that all groups reported reduced symptoms of dizziness, but only the vestibular rehabilitation group showed significant objective improvement in scores obtained from the sensory organization test and other standing balance tests.[15]

MEDICATION TREATMENT FOR BENIGN PAROXYSMAL POSITIONAL VERTIGO

Patients with BPPV often go to the emergency room owing to their sudden symptoms of vertigo and are often treated with vestibular suppressants, anti-emetic agents (anti-nausea and anti-vomiting medications), or medications to improve blood flow.[18]

Medications will not resolve BPPV. According to Halker et al., BPPV can be quickly and effectively treated using canalith repositioning maneuvers. Hence, pharmacological therapies such as antihistamines or benzodiazepines are not recommended for the treatment of BPPV.[19] According to the Clinical Practice Guideline: Benign Paroxysmal Positional Vertigo (Update), BPPV should not be treated routinely with vestibular suppressant medications such as antihistamines and/or benzodiazepines. However, you should refer those with BPPV to clinicians who can treat patients with posterior canal BPPV with canalith repositioning maneuvers.[20]

While vestibular suppressants are not recommended for the treatment of BPPV, the treatment of nausea symptoms to improve patient tolerance of repositioning maneuvers can help a great deal (see Table 14.1). If you are treating a patient who becomes overly nauseous during repositioning, anti-nausea medications often allow for interventions without having the patient's symptoms stop the intervention sessions.

MÉNIÈRE'S DISEASE AND BETAHISTINE

According to Strupp et al., there is no consensus on preventative treatments of Ménière's disease, and presently a stepwise concept is recommended that begins conservatively with betahistine, then

non-destructive techniques such as transtympanic cortisone application, and finally destructive techniques such as labyrinthectomy.[22]

A systematic review of betahistine in Ménière's disease noted that high-quality studies on the effects of betahistine are lacking, with one study finding no evidence of a difference between placebo and betahistine on vertigo.[21] One study found that compared with placebo, betahistine dihydrochloride at a dosage of 16 mg twice daily for 3 months had a significant effect on the frequency, intensity, and duration of vertigo attacks in 144 subjects.[23]

For patients with Ménière's disease, betahistine is frequently ordered as part of their medication regimen. In a 2008 study of 112 patients, it was concluded that higher doses of betahistine dihydrochloride (48 mg three times daily) and a long-term treatment of 12 months seems to be more effective than a low dosage (16 to 24 mg three times daily) and short treatment (Table 14.9).[24]

A combination of orally administered betahistine and the MAO-B inhibitor selegiline was shown to enhance the efficacy of betahistine in a study of thirteen adults achieving the same clinical effect using the combined pharmacotherapy than that of high dosage of betahistine dihydrochloride alone.[25]

NON-PHARMACOLOGIC TREATMENTS OF VESTIBULAR DYSFUNCTION

Non-pharmacologic treatments of vestibular dysfunction may include VRT, vision therapy/optometry, and surgery (e.g., tumor removal or ablative surgeries for Ménière's disease). VRT is indicated for a variety of conditions, including stable vestibular lesions; central lesions from strokes, MS, and Parkinson's disease; mixed (peripheral and central) lesions; head injury; psychogenic vertigo; benign paroxysmal positional vertigo (BPPV); and vertigo/dizziness of uncertain etiology.[26,27] VRT

Table 14.9 Frequency of Attacks of Vertigo after Treatment with Betahistine Dihydrochloride

	LOW DOSE (16–24 MG T.I.D.)		HIGH DOSE (48 MG T.I.D.)	
	Initial	12 months	Initial	12 months
Mean	7.6	4.4	8.8	1.0
Median	4.5	2.0	5.5	0.0

reduces symptoms and imbalance that often lead to falls, is an effective treatment for peripheral disorders, and has promising indications as a treatment of central disoders.[28]

According to Appeadu and Bordoni, among patients with a recent fall, up to 70% reported fears of falling, and of those 50% may limit or exclude physical or social activity due to that fear, and thereby increasing their fall risk.[29] VRT is an exercise-based treatment designed to promote vestibular function, and the use of substitution when the vestibular system is unable to adapt. When needed, habituation is also included to allow for symptom-free body/head motions. Patients are taught to balance under a variety of conditions, which should reduce their fear of falling and increase balance confidence. Recovery times vary depending on the extent of damage and whether the patient is taking a vestibular suppressant. Patients are typically able to walk within 48 hours and return to normal activities within 2–6 weeks, with a return to "normal" after 3 months.[1] If patients who have a permanent vestibular loss stop their VRT exercises, they will decompensate and once again have symptoms of disequilibrium and dizziness. Alghadir et al. identified other prognostic factors for negative outcomes:[2]

- History of migraines
- Inability to move the head or body
- Distal sensory impairment
- Visual dysfunction
- Memory impairment
- Fear of falling
- Anxiety/psychiatric comorbidities

VRT has evolved to be known for not only vestibular treatments, but also treatments of dizziness not of vestibular etiologies, as well as gait and balance training. There are three basic categories of non-pharmacologic treatments for vestibular deficits:

- *Habituation exercises*: These decrease symptoms by systematically provoking them in a repetitive manner.
- *Adaptation exercises*: These induce changes in the neuronal response to retinal slip using head motions while looking at a visual target. That is to say, as a patient attempts to maintain gaze on a target while their head is moving (called gaze stability), due to the vestibular loss the eye will not be able to stay fixated and the image on the retina will "slip" off of it. When this happens, the brain is forced to attempt to increase the gain of the vestibular canal(s) that are not working hard enough. For chronic vestibular conditions, these exercises will work as long as the patient continues to do them. The system will decompensate if left unchallenged. For spontaneous nystagmus caused by an acute unilateral vestibulopathy, adaptation exercises have been shown to aid in the reduction of the time to the normalization of nystagmus.[30]
- *Substitution exercises*: The patient performs exercises that teach them to use alternative strategies to replace permanent vestibular deficits (e.g., training the use of saccades).

VESTIBULAR REHABILITATION CLINICAL PRACTICE GUIDELINE

The clinical practice guideline (CPG) for vestibular rehabilitation for peripheral vestibular hypofunction has been updated based on the following evidence.[27]

Based on strong evidence:

- Vestibular physical therapy provides a clear and substantial benefit to individuals with unilateral and bilateral vestibular hypofunction.
- Clinicians should offer vestibular rehabilitation to adults with unilateral and bilateral vestibular hypofunction presenting with impairments, activity limitations, and participation restrictions related to the vestibular deficit.
- Clinicians should not include voluntary saccadic or smooth pursuit eye movements in isolation without head movement to promote gaze stabilization.
- Clinicians should offer supervised vestibular rehabilitation.

Based on moderate-to-strong evidence:

- Clinicians may offer specific exercise techniques to target identified activity limitations and participation restrictions, including virtual reality or augmented sensory feedback.

- Clinicians may evaluate factors, including time from onset of symptoms, comorbidities, cognitive function, and use of medication that could modify rehabilitation outcomes.

Based on moderate evidence:

- Clinicians may prescribe static and dynamic balance exercises for a minimum of 20 minutes daily for at least 4–6 weeks for individuals with bilateral vestibular hypofunction.
- Clinicians may use achievement of primary goals, resolution of symptoms, normalized balance and vestibular function, or plateau in progress as reasons for stopping therapy.

Based on moderate-to-weak evidence:

- Clinicians may prescribe weekly clinic visits plus a home exercise program of gaze stabilization exercises consisting of a minimum of:
  - Three times per day for a total of at least 12 minutes daily for individuals with acute/subacute unilateral vestibular hypofunction.
  - Three to five times per day for a total of at least 20 minutes daily for 4–6 weeks for individuals with chronic vestibular hypofunction.
  - Three to five times per day for a total of 20–40 minutes daily for approximately 5–7 weeks for individuals with bilateral vestibular hypofunction.

Part of the art of vestibular rehab is knowing how much exercise or stimulation can be tolerated to sufficiently challenge the system but at the same time does not make the patient overly symptomatic (e.g., causing nausea, dizziness, or vomiting). While there are studies that suggest the proper amount of therapy as discussed in the CPG, currently there is no standardized way to progress these exercises, and it is easy to inadvertently push the patient too far. Some clinicians tell patients to perform vestibular exercises for longer than 1 minute. Others tell patients to use a nausea or dizziness scale, and to push into symptoms (e.g., "go to 5 out of 10"). An important concept to remember for vestibular exercises is that frequent system stimulation that is *within the patient's tolerances*

is sufficient to induce the needed changes in the brain. The more frequently the patient challenges the system, the better. However, there is no need to perform prolonged exercises that are outside of the patient's tolerance (e.g., 5 minutes of continuous vestibular stimulation), which may lead to sickness. Research has shown that brief periods of stimulation are sufficient to improve patients' function and symptoms. It is likely that even brief periods of stimulation can induce recovery of vestibular function.[1] Patient participation and tolerance of interventions will improve with frequent interventions of short duration that do not create a situation that patients want to avoid. This does *not* mean you should do only 1 minute of vestibular exercises in your treatment sessions. What it *does* mean is that your patient does not need to perform each vestibular exercise or intervention all at once in order for them to work. Following interventions that stir patient symptoms, it is important to allow some time for recovery before proceeding to more exercises or interventions, even within the same treatment session. Just as we tell our orthopedic patients that interventions are not always "pain-free," vestibular exercises are likewise not completely benign with regard to symptoms of dizziness and nausea. Tell patients to expect some symptoms when they are performing these exercises. Patients should report any increase in dizziness or nausea while performing the exercises (these are completely normal and expected) but should avoid a level of exercise that induces symptoms that are more severe. A common rule of thumb is that if exercises induce symptoms that last longer than a few minutes, you may want to reduce the duration of the exercise.

Two exercises form the mainstay of vestibular stimulation exercises: VOR ×1 and VOR ×2. They are named ×1 and ×2 based on the speed of the image moving across the retina, with ×2 being twice as fast as ×1. However, it is easier to remember and to explain to patients that during the VOR ×1 exercise only one thing is moving: the patient's head. During VOR ×2 exercises, two things are moving: the patient's head and the visual target (in opposite directions).

Traditionally, VOR exercises involves the patient constantly shaking their head yes or no while maintaining fixation on a target. Recent research, however, has found that adaptation does not actually occur unless there is enough contrast between the fixation target and the background. Furthermore, it has been recommended that VOR ×1 is not sufficient to cause adaptation, but instead likely improves the patient's symptoms by improving saccades, and also habituates to motion.[31] The researchers recommend VOR ×2 for actual adaptation. While the traditional VOR ×2 exercise boosts VOR gain on the deficient side, it also boosts it on the intact side. Therefore, the researchers suggest that the quick head shake motion of the exercise only be toward the deficient ear.[31,32]

GAZE STABILIZATION EXERCISES

Gaze stabilization using the VOR has been the core of vestibular exercises. The exercises are said to work due to the retinal slip of the image while the head is moving that causes the need for the body to respond to improve gaze stability.

Visual Targets/Backgrounds

Visual targets and target backgrounds are important considerations. Anything may be used as a visual target for VOR exercises; however, some are better than others. There are several factors that are involved with visual targets and VOR adaptation, including visual contrast and spatial frequency (the rate at which a stimulus changes across space). A study by Mahfuz et al. found that a contrast that is 60 times higher than provided by typical room lighting must be surpassed for "robust active and passive VOR adaptation." In their study, they used a laser pointer and varied the room light and found that VOR gain training using a bright target (e.g., a typical laser pointer) can occur in moderate ambient lighting of 0.5–1 lx (which is the typical lighting of a room with the curtains closed and lights turned off).[32] It is common for physiotherapists to use a black target on a white background when first starting and in room light. As VOR gain improves, it is important to point out that the study by Mahfuz et al. stated that the contrast was needed for "robust" adaptation. If the patient has something of interest, and it is a high-contrast image, it may be used as a target as long as it is not too large.

Traditional VOR Exercises (VOR ×1, VOR ×2)

VOR ×1 EXERCISE

Vestibular hypofunction intervention (VOR ×1) is an exercise of the VOR where only one thing is moving: the patient's head. The patient chooses a stationary visual target that is either held in the hand or in the environment. Targets that are closer are preferred, as that image moves faster across the retina. The visual target is stationary while the patient is instructed to maintain visual fixation on it as they shake their head yes (pitch) for about 1 minute and then no (yaw) for about 1 minute (Figures 14.1 and 14.2). Keep in mind that some symptom provocation is not only expected but normal. Instruct the patient to take a break if they become overly dizzy or nauseous. When first giving VOR ×1 as an intervention, begin using a stationary target with a solid background; later this may be progressed to a visual target with a busy background, such as a checkerboard. First, patients are instructed to perform these exercises in a sitting position, but later they may progress to performing them standing, standing on foam, or while moving

VOR ×2 EXERCISE

VOR ×2 is similar to VOR ×1. The patient is instructed to maintain visual fixation on a visual target while shaking their head. What makes VOR ×2 different from VOR ×1 is that with VOR ×2, two things are moving. The head shakes yes (pitch) or no (yaw), while the target moves in the *opposite direction* of head motion but at exactly the same speed (Figures 14.3 and 14.4). These exercises are repeated with vertical (1 min.) and horizontal motions (1 min) taking breaks as needed and may be performed sitting or standing still. More advanced VOR exercises have the patients perform VOR ×2 while standing on balance foam or walking. Increase the duration of the exercise from 1 to 2 minutes or longer as tolerated.

VOR EXERCISE VARIATIONS

There are a number of ways to challenge the patient using VOR exercises by changing the conditions under which they are performed. You may change

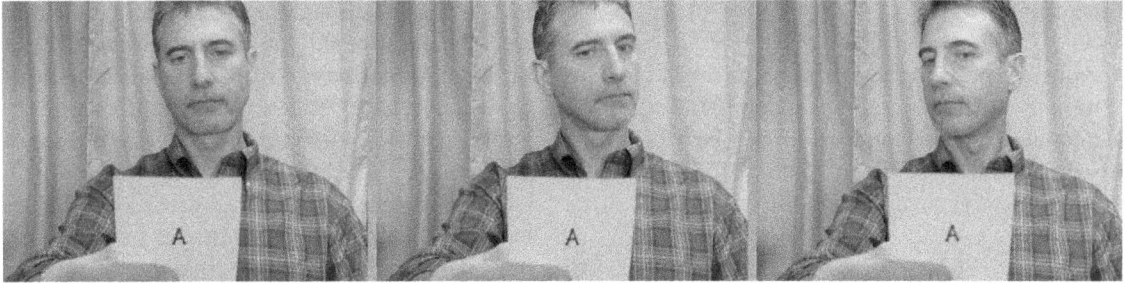

Figure 14.1 VOR x1, Yaw

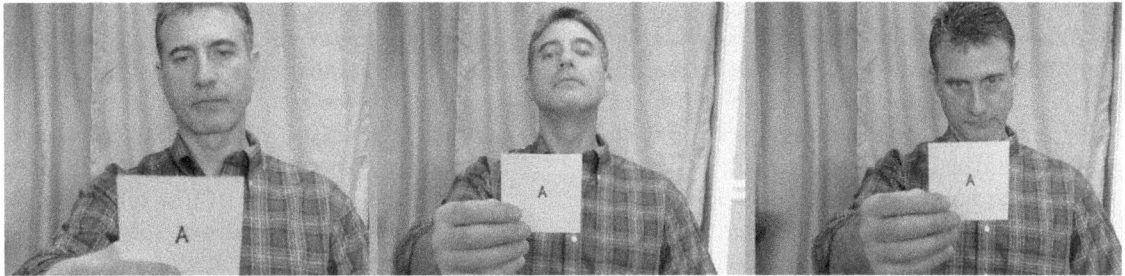

Figure 14.2 VOR x1, Pitch

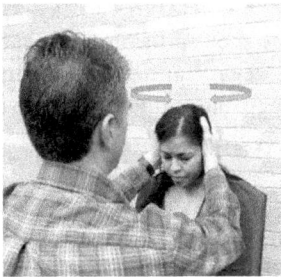

Figure 14.3 VOR x2, Yaw

the task, environment, or the way the person is performing the exercise.

Task:

- Add a dual-task activity such as walking (or, for the athlete, running) while performing the VOR exercise
- Add a mental task (e.g., counting backward by threes)

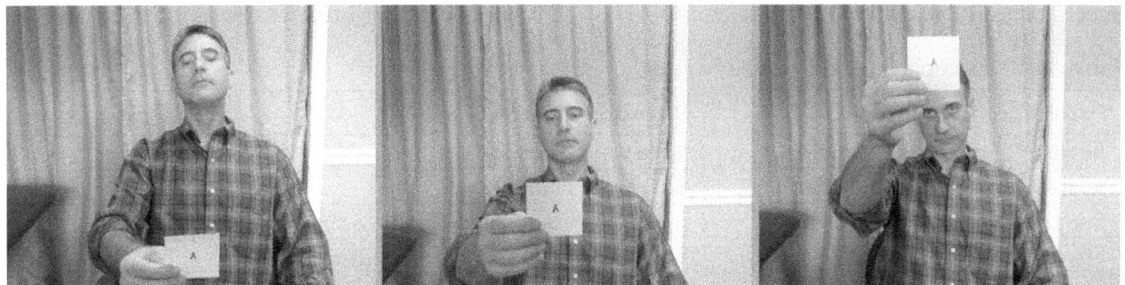

Figure 14.4 VOR x2, Pitch

Environment:

- Position in which the patient performs the exercise (sitting, standing, tandem standing)
- Standing on the floor, foam, rocker board
- Visual target
- Visual background (behind the target)

Person:

- Speed of exercise
- Vary stance width

VOR exercises typically begin with the visual target against a solid-colored background. Later this may be progressed to a visual target with a busy background, such as a checkerboard, or if the patient holds the target with a visually busy room in the background. We honestly don't know if this makes a significant difference in the progression of the VOR gain, but when the vestibular system first begins to adapt, patients will more easily tolerate less challenging visual environments and exercise target backgrounds. In general, when the vestibular system is uncompensated, busier backgrounds tend to make patients more nauseous owing to the added visual stimulation. Typical progressions include using a plain background and then moving to a busier background to increase visual stimulation during the exercise.

TYPICAL VOR EXERCISE PROGRESSION

An example of VOR exercise progression is listed in Table 14.10.

VOR EXERCISE SPEED

The speed of the VOR exercises makes a difference. The head shake should be between 1 to 2 Hz.

Recall that 1 Hz is equal to 360 degrees of motion per second. How do you estimate what 1 Hz of head motion for your patient would be? We typically do not have patients perform these exercises with large head rotations, but *imagine* a pace of head motion where the patient moves from full left cervical rotation to full right rotation and then back to full left again, doing this in 1 second. It is important to realize, however, that the patient does not need to use the entire range of motion while performing the exercise. Now, keeping this speed of head motion in mind, instruct the patient to perform the VOR exercises at that pace but without actually going to full rotation to each side. A simple instruction that helps convey this is to tell the patient to do the exercise "as fast as you can as long as the target is still visually clear." Generally, this verbal cue is enough to get the patient to move at or above the 1 Hz mark. If it is not, you may wish to demonstrate the correct speed and use verbal cues or the auditory cues of a metronome to increase head speed as the patient performs the exercise. Many metronome phone and tablet apps are available; set it to beat at or above 60 beats per minute (bpm) for 1 Hz. There was one study using monkeys that showed using different frequencies seems to be beneficial and should include some high-velocity stimulus (metronome of 120 bpm, or >2 Hz).[33]

Impulse Gaze Stabilization Exercises

The impulse method of gaze stabilization exercises does not include the constant head shaking of traditional VOR exercises, but instead involves the quick, impulsive movement of the head toward the deficient ear while fixating on a visual target. Once the head is turned as far as it can go, and the

Table 14.10 Example of VOR Exercise Progression (Easier to More Difficult)

Patient Position	VOR Type	Background/Activity
Seated	VOR x1	Solid visual background
Seated	VOR x1	Busy background
Standing	VOR x1	Busy background, standing on a solid surface (floor)
Standing	VOR x1	Busy background, standing on foam
Standing	VOR x2	Busy background, standing on a solid surface (floor)
Standing	VOR x2	Busy background (or room as background), foam
Walking	VOR x2	Busy background (room)

visual target can still be seen, the exercise stops. The patient then resets to the starting position and repeats the exercise. There currently is no research on the benefits of impulse VOR exercises. These were adapted from the study on visual contrast for VOR adaptation by Mahfuz et al.[32]

IMPULSE VOR x1 EXERCISE

1. While fixating on a high-contrast, nonmoving target, make impulsive, quick head motions toward the deficient ear.
2. When the head is turned toward the deficient ear as far as it can go while still observing the target, the patient resets and repeats the exercise.
3. Do this to toleration up to ~15 minutes at a time.

IMPULSE VOR x2 EXERCISE

1. Start position: Instruct the patient to turn their head slightly away from the deficient ear while maintaining fixation on a high-contrast fixed visual target that is held at the extreme opposite direction, as long as it still can be seen.
2. Make impulsive, quick head motions toward the deficient ear as far as it can go, as long as the target may be seen. Simultaneously, move the target at the same speed in the opposite direction. The patient resets and repeats the exercise.
3. Do this to toleration up to ~15 minutes at a time.

OPTOKINETIC STIMULATION

Optokinetic stimulation (OKS) was briefly described in Chapter 13. A systematic review with meta-analysis was done by Obrero-Gaitán et al.,[34] who found that OKS may improve the dizziness intensity measure with a visual analog scale, or dynamic balance (measured using a Timed Up and Go (TUG) test and Sensory Organization Test) in patients with balance disorders not due to a vestibular deficit. Further, there is low and very low evidence that OKS is not better than other interventions or no intervention for the improvement of disability due to dizziness or the subjective perception of dizziness in subjects with vestibular and balance disorders. The quality of evidence was

rated low or very low due to the small number of included studies.

You may wish to consider using OKS for those who are found to have deficient optokinetic nystagmus (OKN), for those with motion sickness, or those who are unable to move their neck (e.g., patients with cervical range of motion restrictions). You may have the patient watch the OKS for a few minutes, stopping as needed for nausea.

BENIGN PAROXYSMAL POSITIONAL VERTIGO INTERVENTIONS

Prior to performing any BPPV interventions, you must know your patient's physical limitations and restrictions (as was true in examining the patient for BPPV). Make sure that the patient does not have any contraindications to testing or treatment, such as the following:

- Acute fractures that prevent the patient from lying down quickly or rolling
- Arnold–Chiari malformation
- Recent neck fracture, surgery, or instability
- History of vertebral dissection or unstable carotid disease
- Recent retinal detachment
- Unstable heart disease

If the patient has a condition that you believe is safe to perform repositioning maneuvers, but you are unsure, first get permission from a physician and have them write a prescription for the maneuver.

There are a number of different maneuvers to move crystals back to the utricle. The choice of repositioning maneuver may change depending on your practice location, the size of your patient, which canal is involved, and clinician preference. The canal that is involved will limit your options, but there are still many personal preference choices available.

We refer to the process of moving crystals from the canal back to the utricle as "*canalith repositioning maneuvers.*" This is the term you should use in your plan of care. Do not specify one repositioning maneuver, such as the Epley maneuver, as your plan. If you do, it will lock you into using only that maneuver unless you change your plan. However, if you use "*canalith repositioning*" as your plan, then you may use any repositioning maneuver, which you would specify in your treatment documentation.

Some repositioning maneuvers use patient positioning and gravity as a means of moving crystals. Others involve forcefully moving the patient's head to create a flow of the endolymph toward the utricle; imagine a river sweeping toward the utricle that carries the crystals along with it. In the case of crystals that are stuck (either adhered to the cupula or in a canalith jam), as in cupulolithiasis, forceful movements may be used to break the crystals free (or liberate them) from the cupula or to clear the canalith jam. As a group, we refer to these forceful interventions as *liberatory maneuvers*. At times simple positioning will accomplish the job of moving otoconia, as in cases where prolonged positioning uses gravity to liberate the otoconia.

While using gravity as a means of moving otoconia for testing or repositioning, the position of the patient's head with respect to gravity is most important. If you need to restrict the patient's head or neck movements because of a medical condition or discomfort, keep the patient in a neck-neutral position and move the entire body to position the head. With respect to the ear and its position relative to the ground, there is no difference between lying supine with the head rotated 90 degrees to the right or keeping the neck in neutral and log rolling the entire body *en bloc* to the right. In both instances, the ear is in exactly the same position. In the first example, the ear is positioned by rotating the neck; in the second, the ear is positioned by rolling the entire body. Both positioning methods accomplish the same task, positioning the right ear to the ground. Know your patient's physical restrictions prior to performing any type of canalith repositioning and make modifications as needed.

No matter which repositioning technique you use, keep in mind that most patients will have symptom resolution within just a few treatments. If signs and/or symptoms persist after a few treatment visits, consider referring the patient for further clinical testing to confirm BPPV and rule out other pathologies that may mimic BPPV.

Clinicians new to vestibular interventions for BPPV commonly ask whether canalith repositioning is safe to perform with geriatric patients. If performed properly, this type of intervention is safe and well tolerated by most patients. Always

remember to know your patients' physical limitations, medical precautions, and cervical ranges of motion. Most patients are able to perform testing and interventions for BPPV with very few modifications. If you are ever in doubt, get medical clearance from those specialists who can best address your concerns. Remember, you can always keep the patient in neutral and move/rotate the entire body to reposition crystals.

Resolution Rates for Canalith Repositioning Maneuvers (CRM)

According to Helminski, "CRM is safe with no serious complications."[35] What kind of success should you expect from repositioning maneuvers? A study of 50 people with BPPV found the following resolution "cure" rates using the Epley maneuver after two maneuvers:[36]

- Post-trauma: 52%
- With idiopathic BPPV: 92%

Another study looking at the treatment of BPPV with CRM following mild-to-moderate traumatic brain injury (TBI) found that CRM resulted in significant symptom resolution and improvement in perceived physical health status.[37]

Post-Maneuver Restrictions

There is overwhelming evidence that post-maneuver restrictions (such as sleeping in a chair or with the head elevated) are not necessary. Some physicians still recommend some restrictions, despite the evidence they are not needed.[38–41]

Nausea with CRM

Often patients with BPPV become nauseous and occasionally vomit when they experience vertigo. It is always good practice to ask patients whether the positional vertigo has previously made them vomit previous to coming to you. If the patient has vomited from BPPV, chances are good that they will vomit while you are performing a test for BPPV or even during repositioning maneuvers. Have a plastic bag or bucket ready for this eventuality. An ice-cold wet towel placed across the back of the neck reduces nausea and may improve the patient's tolerance to testing/treatment. If the patient becomes overly nauseous, ask the referring physician to prescribe some type of anti-nausea medication prior to performing repositioning maneuvers. This will help the patient tolerate the interventions and increase their willingness to participate.

Latency of Nystagmus Onset

According to Hain,[42] cupulolithiasis has no latency, and canalithiasis has a latency of 5–30 seconds.

Maneuver Hold Times

Hold times for different repositioning maneuvers vary depending on the researcher. The hold times for gravity-driven maneuvers are basically just the time it takes for crystals to fall toward the ground inside the canal. You want to be sure to give the crystals enough time to move to the lowest possible position within the canal. Keeping this in mind, most hold times range from 30 seconds to 2 minutes. A common practice for testing (e.g., with Dix–Hallpike) is to wait at least 45 seconds in the test position before calling a BPPV test negative. For repositioning techniques, a common practice is to wait for nystagmus/dizziness to end and then add another 30 seconds to the hold time. Remember, holding longer won't affect the outcome, but if you don't hold the position long enough, you may not allow enough time for the crystals to move before you move into the next position of any maneuver. If you proceed through the maneuvers too quickly, the crystals may move (or fall back) in the wrong direction, and the maneuver will need to be repeated. Take your time! Slower is better than faster for gravity-driven tests and maneuvers.

Hand Position and Patient Instructions

During testing and repositioning maneuvers, the position of the vestibular system within the head with respect to the ground is key, and not so much the position of the rest of the body. As a general rule,

if patients can move, turn, or position without assistance, *let them*. This gives them a sense of control. When you are performing repositioning maneuvers, the same holds true. We do not always need to grab someone's head and turn it. Most people have head and neck control, and it is much friendlier to simply ask someone to turn their head and then guide or make corrections only as needed. Keep this in mind during repositioning maneuvers. When instructions call for the head to be turned or rotated, can the patient do that without *you* touching or moving their head? In some cases, the position changes are quick, and the clinicians need a more hands-on approach. For gravity-driven maneuvers, however, it is easy to simply direct the patient to move into the desired position with as little hands-on help as possible unless safety, maneuver requirements, or patient confusion require it.

Multiple-Canal Benign Paroxysmal Positional Vertigo

The incidence of multiple-canal BPPV varies depending on the research study and ranges from 4.7% to 12.2%.[43–46] Patients with multiple-canal involvement may have BPPV occurring in multiple canals of one ear or in both ears simultaneously. Which ear do you treat first? At least one study suggests treating the more symptomatic side first, since symptoms of bilateral involvement may be erroneous, possibly caused by incorrect head positioning during testing.[47] If bilateral symptoms disappear after treatment of the more symptomatic side, it is likely that the patient did not truly have bilateral BPPV. In cases of multi-canal involvement, the sequence of which canal is treated first is not critical and should not affect the outcomes of interventions. However, if you treat the more symptomatically bothersome canal first (followed by the next most bothersome), the patient may have improved tolerance during your interventions.

Patient and Clinician CRM

Repositioning maneuvers done by a clinician in combination with self-administered repositioning are more effective than CRM performed by a clinician alone. For self-administered treatments,

CRMs were more effective than liberatory maneuvers; the Brandt–Daroff was the least effective self-administered treatment.[48]

Canalith Repositioning Maneuvers

There are many CRM. Here we give instructions on the most common maneuvers. To treat the anterior or posterior canal (called the vertical canals) use the modified Epley maneuver, Semont liberatory maneuver, or the Brandt–Daroff maneuver. To treat the lateral canals, you may use the log roll maneuver, barbecue roll maneuver, or Gufoni maneuver.

MODIFIED EPLEY MANEUVER (TREATMENT FOR ANTERIOR/POSTERIOR CANALS)

1. The patient is instructed to long-sit on the bed/table, bending the knees if needed for back comfort. The clinician stands behind the patient. Once in the long-sitting position, tap the patient's shoulder on the side you wish to treat as a tactile cue, and have your other hand prepared to catch the patient's head.
2. Instruct the patient, "Turn your head half-way to this side." If needed, use your hands to correct head position. Instruct the patient, "Keep your head turned and eyes open, then lie back as quickly as you can so your head is hanging over the edge of the bed. Tell me if you feel dizzy or nauseous." As the patient moves into supine use verbal cues for head rotation. Ultimately the patient's head should be in 20 degrees to 30 degrees of extension over the end of the treatment surface. As the patient moves into supine, the clinician releases touch to the shoulder with one hand and catches the patient's head with the other hand guiding it as they lie back. The hand not supporting the head is now free to open the patient's eyelids (using your thumb) if it is closed owing to symptoms of vertigo. Hold this test position 45 seconds, or after nystagmus stops add another 30 seconds in this position. If nystagmus continues past 1 minute, return the patient to

sitting, and after testing all canals, attempt a liberatory maneuver.
3. Keeping head in extension, instruct the patient to rotate it to 45 degrees past neutral to the other side. (Note, this is a 90-degree turn in total, from 45 degrees on one side to 45 degrees on the other.) Hold the position until the nystagmus stops and add 30 more seconds. If no nystagmus is observed, wait 30 seconds before continuing to the next step.
4. Keeping the head rotated, instruct the patient to roll away from the treatment ear onto their side so that the head is angled nose-down toward the ground at 135 degrees from supine. (Remember, the head was already turned 45 degrees, so when the patient rolls onto their side and the head remains turned, they have just moved it another 45 degrees.)

   During the verbal instructions, the clinician taps the patient's shoulder as a tactile cue to indicate the side toward which the patient should roll. As the patient rolls onto that side, allow their head to roll off the supporting hand. Adjust the patient's head position as needed so that he is looking at the ground at about a 45-degree angle. If the patient has head control, you do not have to hold their head in this position.

   Keep in mind that you can rotate the trunk to accommodate a lack of cervical range of motion. Unless the patient lacks head control or has special cervical issues, you do not need to hold the head during this motion. While allowing the patient's head to roll off your supporting hand as he turns onto his side, place a hand on the patient's uppermost shoulder and move to stand to guard against rolling off the treatment table.

   Hold position until the nystagmus stops and add 30 more seconds. If no nystagmus is observed, wait 30 seconds before continuing to the next step. If you are not using video Frenzel goggles, it is difficult to see the patient's eyes. You may simply ask the patient if they are experiencing vertigo and to tell you when it stops.
5. Keeping the head turned, instruct the patient to return to sitting (on the side of the treatment table). Once sitting, the patient may turn the head to neutral. Guard the patient for at least 30 seconds, as otoconia may still be falling toward the otolithic matrix.

6. After a minute, retest, and repeat the procedure as needed.

Pictures of the progression of the modified Epley maneuver are shown in Figures 14.5 to 14.10.

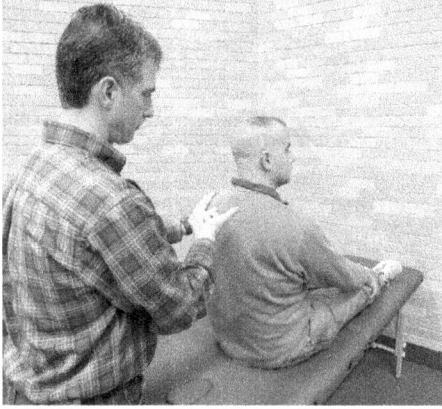

Figure 14.5 Modified Epley Maneuver Progression, Step 1

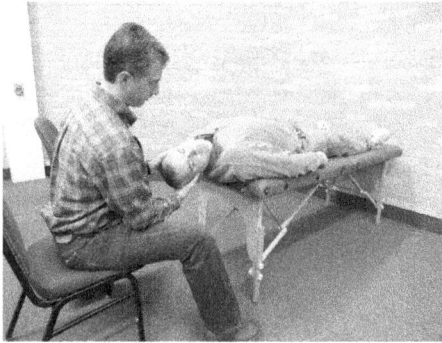

Figure 14.6 Modified Epley Maneuver Progression, Step 2

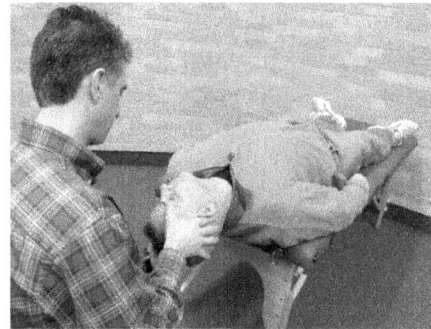

Figure 14.7 Modified Epley Maneuver Progression, Step 3

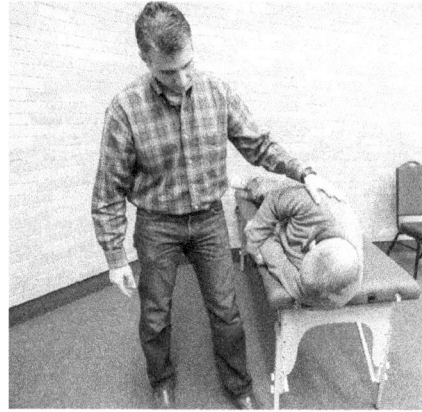

Figure 14.8 Modified Epley Maneuver Progression, Step 4

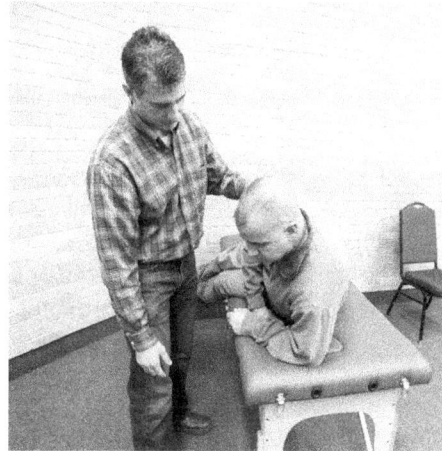

Figure 14.9 Modified Epley Maneuver Progression, Step 5

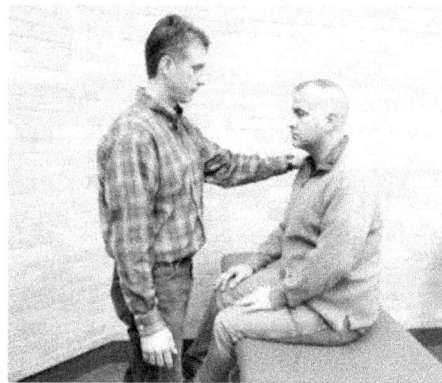

Figure 14.10 Modified Epley Maneuver Progression, Finish

SEMONT LIBERATORY MANEUVERS (TREATMENT FOR ANTERIOR/ POSTERIOR CANALS)

Technically, when treating a posterior canal, the maneuver is called the Semont, and when treating the anterior canal, it is called the reverse Semont.

1. While sitting on the side of the table/bed, the patient is instructed to rotate the head 45 degrees. They turn the head away from the ear to be treated for the posterior canal and toward the ear to be treated for the anterior canal. (Tap the shoulder in the direction you wish the patient to turn the head as a tactile cue.)
2. With the head rotated, the patient moves into side-lying onto the side of suspected involvement. (The patient should now be side-lying on the involved side with the nose rotated up to the ceiling 45 degrees to treat a posterior canal or rotated toward the ground 45 degrees to treat an anterior canal.)

If you are assisting/guiding the maneuver, your hands will be on each side of the patient's head at ear level while the patient crosses the arms in front of their chest and holds your forearms to assist during the moving parts of the maneuver.

3. While maintaining the head position, move the patient rapidly and forcefully into side-lying on the opposite side without stopping in the upright sitting position. When the patient comes to rest, they should be side lying on the other side, head still rotated in the same direction as in step 1. If the nose was up when starting, it should be down when finishing. If the nose was down when starting, it should be up when finishing. This is because the patient does not turn the head during the flip from one side to the other.
4. Hold this position. Hold times vary from 30 seconds to 2 minutes.
5. The patient maintains head rotation while returning to a sitting position.
6. Once seated, the head may return to a neutral position. The clinician should keep a hand on the patient's shoulder for about 30 seconds once seated to guard in case of vertigo.

There is also a reverse Semont maneuver to address anterior canal BPPV.

Photo examples of the Semont liberatory maneuver (SLM) are shown in Figures 14.11 to 14.16, without the clinician.

Photo examples of the reverse Semont liberatory maneuver (RSLM) are shown in Figures 14.17 to 14.20.

For the reverse Semont liberatory maneuver, in step 1, the patient is positioned side-lying with the affected anterior canal rotated toward the ground (head rotated 45 degrees). Next (step 2), instruct the patient to flip quickly and forcefully to side-lying on the opposite side with the affected anterior canal now toward the ceiling (the head does not move throughout the flipping motion). The patient maintains this position for 30 seconds to 2 minutes (step 3). The patient maintains head turn while returning to sitting. Once sitting, the patient may straighten the head.

BRANDT–DAROFF MANEUVER

This is a nonspecific maneuver and does not work as well as more specific maneuvers. However, it is a good maneuver to give as home instruction for those who cannot follow the instructions to perform specific maneuvers (e.g., modified Epley) or if the patient has osteoporosis, as they can perform this on their own.

1. The patient sits on the edge of a treatment table or bed and rotates their head to the left 45 degrees and quickly lies down on their right side. Hold this position for 30 seconds after vertigo stops (or 30 seconds if no vertigo is present).
2. The patient returns to sitting, and the head returns to a neutral position (hold 30 seconds).
3. The patient rotates his head to the right 45 degrees and quickly lies down on his left side, holding this position for 30 seconds after the vertigo stops (or 30 seconds if no vertigo is present).
4. The patient returns to sitting, and head returns to a neutral position (hold 30 seconds). This completes one cycle.
5. Do five cycles in a row, three times daily until symptoms resolve.

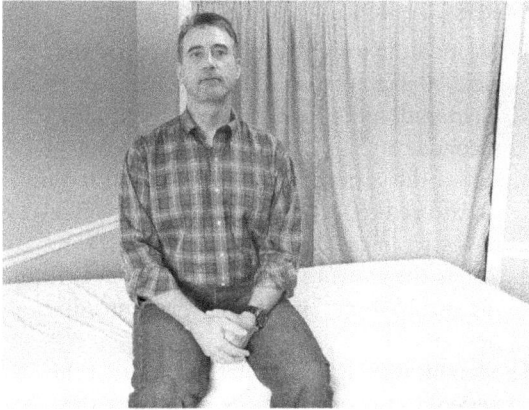

Figure 14.11 SLM, Beginning

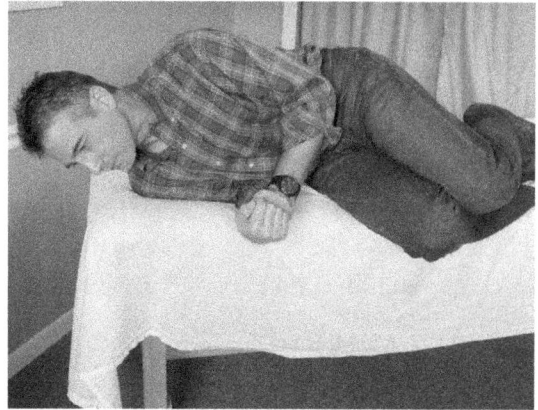

Figure 14.14 SLM, Step 4

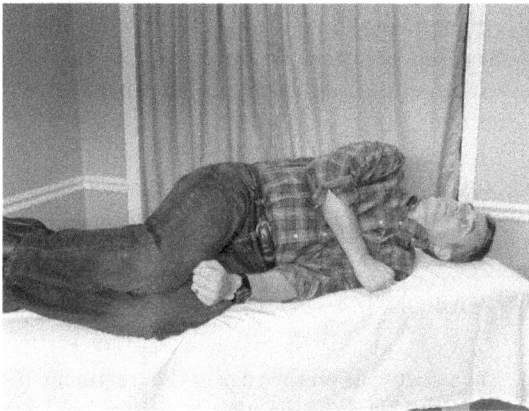

Figure 14.12 SLM, Step 2

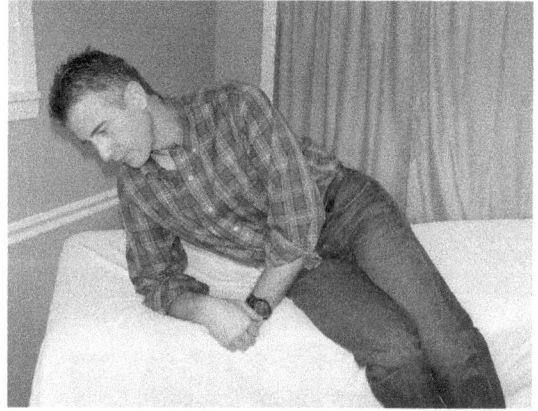

Figure 14.15 SLM, Step 5

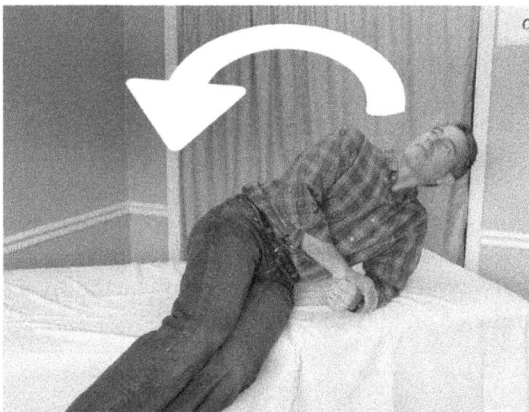

Figure 14.13 SLM, Step 3

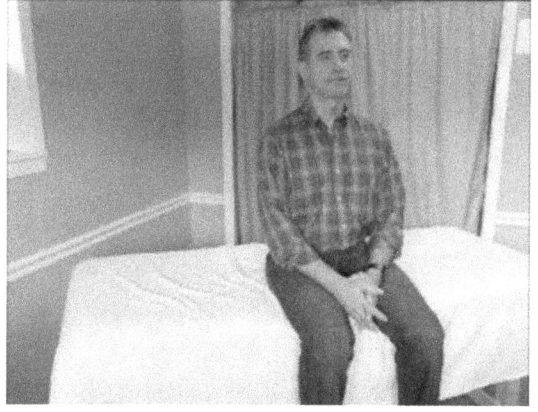

Figure 14.16 SLM, Step 6

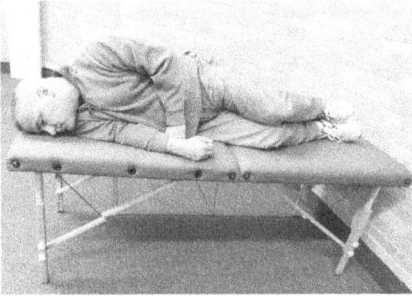

Figure 14.17 RSLM, Step 1

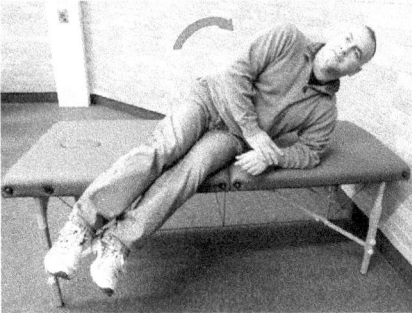

Figure 14.18 RSLM, Step 2

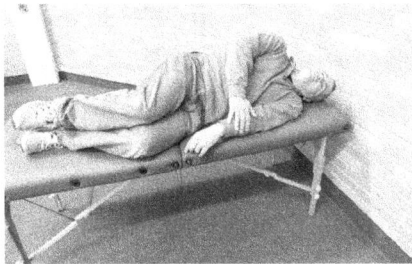

Figure 14.19 RSLM, Step 3

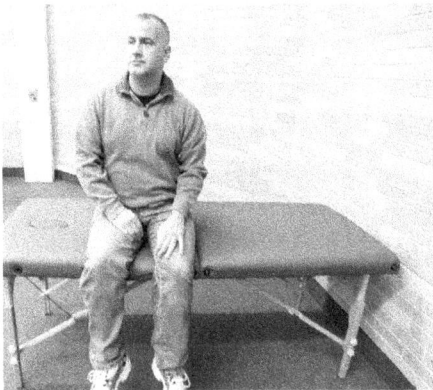

Figure 14.20 RSLM, Step 4

BARBECUE ROLL

1. Position the patient supine, then rotate the head 90 degrees toward the involved ear. Hold until nystagmus/dizziness stops plus 30 seconds.
2. Rotate the patient's head back to neutral (nose toward ceiling). Hold until nystagmus/dizziness stops plus 30 seconds.
3. Rotate the patient's head 90 degrees away from the involved ear. Hold until nystagmus/dizziness stops plus 30 seconds.
4. Maintaining the head rotation, instruct the patient to roll onto the side away from the involved ear until the nose is directly toward the ground. Hold until nystagmus/dizziness stops plus 30 seconds.
5. Maintaining the head position, instruct the patient to push into sitting. Once sitting, the head may return to a neutral position. The examiner should then guard the patient for 30 seconds.

Photos of the barbecue roll are shown (treating BPPV of the right lateral canal) in Figures 14.21 to 14.24.

GUFONI MANEUVER

1. The patient sits on the edge of the treatment table/bed, arms by the sides.
2. Instruct the patient to move quickly into side-lying with the head in a neutral position onto the unaffected (healthy) side. One side-lying, the head is immediately rotated 45 degrees toward the floor (nose down).
3. Hold for 2 minutes.
4. Keeping the head turned, the patient returns to sitting. Once sitting, the head may return to a neutral position.

Videos of other maneuvers (Lempert, Vannucchi–Asprella, Kim's deep head hang for anterior canal BPPV, and apogeotropic conversion methods) are included on the publisher's website.

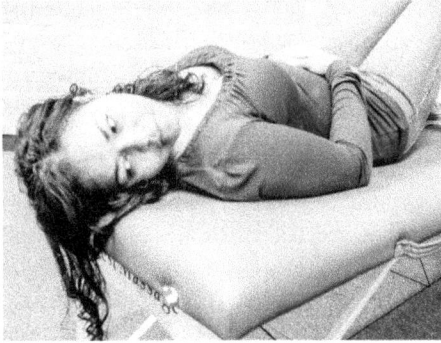

Figure 14.21 Barbecue Roll, Step 1

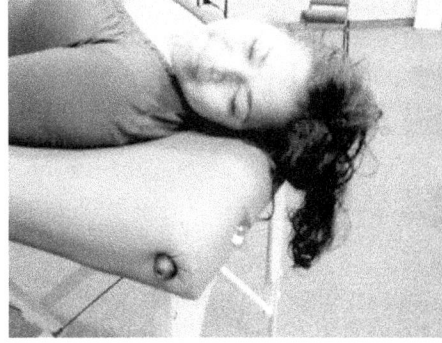

Figure 14.23 Barbecue Roll, Step 3

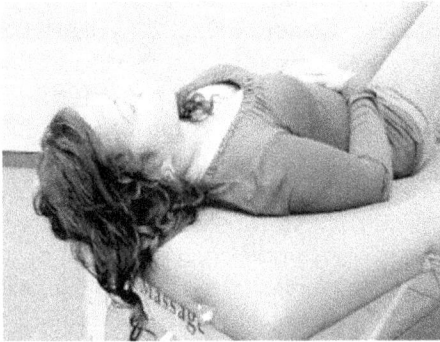

Figure 14.22 Barbecue Roll, Step 2

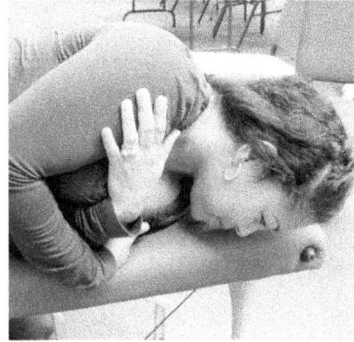

Figure 14.24 Barbecue Roll, Step 4

MOTION HABITUATION

Motion habituation is the repetition of a motion that provokes symptoms until the motion is no longer bothersome. This is done over time, and the patient must be given time to recover from symptoms provoked by the offending motion(s) until it is repeated. According to Whitney et al., habituation exercises are most apt for the treatment of persistent postural–perceptual dizziness (PPPD).[49] You may use motions that provoke symptoms on the Motion Sensitivity Quotient/Test or the Modified Motion Sensitivity Test as treatment motions. You may readminister these tests every week to assess changes to motion sensitivity, adjusting the exercises as needed. When choosing motions to use as treatment, do not use motions that are least or most bothersome, but instead choose motions that are moderately bothersome. Many patients presenting with vestibulopathy may also test positive for motion sensitivities.

BALANCE EXERCISES

The physical therapist can provide balance retraining, while the occupational therapist can apply controlled movement to functional activities. There are crossover responsibilities between these two disciplines regarding balance interventions. While audiologists treat balance as it relates to the vestibular system, they should refer patients to physical and occupational therapists when comorbidities beyond the vestibular system are involved or when a patient has functional deficits with gait and ADLs. The team approach typically yields the best outcomes for functional movement.

Typical progressions of balance interventions go from a focus on stability to that of mobility. When designing a balance intervention program, it is important to keep each individual patient's needs in mind. The 90-year-old patient's balance needs are, not surprisingly, different from those of the college or professional athlete. By considering the individual functional needs of each patient, it becomes easier to choose the appropriate interventions, activities, and exercises. In the case of the geriatric patient, a helpful strategy is to start with basic stability exercises, such as standing postures with a variety of feet positions. From there you can move to trunk sways, reaching, weight-shifting activities, stepping, and then more dynamically moving activities. Younger patients who are more active may only require dynamic activities and exercises. You will decide this after your evaluation. For athletes, treatment focus depends upon whether they are patients or clients. When they have been injured, treatment will first have to address the physical impairments and deficits and later progress to more dynamic interventions. For clients, perform a physical assessment to test their abilities, and plan training strategies around any deficiencies or the athlete's sport or position within a sport.

ANKLE PROPRIOCEPTION INTERVENTIONS

It is impossible to train balance without also affecting proprioception and strength. Training of proprioception is often called *neuromuscular reeducation/exercise/training*. What constitutes a neuromuscular or proprioception exercise? Generally, these are exercises that include joint movement. This is a very broad way to categorize these exercises; after all, we move our joints in walking, weight shifting, or weight lifting. It seems that proprioceptive exercises are those that include joint motion for the purpose of improving somatosensation. Finding research on this subject is sometimes challenging for the simple fact that proprioception is

not always measured or described in the same way. Results of various studies are mixed as to the efficacy of such exercises to improve proprioception. If you are having the patient perform standing balance exercises/activities, make sure you have them wear a gait belt and have your hand on it. You can do this without providing proprioceptive feedback.

There have been a few studies showing improvement using proprioceptive exercises. While tai chi has been widely discussed in the literature as a balance exercise, it is not designed to be a proprioceptive exercise per se. However, owing to the constant weight shifting involving joint motion, weight bearing, and turning, it is a great proprioceptive exercise for the lower extremities by nature.

In a review of studies that used tai chi as an intervention for balance and postural control in people with peripheral neuropathy, the authors found tai chi was associated with significant increases in plantar vibration and tactile sensitivity.[50] A different tai chi study compared proprioceptive exercises to the effects of tai chi on ankle strength and proprioception (ankle joint position sense). The proprioceptive exercise included both static and dynamic balance tasks and transitions. This study ($n = 60$) found that both proprioception exercises *and* tai chi significantly improved ankle proprioception in the elderly, with no significant difference between these groups.[51] In a therapy scenario, we do not perform tai chi forms but rather incorporate the weight-shifting exercises and activities, which are integral components of tai chi, into our plans of care.

A study on the effectiveness of a sensorimotor exercise program on proprioception, balance, muscle strength, functional mobility, and risk of falls in older people ($n = 56$) found that these exercises improved balance and confidence in this patient population.[52] After reading the sensorimotor interventions listed next, you can see that it involves more than proprioception. The intervention included strengthening, as well as the following sensorimotor exercises (four exercises with four levels of difficulty):

1. *Adhesive star*: The patient stands in the center of an eight-pointed star on a non-slip mat, with the points 40 cm distant from the center. The

patient is instructed to slide a foot toward the points (which were numbered) upon a verbal cue. Progression is from a four-pointed star to an eight-pointed star.

2. *Colored path*: Seven swatches of white paper and seven swatches of blue paper are alternately laid out on a non-slip mat in a zigzag pattern. Patients are instructed to first walk up and down the mat on one color. Then, down the mat using one color and back with the other. Next, they alternate colors, and finally, step on colors called out by the therapist.

3. *Rubber step*: Patients attempt to balance on a step. Have the patient stand on a 5 cm step and toss a light ball upon a verbal cue. Next, the patient ascends/descends the 5 cm step and then tosses the ball again. Repeat the task using a 10 cm step.

4. *Obstacles on the path*: The subjects walk on a non-slip mat over 3.6 m and perform dorsiflexion, hip flexion, and knee flexion whenever encountering an obstacle. Progressions include different heights of obstacles, navigating cones, and a mix of obstacles.

Ankle-Specific Proprioception Exercises

- *Supine*: Prop the lower limb on a pillow with the ankle and foot hanging off the edge. Instruct the patient to trace the alphabet with each ankle with as big movements as possible.
- *Sitting*: Place a tennis ball under the patient's foot and instruct the patient to trace the alphabet with each ankle with as big movements as possible.
- *Static standing exercises*: First, allow the patient to touch a refence surface, and later progress to standing without the added touch. Attempt these exercises for 30 seconds to 1 minute.
  - Stand on a firm surface with feet together and eyes open. Progress to eyes closed, then to standing on foam with eyes open/closed.
  - Stand in semi-tandem with the eyes open and arms by the sides or across the chest. Progress to eyes closed or full tandem.
  - Stand on one leg and eyes open on a firm surface. Progress to standing on foam.

VARYING EXERCISES

How can we vary exercises? According to Shumway-Cook, three things influence our movement: the individual, the task, and the environment.[53] By changing one or more of these, the exercise or activity may require more concentration or the recruitment of different systems in order to complete the task at hand. By varying the conditions or tasks, we challenge the body to respond and perform under a wider variety of circumstances requiring balance. The take-home message is that you can avoid repetitively using the same exact interventions by varying the conditions and, in the process, challenge the body in new and different ways. As patients progress with their abilities to succeed with one intervention or task, you may vary the environment, task, or person to further challenge the body to improve. Ways to advance an intervention include the following:

- Varying environments (e.g., standing surface, noise, light).
  - We may change the environment by varying the surface the patient is standing on. For example, more firm surfaces (such as wood, tile, or concrete) are generally easier to stand on because they are stable and noncompliant (i.e., they do not deform under the patient's weight). A softer, more compliant surface—such as a thick carpet or grass outdoors—provides a greater challenge. Even more compliant surfaces, such as high-density foam, or unstable surfaces, such as rocker boards, add maximal challenges.
- Varying tasks (e.g., static vs. dynamic, stability vs. mobility).
  - We may vary the way in which the patient performs a task. Stable tasks may use a wider base of support or allow for additional proprioceptive input by allowing the patient to touch a wall, counter, or assistive device. We may increase the challenge provided to the patient during a task by reducing the allowance to use the

hands for added touch proprioception or by reducing the base of support. Further progression may lead to moving or reaching tasks within and then outside the base of support.

- For upper extremity tasks performed while standing, we may change the task by changing the objects to be manipulated (e.g., using a variety of object contact surfaces: slippery, smooth, coarse). The weight or size of objects can also be varied.
- For upper extremity use while standing, we may vary the angle to which the patient must reach (e.g., overhead, lower than the waist, or movements that require trunk rotation).

- Varying something about the individual (e.g., single- vs. dual-task concentration).
  - Consider the patient's cognition, attention, motivation, emotion, and the sensory and motor abilities of the individual.
  - Adding a mental task to the physical task is an example of dual tasking. We are asking the patient to do two or more things at once, such as balancing on a piece of high-density foam while counting backward by twos. Another example of dual tasking combines changing the individual and the task by having the patient carry an object while walking or move objects from one pants pocket to another while walking. When we divide concentration between more than one task, patients are challenged. There may be times when we decide that dual tasking is a beneficial activity, and at other times we may instruct the patient to *avoid* dual tasking, as it may prove to be too challenging and thus present a safety hazard. A commonly seen example is that some elderly patients lack sufficient cognition to safely talk while walking. When they do attempt this, you notice that their steps become smaller, and some may even stumble. Use your clinical judgment to decide when dual tasking is appropriate as an intervention or when you should advise against it.

SITTING BALANCE

Most therapists are very familiar with training sitting balance, from managing sitting on a firm to soft surface and then reaching within and outside of the base of support. You may challenge sitting balance as a progression by moving from sitting on a firm surface to a soft surface, to sitting on a large ball. You may remove a foot surface—that is, do not let the patient's feet touch the floor while sitting on a firm or soft surface. Start with added stability by allowing the patient to use their hands to help maintain seated balance or to touch a reference object. Later, you may limit or eliminate the use of the upper extremities for the assistance in sitting balance.

For more advanced sitting balance challenges, you may wish to incorporate sitting on a wobble board or inflatable therapy ball. Once patients have acquired the skill to sit on stable surfaces, they may further be challenged by adding reaching tasks or seated marching while sitting. Using reaching activities beyond the patient's arm length is an effective way to improve reach speed and distance as well as increasing load through a stroke-affected foot and activation of the affected leg muscles. The patient should be wearing a gait belt and guarded against falling.

STANDING *BALANCE*

Listed next are balance interventions that are in order from *more stable* to *less stable,* or *more mobile*.

Static Standing

- Static standing on a firm surface with eyes open (wider base → narrow base) → static standing with eyes closed → standing eyes open/closed on a soft surface.
  - Typically, wider bases of support are easier to maintain. As the patient becomes more skilled at balancing with a certain stance width, you may make the task or exercise more challenging by narrowing the base of support used while performing it. Many

therapists also have patients stand in tandem (heel to toe) or partial tandem (feet closely side by side with one foot somewhat advanced). This may occur within the same treatment session or over numerous sessions.

- Standing with the eyes closed removes a lot of information used to balance and also trains balance in low-light environments. You may time the patient's ability to perform these tasks to show how long they can stand with their eyes closed. Documenting these times will help show the patient's progress in balance ability.
- Standing on high-density balance foam simulates standing on other compliant or unstable surfaces, such as thick carpeting, grass, or gravel. Patients who have difficulty standing on balance foam will likely have difficulty while standing on these real-life examples. Since the task of standing on foam is similar to standing on these other environments, there will be crossover improvement for balancing on them when you train the patient on foam.
- Standing on one foot.

Dynamic Standing

Using the variations from the "static standing" list, we can begin challenging standing–moving tasks by using different techniques, such as trunk sways, weight shifting, balance challenges, balancing while performing an upper extremity task such as reaching within and outside of the limits of stability, and adding unilateral stance activities.

TRUNK SWAYS

Trunk sways are a great starting place for dynamic motions for those who are challenged by ADLs that require standing, such as grooming, brushing teeth at the sink, cooking at the stove, and standing at the bus stop. While using trunk sways as an intervention, the patient is instructed to stand with their feet together or with a close-stance width. While performing the trunk sway, do not allow bending at the waist in any direction

(e.g., no forward flexing or side bending), and instruct the patient to stand as straight as possible. Instruct the patient to lean their entire body (keeping the back straight) to the farthest point of trunk excursion possible to the limits of their stability as long as the patient's feet (heels or toes) do not lift from the floor. Progress the patient from only swaying in one direction to tracing a box around themselves.

You may assess balance control and limits of stability by instructing the patient to use trunk sways to trace a box pattern around the base of support. As they move the trunk (again, without bending at the waist) observe any areas around the base of support the patient avoids. You may also use trunk sways as a balance exercise, swaying toward areas over which the patient has less control to improve stability. You may also instruct the patient to sway as if they were standing in the center of a clock drawn on the floor, calling out the number to which they should sway. An example of an anterior trunk sway is shown in Figures 14.25 and 14.26.

UNILATERAL STANCE WITH DYNAMIC CONTRALATERAL LOWER EXTREMITY ACTIVITY

Standing on one leg is needed to perform many functional movements, from putting a leg through a pant leg while getting dressed to bearing weight on one limb while stepping into a bathtub or up a stair step. How many activities can you imagine with which to practice unilateral weight-bearing stance? You may simply challenge your patients to stand on one foot while being timed. To keep the patient's interest, incorporate unilateral leg stance into other games or activities. One example is to draw a large number pad (as on a phone) and place it on a step. While the patient stands on one leg, they are instructed to type out numbers with the contralateral foot (e.g., phone numbers of friends or family, birth dates of family members). When the activity is meaningful in some way, the patient will be more interested in participating.

DYNAMIC STANDING ON FOAM

Ask the patient to perform upper extremity tasks such as reaching (both inside and outside the base

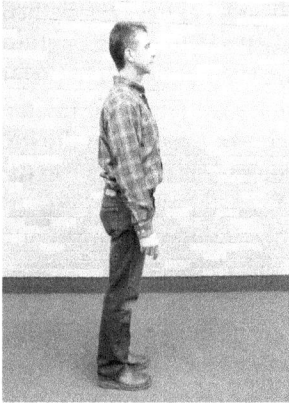

Figure 14.25 Trunk Sway 1

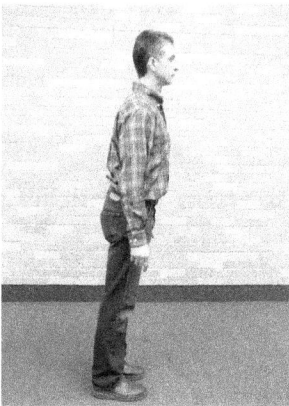

Figure 14.26 Trunk Sway 2

of support), tossing a ball, or hitting a balloon. You may further challenge the patients by having them perform a mental task (e.g., counting backward by threes), or by changing the environment by having them close their eyes to eliminate visual input. For more advanced exercises, you may include stepping on and off the foam.

WEIGHT SHIFTING

Patients may be taught awareness and control of their centers of gravity by performing lateral and diagonal weight shifting. Weight shifting challenges the patient to transfer, in a controlled manner, weight from one supporting foot to the other. Such activities are needed to step into a bathtub, put on pants while standing, and walk.

For lateral weight shifting, begin with the feet close together but not touching (~6 inches or 15 cm apart, or wider if needed) while the weight is shared equally between the feet (Figure 14.27).

Next, instruct a weight shift to place more weight through one foot, called *asymmetrical standing* (Figure 14.28).

This asymmetrical stance position is held for a few seconds, and the therapist should count out loud, after which the patient returns to a more symmetrically balanced stance. Using a phrase such as "Pretend you are preparing to place your foot on a step" will help the patient visualize how far they need to shift their weight. When first performing lateral weight shifts, patients with poor balance will usually avoid an asymmetrical stance, preferring instead to keep either their hips or head closer to the base of support. For example, while performing lateral weight shifting, balance-impaired patients typically either lean their heads sideways (trunk side flexion) while keeping the hips centered or they keep their heads centered over the base of support while pushing their hips out sideways in an attempt to perform the weight-shifting tasks as instructed. These patients do not realize they are making these compensatory movements; therefore, the therapist needs to use verbal, visual, and tactile cues to draw attention to and correct these compensations. For the first few treatment sessions, a full-length mirror is a helpful way to provide visual feedback. However, do not overly use this during your intervention, as the goal is for the patient to begin relying more on proprioceptive feedback for trunk position and not too much on vision for balance. Examples of compensations are shown in Figures 14.29 and 14.30.

If needed, allow the patient to touch the wall or some other support surface such as a chair-back, countertop, or even you for proprioceptive feedback. Patients are not allowed to lean on support surfaces, but just to touch them. As patients improve their ability to weight shift from one foot to the other while maintaining good posture (without excess leaning to compensate for a lack of control), begin limiting or removing the support surfaces. Examples of using support surfaces

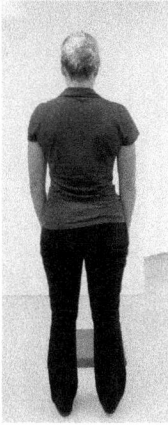

Figure 14.27 Weight Shift, Center

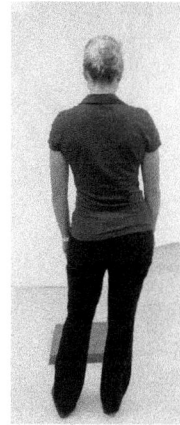

Figure 14.29 Weight Shift Compensation 1

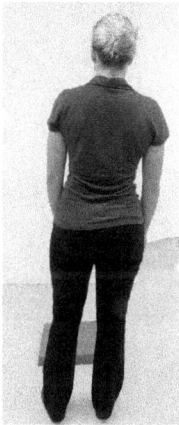

Figure 14.28 Weight Shift, Asymmetrical Standing

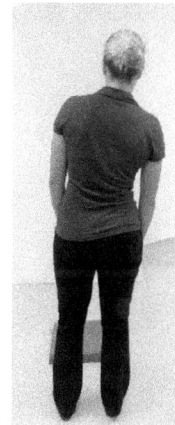

Figure 14.30 Weight Shift Compensation 2

for proprioceptive feedback can be seen in Figures 14.31 and 14.32, which depict a patient using a wall for proprioceptive feedback. Figure 14.33 depicts a patient holding a chairback for proprioceptive feedback.

As an example, the therapist instructs the patient to place their hands on either the therapist's forearms or hands for proprioceptive feedback. Next, the therapist instructs the patient to step and shift weight (one step at a time) with constant verbal cues for step length and body position (Figures 14.34 and 14.35).

This technique is the same for lateral and diagonal weight shifts, as if taking a step forward or back. Diagonal weight shifting begins with the patient standing with their feet a comfortable distance apart and instructing them to take a step forward with one foot without completely picking up the foot of the trailing leg, making sure the toes of the training leg stay on the ground (Figure 14.36).

As the patient shifts to bear weight primarily on the front (advanced) foot, the heel of the back foot lifts off the ground, as in the pre-swing position of gait (Figure 14.37).

It is common for patients to avoid shifting completely to the advanced front foot in first attempting this exercise. This may be secondary to the patient's perception of weakness or a fear of falling. They typically shift partway, leaving their center of gravity directly between their two feet,

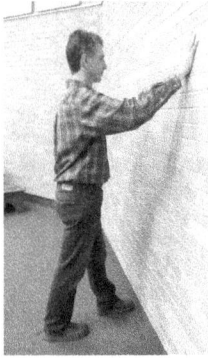

Figure 14.31 Diagonal Step 1, Touching a Wall

Figure 14.32 Diagonal Step 2, Touching a Wall

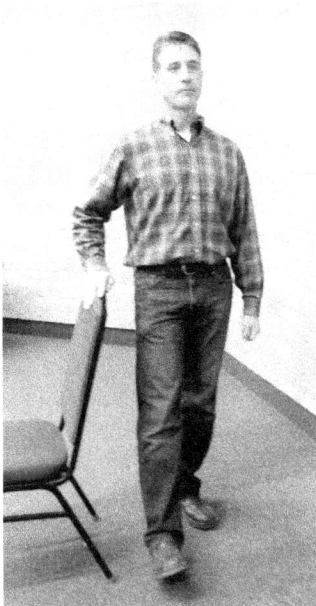

Figure 14.33 Diagonal Step 3, Touching Chairback

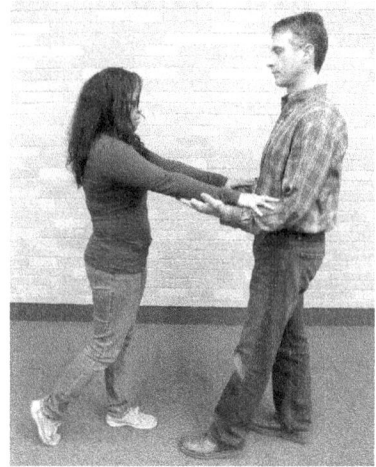

Figure 14.34 Weight Shift, Handhold 1

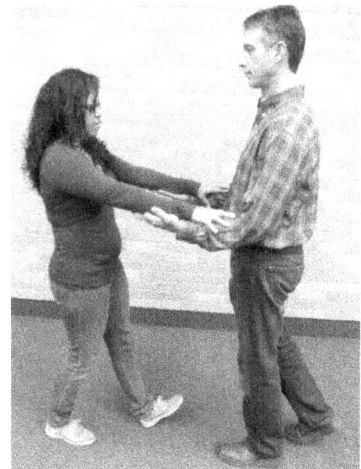

Figure 14.35 Weight Shift, Handhold 2

and then lean the trunk forward over the front foot. Patients are usually not aware they are doing this until the therapist tactilely cues their hips and torso to line up over the front foot. For this reason, it is helpful to perform weight-shifting exercises/activities in front of a full-length mirror so that the patient has a visual cue to reference. The goal is to get the body's weight supported by the front foot. When done properly, they should be able to lift the trailing foot off the floor without losing balance.

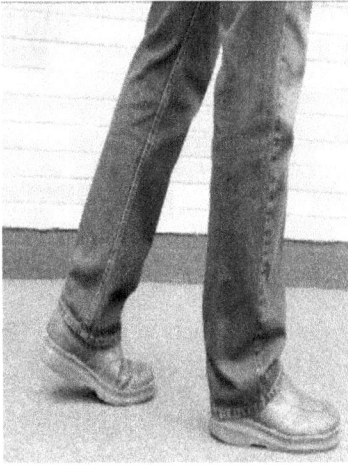

Figure 14.36 Standing with Foot Advanced

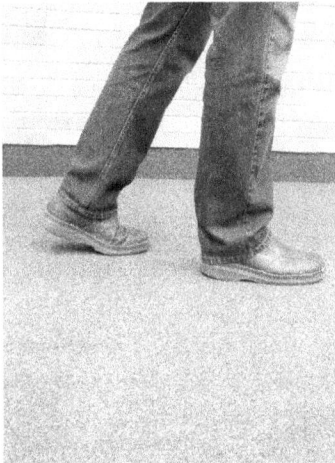

Figure 14.37 Weight Bearing on Advanced Foot

STEP-UPS

There are a variety of ways to perform stepping activities to incorporate weight shifting. For example, you may have the patient step up and down from a stair step or balance platform while giving verbal cues to weight shift, first laterally and then after placing the foot on the step, diagonally weight shifting onto the step. Correct any excessive leaning laterally past the supporting foot while shifting laterally. Do not allow patients to perform compensatory motions such as attempting to move quickly and "power" their way while stepping or changing positions. Instead, cue controlled and deliberate, slow movements. To return to standing

on the floor, perform the same motions given to step up, only in reverse order. Repeat this activity by alternately stepping up with each leg. Repeat alternating steps several times as tolerated. While the patient is learning to pay attention to the proprioceptive inputs, the slow movements also help strengthen the muscles and increase the stability needed to perform these motions. Use a gait belt and guard the patient during balance exercises. Verbally and tactilely cue the patient constructively to provide feedback during the motions. The feedback should be accurate to either commend correct motions or correct undesired movements or compensations. Make sure that at the end of each weight shift, the head and hips are over the supporting foot (base of support). Weight-shifting exercises and activities should form the core of your balance interventions.

CLOCK STANDING

Have the patient imagine that they are standing in the center of a clock, facing 12. Have the patient step toward the 12 with their right leg and stand on the right leg, with the left leg trailing and left toes on the floor and heel off, stay in the standing position 1–3 seconds, and then return to the center. Do this with the right leg for each number on the right side of the clock, and the left leg for each number on the left side of the clock. Each leg will step toward numbers 12 and 6 (alternately). Patients with slight dementia have difficulty imaging a clock, so in these cases either have them facing an actual clock that they may use as a reference or put tape on the floor.

Some elderly patients become visually dependent. Many patients who have balance deficits rely not only on vision to improve their balance but also actively seek increased somatosensory information through light touch. You may have had the experience of seeing a balance-impaired person touching anything within reach as they walk, such as furniture, walls, or other people. These people are not necessarily leaning on these objects but instead are collecting information through their hands to aid balance. When they touch the wall or furniture, for example, they have a reference to the location of the floor. This information helps to provide a frame of reference in which they can determine their own location in space and plan to balance against gravity. Studies have demonstrated that sensory input to the hand and arm through contact can reduce postural sway in people who do not have balance impairments as well as in those with vestibular deficits even when the contact is not used to physically support the body (that is, it is only used for touch).[54]

The very act of touching things within reach while standing or walking is a red flag, letting you know that the person likely does not have enough information with which to balance. How could this be useful? First, we know that some patients who are balance-compromised may benefit from the use of an assistive device. The added somatosensory information gained by touching a cane to the floor may be enough to increase function and decrease fall risk. Further, we may use the sense of touch during balance training. When a patient's ability to balance is compromised, we may choose to start balance interventions while allowing the patient to touch (not lean on) a counter, wall, chair, etc. The purpose would be to give them more somatosensory information to aid in training. As patients progress in their ability to balance (whether statically or dynamically), you may reduce touch information to increase the challenge of balance interventions. For example, when you begin, the patient may be allowed to touch another object with both hands. Later, you may restrict their touch to only one hand. You may further challenge the patient by reducing the touching of a reference object to just one or two fingers. Ultimately you may wish to eliminate the allowance of using touch as a balance aid. Through this process, the patient can learn to use more information during balance training as well as having an increased sense of security.

OTHER DYNAMIC BALANCE EXERCISES

Once patients gain control of weight shifting, you may progress them to more dynamic exercises and activities. Some examples include side-stepping, walking backward, stepping up/down from a raised surface, picking up objects from the floor (with squats and pendulum [golfer's lift] techniques), stepping in a variety of directions, or stepping while performing other tasks (e.g., turning the head, carrying an object, or performing mental tasks).

While performing side-stepping, make sure to prevent compensatory movements of trunk/hip rotation or external leg rotation and flexion. An easy way to do this is to use a gait belt to physically restrain the patient from rotating the hips during the side-step. Perform this exercise/activity at both a comfortable patient-selected pace and also a quick pace to help train quicker reactions that guard against falling. It is an exercise that strengthens hip abductors, and an activity used in ADL and also for protective responses. Do not do this exercise too many times a day with different patients, or you may give yourself bursitis!

Backward walking is a very dynamic and difficult activity, especially if performed slowly. Typically, the patient will need some tactile assistance by placing their hands on the therapist's forearms (who is holding the gait belt), as well as verbal cues when first attempting this activity. For the balance-impaired patient, perform each step deliberately and slowly, reinforcing weight shifting as they step. Athletes involved in more advanced training can run backward as part of their training.

Perturbations are another way to add balance challenges. In terms of balance, a perturbation occurs when we introduce an external force like a nudge or pull to move the patient's center of gravity away from the base of support. The patient's task is to regain control of the center of gravity. You may use perturbations during sitting, standing, or walking balance tasks.

Reaching activities challenge balance control in sitting and standing. These activities may be as simple as reaching within the base of support or more challenging by reaching outside the base to touch or grasp an object. The following are some examples of reaching activities:

- Reaching (sitting or standing) to hit a balloon back and forth to the therapist
- Reaching to move items along a counter from one side of the patient to the other
- Picking up objects from the floor
- Removing items placed on an overhead shelf
- Performing a ball toss

Sometimes, having the patient perform an ADL while standing challenges balance, such as the following:

- Grooming in front of a mirror
- Performing upper and lower body dressing while standing
- Weight shifting to an advanced foot to hang clothes in a closet
- Weight shifting laterally or diagonally to put dishes/glasses into a kitchen cupboard

If you want to further challenge the patient, remember to vary the individual, task, or environment. While the physical therapist may instruct weight shifting as an exercise to improve control of balance, proprioceptive awareness, and lower extremity strength, the occupational therapist may have the patient perform the same weight shifts while performing functional activities, such as putting dishes in a cupboard, getting clothes out of the closet, or stepping into a bathtub. This would not be a duplication of service, since each discipline is performing the weight shift for different reasons.

In summary, proprioceptive and balance interventions may include joint-specific proprioception exercises, such as wobble boards, to standing activities (both static and dynamic) that incorporate ankle, knee, and hip movements. Finally, we may use light touch as a somatosensory balance aid in retraining balance. Addressing muscle weakness and range of motion limitations of the hips and lower extremities will improve the patient's stability.

If you plan to have strengthening-specific exercises in the same treatment session as functional or balance activities, perform the balance and functional interventions first, so you do not retrain balance and function with fatigued or overworked lower extremity muscles. Plan for the patient to have a rest period after strengthening prior to leaving the clinic/treatment session.

REFERENCES

1. Han BI, Song HS, Kim JS. Vestibular rehabilitation therapy: review of indications, mechanisms, and key exercises. *J Clin Neurol.* Dec 2011;7(4):184–96. doi:10.3988/jcn.2011.7.4.184

2. Alghadir AH, Iqbal ZA, Whitney SL. An update on vestibular physical therapy. *J Chin Med Assoc.* Jan 2013;76(1):1–8. doi:10.1016/j.jcma.2012.09.003

3. Dougherty JM, Carney M, Hohman MH, Emmady PD. *Vestibular Dysfunction.* StatPearls Publishing; Updated 2023. https://www.ncbi.nlm.nih.gov/books/NBK558926/

4. Chen J, Liu Z, Xie Y, Jin S. Effects of vestibular rehabilitation training combined with anti-vertigo drugs on vertigo and balance function in patients with vestibular neuronitis: a systematic review and meta-analysis. *Front Neurol.* 2023;14:1278307. doi:10.3389/fneur.2023.1278307

5. Ismail EI, Morgan AE, Abdel Rahman AM. Corticosteroids versus vestibular rehabilitation in long-term outcomes in vestibular neuritis. *J Vestib Res.* 2018;28(5–6):417–424. doi:10.3233/ves-180645

6. Hidayati HB, Imania HAN, Octaviana DS, et al. Vestibular rehabilitation therapy and corticosteroids for vestibular neuritis: a systematic review and meta-analysis of randomized controlled trials. *Medicina (Kaunas).* Sep 5 2022;58(9):1221. doi:10.3390/medicina58091221

7. Lawson B. Dizziness in the older person. *Rev Clin Gerontol.* 2005;15:187–206.

8. Furman J, Raz Y, Whitney S. Geriatric vestibulopathy assessment and management. *Curr Options Otolaryngol Head Neck Surg.* 2010;18:386–391.

9. Rogers TS, Noel MA, Garcia B. Dizziness: Evaluation and management. *Am Fam Physician.* 2023;107(5):514–523.

10. Muncie HL, Sirmans SM, James E. Dizziness: Approach to evaluation and management. *Am Fam Physician.* 2017;95(3):157.

11. Rascol O, Hain TC, Brefel C, et al. Antivertigo medications and drug-induced vertigo. A pharmacological review. *Drugs.* 1995;50(5):777–791.

12. Shepard N, Telian S, Smith-Wheelock M. Habituation and balance retraining therapy: A retrospective review. *Neurol Clin.* 1990;8(2):459–475.

13. Shepard NT, Telian SA. Programmatic vestibular rehabilitation. *Head Neck Surg.* 1995;112:173–182.

14. Shepard NT, Telian SA, Smith-Wheelock M, Raj A. Vestibular and balance rehabilitation therapy. *Ann Otol Rhinol Laryngol.* 1993;102(3 Pt 1):198–205.

15. Horak F, Jones-Rycewicz C, Black F, Shumway-Cook A. Effects of vestibular rehabilitation on dizziness and imbalance. *Otolaryngol Head Neck Surg.* 1992;106(2):175–180.

16. Hillier SL, McDonnell M. Vestibular rehabilitation for unilateral peripheral vestibular dysfunction. *Cochran Database Syst Rev.* 2011;16(2):CD005397. doi: 10.1002/14651858.CD005397.pub3

17. Kulcu D, Yanik B, Boynukali S, Kurtais Y. Efficacy of a home-based exercise program on benign paroxysmal positional vertigo compared with betahistine. *Otolaryngol Head Neck Surg.* 2008;37(3):373–379.

18. Do Y-K Kim J, Yang H-S, et al. The effect of early canalith repositioning on benign paroxysmal positional vertigo on recurrence. *Clin Exp Otorhinolayngol.* 2011;4(3):113–117.

19. Halker R, Barrs D, Wellik K, Wingerchuck D, Demaerschalk B. Establishing a diagnosis of benign paroxysmal positional vertigo through the Dix-Hallpike and side-lying maneuvers. *The Neurologist.* 2008;14:201–204.

20. Bhattacharyya N, Gubbels SP, Schwartz SR, Edlow JA, El-Kashlan H, Fife T, Holmberg JM, Mahoney K, Hollingsworth DB, Roberts R, Seidman MD, Steiner RW, Do BT, Voelker CC, Waguespack RW, Corrigan MD. Clinical practice guideline: Benign Paroxysmal positional vertigo (Update). *Otolaryngol Head Neck Surg.* 2017;156(3_suppl):S1–S47. doi: 10.1177/0194599816689667

21. Strupp M, Dlugaiczyk J, Ertl-Wagner BB, Rujescu D, Westhofen M, Dieterich M. Vestibular disorders. *Dtsch Arztebl Int.* 2020;117(17):300–310. doi: 10.3238/arztebl.2020.0300

22. Van Esch B, van der Zaag-Loonen H, Bruintjes T, van Benthem PP. Betahistine in Ménière's disease or syndrome: A systematic review. *Audiol Neurootol.* 2022;27(1):1–33. doi: 10.1159/000515821

23. Guidetti ME, Ghilardi L, Fattori B, et al. Betahistine dihydrochloride in the treatment of peripheral vestibular vertigo. *Eur Arch Otorhinolaryngol.* 2003;260(2):73–77.

24. Strupp M, Huppert D, Frenzel C, et al. Long-term prophylactic treatment of attacks of vertigo in Ménière's disease: Comparison of a high with a low dosage of betahistine in an open trial. *Acta Otolaryngol (Stockh).* 2008;128:620–624.

25. Strupp M, Kraus L, Schautzer F, Rujescu D. Menière's disease: Combined pharmacotherapy with betahistine and the MAO-B inhibitor selegiline-an observational study. *J Neurol.* 2018;265(Suppl 1):80–85. doi: 10.1007/s00415-018-8809-8. Retraction in: *J Neurol.* 2020;267(4):1225. doi: 10.1007/s00415-020-09791-7

26. McDonnell MN, Hillier SL. Vestibular rehabilitation for unilateral peripheral vestibular dysfunction. *Cochrane Database Syst Rev.* Jan 13 2015;1(1):Cd005397. doi:10.1002/14651858.CD005397.pub4

27. Hall CD, Herdman SJ, Whitney SL, Anson ER, Carender WJ, Hoppes CW, Cass SP, Christy JB, Cohen HS, Fife TD, Furman JM, Shepard NT, Clendaniel RA, Dishman JD, Goebel JA, Meldrum D, Ryan C, Wallace RL, Woodward NJ. Vestibular rehabilitation for peripheral vestibular hypofunction: an updated clinical practice guideline from the academy of neurologic physical therapy of the american physical therapy association. *J Neurol Phys Therapy.* 2022;46(2):118–177. doi:10.1097/NPT.0000000000000382

28. Edwards C, Franklin E. *Vestibular Rehabilitation.* StatPearls Publishing; Updated 2023. https://www.ncbi.nlm.nih.gov/books/NBK572153/

29. Appeadu MK, Bordoni B. *Falls and Fall Prevention in Older Adults.* StatPearls Publishing; Updated 2023. https://www.ncbi.nlm.nih.gov/books/NBK560761/

30. Lacour M, Lopez C, Thiry A, Tardivet L. Vestibular rehabilitation improves spontaneous nystagmus normalization in patients with acute unilateral vestibulopathy. *Front Rehabil Sci*. 2023;4:1122301. doi:10.3389/fresc.2023.1122301

31. Schubert M. Personal communication. In: Plishka C, ed. 2024.

32. Muntaseer Mahfuz M, Schubert MC, Todd CJ, Figtree WVC, Khan SI, Migliaccio AA. The effect of visual contrast on human vestibulo-ocular reflex adaptation. *J Assoc Res Otolaryngol*. Feb 2018;19(1):113–122. doi:10.1007/s10162-017-0644-6

33. Clendaniel RA, Lasker DM, Minor LB. Differential adaptation of the linear and nonlinear components of the horizontal vestibuloocular reflex in squirrel monkeys. *J Neurophysiol*. Dec 2002;88(6):3534–3540. doi:10.1152/jn.00404.2002

34. Obrero-Gaitán E, Sedeño-Vidal A, Peinado-Rubia AB, Cortés-Pérez I, Ibáñez-Vera AJ, Lomas-Vega R. Optokinetic stimulation for the treatment of vestibular and balance disorders: a systematic review with meta-analysis. *Eur Arch Otorhinolaryngol*. Sep 2024;281(9):4473–4484. doi:10.1007/s00405-024-08604-1

35. Helminski JO. Effectiveness of the canalith repositioning procedure in the treatment of benign paroxysmal positional vertigo. *Phys Ther*. Oct 2014;94(10):1373–1382. doi:10.2522/ptj.20130239

36. Maciejewska B, Maciejewska-Szaniec Z, Pilarska A, Mehr K, Michalak M, Wiskirska-Woznica B. Effectiveness of the canalith repositioning procedure in idiopathic and posttraumatic benign paroxysmal positional vertigo. *Family Med Primary Care Rev*. 2016;3:278–184.

37. Ouchterlony D, Masanic C, Michalak A, Topolovec-Vranic,Rutka JA . Treating benign paroxysmal positional vertigo in the patient with traumatic brain injury: effectiveness of the canalith repositioning procedure. *J Neurosci Nurs*. 2016;48(2):90–99.

38. Papacharalampous GX, Vlastarakos PV, Kotsis GP, Davilis D, Manolopoulos L. The role of postural restrictions after BPPV treatment: real effect on successful treatment and BPPV's recurrence rates. *Int J Otolaryngol*. 2012;2012:932847. doi:10.1155/2012/932847

39. Fyrmpas G, Rachovitsas D, Haidich AB, et al. Are postural restrictions after an Epley maneuver unnecessary? First results of a controlled study and review of the literature. *Auris Nasus Larynx*. Dec 2009;36(6):637–643. doi:10.1016/j.anl.2009.04.004

40. Toupet M, Ferrary E, Bozorg, Grayeli A. Effect of repositioning maneuver type and postmaneuver restrictions on vertigo and dizziness in benign positional paroxysmal vertigo. *Scientific World J*. 2012:162123. doi:10.1100/2012/162123

41. Devaiah AK, Andreoli S. Postmaneuver restrictions in benign paroxysmal positional vertigo: an individual patient data meta-analysis. *Otolaryngol Head Neck Surg*. Feb 2010;142(2):155–159. doi:10.1016/j.otohns.2009.09.013

42. Hain TC. *Cupulolithiasis, Canalithiasis and Vestibulithiasis*. Dizziness-and-balance.com; 2024. https://dizziness-and-balance.com/disorders/bppv/cupulolithiasis.htm

43. Tomaz A, Ganança MM, Ganança CF, Ganança FF, Caovilla HH, Harker L. Benign paroxysmal positional vertigo: concomitant involvement of different semicircular canals. *Ann Otol Rhinol Laryngol*. Feb 2009;118(2):113–117. doi:10.1177/000348940911800206

44. Balatsouras DG. Benign paroxysmal positional vertigo with multiple canal involvement. *Am J Otolaryngol*. Mar–Apr 2012;33(2):250–258. doi:10.1016/j.amjoto.2011.07.007

45. Soto-Varela A, Rossi-Izquierdo M, Santos-Pérez S. Benign paroxysmal positional vertigo simultaneously affecting several canals: a 46-patient series. *Eur Arch Otorhinolaryngol*. Mar 2013;270(3):817–822. doi:10.1007/s00405-012-2043-2

46. Shim DB, Song CE, Jung EJ, Ko KM, Park JW, Song MH. Benign paroxysmal positional vertigo with simultaneous involvement

of multiple semicircular canals. *Korean J Audiol.* 2014;18(3):126–130. doi:10.7874/kja.2014.18.3.126

47. Steddin S, Brandt T. Unilateral mimicking bilateral benign paroxysmal positioning vertigo. *Arch Otolaryngol Head Neck Surg.* Dec 1994;120(12):1339–1341. doi:10.1001/archotol.1994.01880360037007

48. Helminski JO, Zee DS, Janssen I, Hain TC. Effectiveness of particle repositioning maneuvers in the treatment of benign paroxysmal positional vertigo: a systematic review. *Phys Ther.* May 2010;90(5):663–678. doi:10.2522/ptj.20090071

49. Whitney SL, Alghwiri AA , Alghadir A. An overview of vestibular rehabilitation. *Handb Clin Neurol.* 2016;137:187–205. doi:10.1016/B978-0-444-63437-5.00013-3

50. Yang M, Shao C, Shao C, Saint K, Wayne PM, Bao T. Tai Chi for balance and postural control in people with peripheral neuropathy: A scoping review. *Complement Ther Med.* Nov 2024;86:103089. doi:10.1016/j.ctim.2024.103089

51. Liu J, Wang XQ, Zheng JJ, *et al.* Effects of Tai Chi versus proprioception exercise program on neuromuscular function of the ankle in elderly people: a randomized controlled trial. *Evid Based Complement Alternat Med.* 2012;2012:265486. doi:10.1155/2012/265486

52. Freire I, Seixas A. Effectiveness of a sensorimotor exercise program on proprioception, balance, muscle strength, functional mobility and risk of falls in older people. *Front Physiol.* 2024;15:1309161. doi:10.3389/fphys.2024.1309161

53. Shumway-Cook A WM, Rachwani J, Santamaria V. *Motor Control: Translating Research into Clinical Practice.* 6th ed. Wolters Kluwer; 2023.

54. Jeka JJ. Light touch contact as a balance aid. *Phys Ther.* May 1997;77(5):476–487. doi:10.1093/ptj/77.5.476.

15

Parkinson's, Multiple Sclerosis, and Stroke

Chapter Goals

1. Define Parkinson's disease (PD)
2. List treatment interventions for PD
3. Define multiple sclerosis (MS)
4. List treatment interventions for MS
5. Define stroke/cerebrovascular accident (CVA)
6. List treatment interventions for CVA

PARKINSON'S DISEASE

Also known as paralysis agitans, Parkinson's disease (PD) was first described in 1817 as the "shaking palsy" and is characterized by a loss of the cells producing the neurotransmitter dopamine in the substantia nigra pars compacta. Dopamine is produced in the substantia nigra pars compacta, the ventral tegmental area of the brain, and the arcuate nucleus of the hypothalamus. It influences both the direct and indirect pathways of the basal ganglia.

There is no single confirmed etiology, and most cases are idiopathic (of unknown cause). There are some cases that are linked to gene mutation, and it is generally believed that there are genetic predispositions and environmental factors that play roles. When there is a deficiency of dopamine,

movements become delayed or uncoordinated. When there is too much dopamine, repetitive movements called tics occur and can be observed in patients on higher levels of carbidopa/levodopa. Low levels of dopamine are also associated with painful symptoms that frequently occur with PD.

GEEK STUFF

Interesting statistics regarding PD:

- Smokers are 50% less likely to develop PD, while former smokers are 20% less likely.[1]
- Non-coffee drinkers are five times more likely to have PD (than those who have seven or more cups per day).
- PD is rare prior to age 40.
- Men are 1.5 to 2 times more affected.
- Fall rates in the PD population range from 40% to 68%.
- Within the first 10 years after diagnosis, a quarter of people with PD experience fractures.
- Most falls occur when those with PD are most active, during the day while indoors.
- After Alzheimer's disease, PD is the second-most common neurodegenerative disease.

DOI: 10.1201/9781003524441-15

Along with the loss of dopamine, there is also a loss of nerve endings that produce norepinephrine, which is the main neurotransmitter of the sympathetic nervous system, and may explain other symptoms that accompany PD, such as pulse and blood pressure irregularities, and fatigue. Some patients with PD develop *Lewy bodies* in the brain, which are a collection of proteins and are associated with PD dementia. It is unknown why or how they form, or how they are involved in the disease process.

There are three main categories of PD, and they include primary (idiopathic) PD, secondary parkinsonism, and Parkinson's-plus syndrome. The most common subtype is the tremor-predominant, with about one-third of PD patients having the postural instability gait disorder (PIGD) subtype. Young onset is not common and is more common with a family history of PD, and has an incidence of about four percent for those diagnosed before age 50.[1]

PRIMARY PD

Primary PD occurs due to the lack of dopamine-producing cells, and has three subtypes:

1. Tremor predominant
2. Postural instability gait disorder (PIGD)
3. Young onset

There are four main PD symptoms:

1. Resting tremors
2. Bradykinesia
3. Rigidity
4. Postural instability

There is no single test to diagnose primary PD. Things used to support the diagnosis of PD include:

- A good response to levodopa after 4–8 weeks of medication therapy
- When the patient has a resting tremor in addition to one of the other main symptoms, or when resting tremor is absent but the other three main symptoms are present

Tremors

Resting tremors develop in about 70% of patients and typically begin on one side of the body, and later in the disease may occur bilaterally. They are worse on the side of the initial symptoms. These tremors disappear with active motion and may be observed in the legs, chin, mouth, and tongue. Amplitude varies and is usually more pronounced when the patient is under stress. The classic "pill rolling" tremor of the hand is often observed. Postural tremors may also occur in the head and trunk. Action tremors can occur in patients with advanced PD and fluctuate in frequency and intensity.

Intention tremors should not be confused with other types of tremors, such as benign essential tremor or cerebellar tremor. See Table 15.1 to compare and contrast the types of tremors.

Table 15.1 Types of Tremors

PD Tremor	Benign Essential Tremor	Cerebellar Tremor
<ul><li>Caused by PD</li><li>Primarily at rest</li><li>Progresses</li><li>Also have bradykinesia, rigidity (stiffness), balance deficits</li><li>Not affected by alcohol (ethanol [EtOH])</li><li>Treated with Botox, PD medications, deep brain stimulation (DBS), and ablation</li></ul>	<ul><li>Genetic cause</li><li>At rest and with motion, or while holding postures</li><li>Does not progress</li><li>Does not present with bradykinesia, rigidity, or balance deficits</li><li>Improves with alcohol, worse with stimulants (caffeine)</li><li>Treated with a beta blocker (propranolol)</li></ul>	<ul><li>Caused by stroke, MS plaque, or tumors</li><li>Only with action</li><li>Does not progress</li><li>Most present with dysmetria (finger–nose–finger test) or dyssynergia (abnormal heel–shin slide)</li><li>No change with EtOH</li><li>Does not respond well to medication</li><li>Responds to DBS</li></ul>

Bradykinesia

Bradykinesia, or slowness of movement, is often accompanied by difficulty performing simultaneous and repetitive movements such as walking, typing, writing, or playing a musical instrument. These slow movements are also marked by a decrease in amplitude and loss of dexterity.

Rigidity

Eighty-nine percent of patients with PD develop rigidity[2] due to increased muscle tone, and there are two categories: cogwheel and lead pipe. Cogwheel rigidity is characterized by a ratchet-like resistance to passive movement. Lead pipe rigidity, on the other hand, is characterized by sustained resistance to passive movement throughout the entire movement. Rigidity in patients with PD is not velocity dependent. Often asymmetric, especially in early stages of PD, proximal muscles are typically affected first and include the shoulders, neck, face, and extremities. Initially, it usually affects one side of the body, but eventually spreads to both sides and causes the stooped posture observed with advanced PD. It has a direct impact on increasing resting energy expenditure and fatigue levels. It is considered the most disabling symptom.

Postural Instability

Affected by stooped posture and rigidity, postural instability in PD is largely the result of delayed or absent postural reflexes.

Other Motor Symptoms

Other common motor symptoms include:

- *Micrographia*: Small handwriting.
- *Hypophonia*: Soft voice and reduced volume.
- *Palilalia*: Stuttering, stammering, repeating syllables.
- *Hypomimia*: Reduced facial expressions.
- *Dystonia*: Abnormal postures, especially in the morning affecting the feet.
- *Abnormal gait*: Marked by short, shuffling steps, decreased arm swing, freezing episodes (including start hesitation, legs trembling in place, and shuffling/small steps) in new environments or small spaces such as doorways, difficulty changing speeds or transitioning to new surfaces. Patients have decreased stride length, increased double-support time, limited hip and knee extension, decreased plantarflexion following terminal stance, decreased initial knee and hip flexion at the beginning of the gait cycle, decreased clearance in swing phases, and flat-foot initial foot contact.
- *ADLs*: Activity of daily living issues include difficulty using utensils, chewing food, buttoning clothes, and swallowing liquids.
- *Oculomotor*: May have an impaired ability to initiate saccades.

Non-Motor Symptoms

- Depression
- Anxiety
- Autonomic dysfunctions including orthostatic hypotension, drooling, constipation, regurgitation, urinary frequency, incontinence, gastrointestinal dysfunction, sexual dysfunction, excessive sweating, cold/heat intolerance, and integumentary changes
- Visuospatial dysfunction
- Cognitive deficits
- Language deficits
- Long-term memory deficits
- Difficulty with executive functional (e.g., planning, abstract thinking)

Refer to Table 15.2 for symptoms by stage.

SECONDARY PARKINSONISM

Patients with secondary parkinsonism present PD symptoms, but it is not due to the loss of dopamine-producing cells. Etiologies include medications (those that block dopamine receptors, deplete dopamine, certain antiemetic drugs, calcium-channel agonists, certain anti-arrhythmic agents, certain anticonvulsants, and certain mood stabilizers), basal ganglia strokes, cerebrovascular disease or tumors involving the basal ganglia and subcortical white matter, normal pressure hydrocephalus, and other metabolic deficits.

Symptoms present more symmetrically than in primary PD. Tremors are less common than primary PD. Bradykinesia, rigidity, and a flat affect manifest earlier than in primary PD. When caused by drugs, symptoms may take months to develop and may or may not resolve if the drug is stopped. It is treated with anticholinergics, and the use of

Table 15.2 PD Symptoms by Disease Stage

Early	Mid-Stage	Late Stage

• Fine motor task difficulty
• Mild balance/gait deficits
• Bradykinesia
• Substitute passive forms of recreation for active ones
	• On/off stages of medications
	• Dyskinesias
	• Flat affect
	• Swallowing deficits
	• Freezing episodes
	• Bradykinesia is more marked
	• Bradyphrenia (slowness of thought)
	• Hand function issues due to sweating
	• Assistance needed for many ADLs
	• No longer safe to drive
	• Can't work outside of the home
	• Reach/grasp deficits:
	  • Noticeable when fast or accurate movements are needed
	  • Tremors may disrupt force trajectory
	  • Force grip takes longer to develop
	  • Difficulty releasing objects
	  • Excessive force used while lifting objects
		• Often wheelchair bound
		• Increased deficits with cognition, speech, swallowing
		• Increased pain to back, neck, and legs
		• Gradually will require max or total assistance for all activities

dopamine agents may worsen any underlying psychiatric conditions.

PARKINSON'S-PLUS SYNDROMES

Parkinson's-plus syndromes are mostly idiopathic diseases similar in presentation to primary PD, and include progressive supranuclear palsy, multiple system atrophy, corticobasal ganglionic degeneration, striatonigral degeneration, Shy–Drager syndrome, and olivopontocerebellar atrophy. Symptoms present bilaterally and early in the disease, and there is a limited or lack of improvement from the administration of levodopa. Other symptoms may include cranial nerve impairment, apraxia (motor planning deficit), dementia, falling, and a lack of or irregular resting tremor, hallucinations, dysautonomia, gaze palsy, myoclonus, pyramidal tract signs, and alien limb phenomenon. The disease progression is faster than that of primary PD.

The prevalence (all individuals affected by a disease at a particular time) of PD in North America is greater than once thought and has been found to be 572/100,000 of people 45 years of age and older.[3] A study in 2022 found that in the United States, the incidence (new cases over a period of time) of PD increased with age and was higher in males and ranged from 108 to 212 per 100,000 of people aged 65 years and older.[3] There is no single test to diagnose PD, also known as paralysis agitans. It is a neurodegenerative disorder characterized by the loss of the neurotransmitter dopamine-producing cells. Dopamine is used to normalize sequential movements, automaticity of learned movements, and normalize muscle tone. Most cases are idiopathic with no single etiology confirmed, but there are some cases that are genetic.

When there are deficient levels of dopamine, movements become delayed and uncoordinated. When there is too much, the brain causes unwanted and unnecessary movements such as repetitive ticks. As levels of dopamine increase or decrease beyond what is normal, memory, attention, and problem-solving suffer. As dopamine also assists in the processing of pain, low levels are associated with painful symptoms that frequently occur in PD.

PARKINSON'S SYMPTOMS

The four main symptoms of PD are resting tremors, bradykinesia, rigidity, and postural instability.

Tremors

Resting tremors have been described as looking like the patient is "pill rolling," and up to 70% of patients develop it. In early stages, it occurs at rest, disappears with hand motion, is present only on one side of the body, and the amplitude is more pronounced if the patient is under stress. However, with the progression of the disease, it may gradually involve both sides but is typically worse on the side on which it was first noticed.

Bradykinesia

Bradykinesia is the slowness of movement. Along with slowness, the patient may have difficulty performing simultaneous movements and repetitive motor functions of walking, writing, or playing a musical instrument. Patients have difficulty controlling muscle activation and force generation and lose amplitude of normal movements.

Rigidity

Rigidity affects >90% of PD patients and is considered the most disabling symptom. There are two types of rigidity seen in PD: cogwheel and lead pipe. For cogwheel rigidity, the patient's limbs have a ratchet-like, jerky starting-and-stopping resistance to passive movement, whereas lead pipe rigidity has a sustained resistance to passive movement throughout the range of motion. It is not velocity dependent. Rigidity is often asymmetrical, especially in earlier stages of PD, and typically affects proximal muscles first and then muscles of the face and extremities. Eventually, it affects both sides of the body. It greatly impacts resting energy expenditures and fatigue levels.

Postural Instability

Postural instability is affected by rigidity that causes the stooped postures of PD that shifts the patient's center of gravity forward. In addition, the patient's lose their postural reflexes, and if they have them, they are affected by bradykinesia.

Other Motor Symptoms

Other motor symptoms that are seen in PD include small handwriting (micrographia), reduced voice volumes (hypophonia), stuttering/stammering (palilalia), reduced facial expressions (hypomimia), and abnormal postures (dystonia). Gait is affected by decreased stride lengths, increased double-support time, limited hip/knee extension, decreased plantarflexion following terminal stance, absent heel strike, and diminished ankle plantarflexion. Patients have difficulty changing speed, transitioning to different surfaces, and as the disease progresses, they have freezing gait (start hesitation, legs trembling in place [looks like a gallop], and shuffle). Oculomotor function may also be affected with eye movement abnormalities, including hypometric saccades, particularly in the vertical plane, and impaired voluntary saccades compared to reflexive ones.[4] Patients may also exhibit the "round the houses" sign, characterized by a curved trajectory during vertical saccades. Additionally, there can be increased square wave jerks and impaired optokinetic nystagmus (OKN), especially with downward stimuli.[4] These abnormalities can lead to a smaller scanned area and an increased risk of falls.[4]

Deficits with breathing, swallowing, and coughing are common with PD, with aspiration pneumonia being the most common cause of death in patients with PD.[5]

Non-Motor Symptoms

There are many non-motor symptoms, including depression and anxiety, and autonomic dysfunctions: orthostasis, drooling, constipation, regurgitation, urinary frequency, incontinence, excessive sweating, cold/heat intolerance, sexual dysfunction, gastrointestinal dysfunction, visuospatial dysfunction, and deficits with memory, executive functioning, cognitive function, and language.

PD TREATMENT SPECIFICS

The European Physiotherapy Guideline for Parkinson's disease identified the following core areas of physiotherapy treatments:[6-8]

1. Physical capacity (includes neuromuscular and cardiorespiratory systems)
2. Transfers
3. Manual activities
4. Balance
5. Gait
6. Posture

Table 15.3 PD Intervention Recommendations

Intervention	Recommendation
Aerobic exercise	Moderate to high-intensity aerobic exercise to improve VO_2, reduce motor disease severity and improve functional outcomes in individuals
Resistance training	Resistance training to reduce motor disease severity and improve strength, power, non-motor symptoms, functional outcomes, and quality of life in individuals
Balance training	Balance training intervention programs to reduce postural control impairments and improve balance and gait outcomes, mobility, balance confidence, and quality of life in individuals
External cueing	To reduce motor disease severity and freezing of gait and to improve gait outcomes in individuals
Community-based exercise	Recommend community-based exercise to reduce motor disease severity and improve non-motor symptoms, functional outcomes, and quality of life in individuals
Gait training	Gait training to reduce motor disease severity and improve stride length, gait speed, mobility, and balance in individuals
Task-specific training	To improve task-specific impairment levels and functional outcomes for individuals
Behavior-change approach	To improve physical activity and quality of life in individuals
Integrated care	Physical therapist services should be delivered within an integrated care approach to reduce motor disease severity and improve quality of life in individuals

According to the Physical Therapist Management of Parkinson Disease clinical practice guideline from the American Physical Therapy Association (APTA), interventions that are recommended with a high quality of evidence are included in Table 15.3.[9]

There was a moderate quality level of evidence for the delivery of physical therapy via telerehabilitation.

When training one's gait, visual and auditory cues are helpful after patients begin to have freezing episodes. In a study by Hu et al., the authors conclude that carpets with visual cues can improve the gait of PT patients, even those with mild executive dysfunction. Stride length and gait speed were significantly improved and fall risk was significantly mitigated while walking on carpets with chessboard and striped patterns.[10] In a systematic review and meta-analysis of the effectiveness of rhythmic auditory stimulation (RAS) on gait in PD, the authors found that "on average, a gait speed improvement of 0.53 standard deviation (SD) units (95% CI, 0.23 to 0.83; $P = .0005$), a stride length improvement of 0.51 SD units (95% CI, 0.18 to 0.84; $P = .003$) greater than that in the control group."[11] Although the quality of evidence was low, they concluded that RAS may have a beneficial effect on gait speed and stride length in patients with Parkinson's disease.[11]

Clinicians should also address any oculomotor deficits with exercises or optometric interventions.

MULTIPLE SCLEROSIS (MS)

Sclerosis is a medical term referring to distinctive areas of scar-like tissue (also called plaques or lesions).[12] MS is a chronic autoimmune disorder in which the immune system attacks myelin in the central nervous system. MS affects women more often than men, and white people are more likely to have MS than other ethnicities. The disease usually presents in young adults between the ages of 20 and 40 years.

Patients with MS frequently complain of gait and balance disturbance.[13] In a scoping review of falls in the MS population, Kaddoura et al. found the following factors associated with falls in patients with MS: mobility and balance impairment, severity and progression of the disease, fear of falling, bladder dysfunction, fatigue, and cognitive dysfunction, with mobility and balance impairment being identified as the most common cause of falls.[14]

TYPES OF MS

There are five types of MS:[12]

1. *Clinically isolated syndrome*: A single attack causes symptoms followed by a complete, or near-complete, recovery. Clinical tests may show "silent" damage in other places within the central nervous system. When identified, these damaged areas could allow a diagnosis of MS, even after a single attack.
2. *Relapsing–remitting*: Recurrent attacks cause symptoms with total or partial recovery, with periods between attacks called remission. Most are diagnosed with this form of MS initially.
3. *Secondary progressive*: Attacks become less common, and patients develop steady symptoms with deterioration in functioning over time. Attacks are referred to as active MS, while periods without attacks are called non-relapsing.
4. *Primary progressive*: This type of MS is less common and presents with progressively worsening symptoms from the beginning and does not have noticeable attacks. Symptoms may wax and wane.
5. *Radiologically isolated syndrome*: The rarest form of MS in which MRI scans show plaques that look like MS, but the patient does not have symptoms. Symptoms may occur in the future, however.

MS SYMPTOMS

MS symptoms vary between patients depending on where the lesions are located. Early symptoms may include vision problems, muscle weakness or stiffness, paresthesia, clumsiness, balance and gait difficulties, intermittent dizziness, and bladder control problems. Other symptoms include spasticity, ataxia, sexual dysfunction, mental or physical fatigue, mood changes, difficulty with emotional expression, cognitive changes, difficulties with memory or judgment, and problems concentrating, multitasking, thinking, and learning. Symptoms may lead to partial or complete paralysis. Symptoms are worse when exposed to heat, when having a fever, or following common infections.[12]

Vision problems are common in patients suffering from MS and may include blurred or grayed vision, temporary blindness in one eye, loss of color vision, depth perception deficits, partial visual field loss, nystagmus, opsoclonus (involuntary and chaotic conjugate eye motions), and diplopia.[12] Vision therapy exercises, special eyeglasses, and resting the eyes may help.[12]

MS INTERVENTION SPECIFICS

A detailed meta-analysis revealed that physical exercise significantly reduces fatigue in patients with MS and strongly recommended a regular exercise program.[15] In a Cochrane Library review of exercise therapy for fatigue in MS, the authors concluded that "exercise therapy can be prescribed in people with MS without harm."[16] A systematic review performed by Kim et al. found that "exercise guidelines for MS consistently recommended 2–3 days/week of aerobic training (10–30 minutes at moderate-intensity) and 2–3 days/week of resistance training (1–3 sets of 8–15 repetition maximum [RM])."[17]

A 2024 systematic review and meta-analysis concluded, "Exercise had beneficial effects in improving balance, walking ability, walking endurance, fatigue, and quality of life in people with MS. Resistance exercise and aerobic exercise are the most effective interventions for improving fatigue and quality of life in people with MS, respectively. The effect of exercise on improving fatigue was associated with the age of the participants, with the younger age of the participants, the greater the improvement in fatigue."[18]

A systematic review and meta-analysis found that the cooling garments were effective at improving walking capacity and functional mobility, and some studies demonstrated improvements in muscular strength and balance.[19] At the time of writing, the Multiple Sclerosis Foundation's Cooling Program provided cooling vests and other items for free to patients with MS.

STROKE (CVA)

A stroke is when there is loss of blood flow in the brain causing death or damage to brain cells, and is more common in men than women. The lack of blood flow is the result of an occluded blood vessel (called an ischemic stroke) due to a clot or secondary to a bleed (called a hemorrhagic stroke). A transient ischemic attack (TIA) is a temporary blockage of blood flow in the brain that dissipates after a short time. Once the blockage dissipates, symptoms resolve.

There are two varieties of ischemic strokes:[20]

- *Thrombotic*: The most common type. A blood clot forms inside an artery in the brain.
- *Embolic*: Caused when a clot or piece of plaque forms in the heart or an artery that leads to the brain and is pushed through the bloodstream and lodges in narrower brain arteries.

Hemorrhagic strokes also come in two varieties:[20]

- *Subarachnoid hemorrhage*: A bleed that occurs between the skull and brain surface.
- *Intracranial hemorrhage*: A bleed that occurs within the brain, and many are caused by long-term hypertension.

STROKE SYMPTOMS

Symptoms vary depending on the location of the stroke and may include dizziness, nausea, vomiting, severe headache, confusion, disorientation, memory loss, abnormal or slurred speech, loss of vision, loss of balance or coordination, difficulty walking, painless loss of neurologic function, and numbness in an arm, leg, or face (especially on one side).[20] Symptoms may result in paralysis on one side of the body, vision problems, impulsive

behavior, memory loss, speech/language problems, and slow, cautious behavior.[20]

Stroke Symptoms by Location

Presentations of impairments secondary to cerebrovascular accident (CVA) may be different based on the location of the stroke. Here are general symptoms based on CVA location:

- *Frontal lobe*: Contralateral motor impairments, hemiplegia/hemiparesis, problem solving, impaired judgment, behavioral/personality changes, speech changes, impaired memory
- *Parietal lobe*: Contralateral weakness, impaired spatial awareness, impaired language skills (e.g., aphasia), contralateral paresthesia, contralateral inferior quadrantanopia, inability to recognize objects on the left side of space as well as one's own left side of the body as one's own, loss of proprioception, hemispatial neglect/inattention, impulsive and inappropriate behavior, difficulty reading, writing, learning, and with simple math
- *Temporal lobe*: Short-term memory problems, difficulty understanding language or writing (alexia), acalculia (like alexia, but for numbers and math), seizures, severe or frequent feelings of anxiety or pain, confusion, and changes in vision[21] (including contralateral superior quadrantanopia)[22]
- *Occipital lobe*: Cortical blindness, visual hallucinations, prosopagnosia (the inability to recognize faces)
- *Cerebellum*: Dizziness/vertigo, nausea, loss of coordination, balance deficits, ataxic gait, dysarthria, nystagmus, skew deviations of the eyes, and headache
- *Thalamus*: Amnesia, coma, aphasia, loss of alertness, numbness, sensory impairments (touch/temperature), chronic pain, impaired posture/movements
- *Basal ganglia*: Numbness/weakness on one side of the face/body, lack of coordination/balance, difficulty speaking or understanding words, difficulty seeing out of one or both eyes, chorea/ticks, difficulty swallowing, poststroke depression, emotional blunting, future risk of

parkinsonism, impaired executive function, attention, and memory

- *Internal capsule*: (Pure motor stroke) hemiplegia, weakness/numbness on one side of the face/body, facial droop, difficulty with vision, difficulty with ambulation
- *Brainstem (midbrain, pons, medulla)*: Crossed findings where deficits in the face are contralateral to deficits in the body, coma, dysphagia, breathing difficulty, vertigo and disequilibrium (occur together), weakness on one side of the body

Stroke Symptoms by Artery

- *Anterior cerebral artery (ACA)*: Supplies the frontal lobe, prefrontal, primary motor, primary sensory, and supplemental motor cortices corresponding to the lower extremities in the cortical homunculus.[22] Symptoms include contralateral sensory and motor deficits in the lower extremity, while the upper extremity and face are spared.[22,23]
- *Middle cerebral artery (MCA)*: Supplies the frontal, temporal, and parietal lobes, the basal ganglia, and internal capsule. This is the most common artery involved in stroke.[22] Classic MCA presentation includes contralateral hemiparesis, facial paralysis, and sensory loss in the upper extremities and face.[22] Additionally, other symptoms that may be seen include gaze preference toward the side of lesion, dysarthria, hemineglect (inattention), visual field loss, and aphasia.[22]
- *Posterior cerebral artery (PCA)*: Superficially, it supplies the occipital lobe and the medial temporal lobe, while the deep PCA supplies the thalamus and other deep brain structures.[22] The most common cause of PCA infarct is a thrombus in the vertebral artery.[22]
  - Symptoms of superficial PCA strokes include homonymous hemianopia, and rarely with amnesia or cortical blindness.[22,24,25]
  - Symptoms of deep thrombus strokes include hypersomnolence, cognitive deficits, ocular findings hypoesthesia, ataxia, hemisensory loss, and hemiparesis.[22]

- Basilar and vertebral arteries (vertebrobasilar infarcts): The main branches of the vertebral artery are the posterior inferior cerebellar artery (PICA) and the anterior spinal artery. The vertebral arteries merge to form the basilar artery. The basilar artery gives rise to the anterior inferior cerebellar artery (AICA). Along with the superior cerebellar artery (SCA) that arises near the end of the basilar artery, the PICA and AICA supply the cerebellum and brainstem.[22] Symptoms of vertebrobasilar infarcts include ataxia, vertigo, headache, vomiting, oropharyngeal dysfunction, visual field deficits, and abnormal oculomotor findings.[22]

LOCALIZING BRAINSTEM STROKES

When using symptoms to localize strokes, follow the following three points:[26]

1. Use the Rule of 4s as described in Chapter 5. You can use this to help localize a stroke. For example, if someone has an ocular nerve palsy, the lesion is likely in the midbrain, while someone with facial nerve paralysis likely has one of the cranial nerves (CNs) from the pons affected, and a tongue deviation is likely caused by a lesion in the medulla (hypoglossal nerve).
2. Is the lesion medial or lateral? First, think which structures are medial and which are lateral.
   - Medial structures include:
     - Motor pathway going to the body
     - *Medial lemniscus*: Carries fine touch, vibration and proprioception
     - *Medial longitudinal fasciculus*: Controls eye movements
     - *Motor component of CNs*: Includes the CNs controlling eye movements (III, IV, VI) and the hypoglossal nerve (CN XII) that controls the tongue
   - Lateral (side) structures include:
     - Spinocerebellar pathway
     - *Spinothalamic tract*: Carries crude touch, temperature, and pain sensation information
     - *Sympathetic pathway*: Traveling to the face

- *Sensation from the face*: Information coming from the face via the trigeminal nerve

3. Deficits to the face will be ipsilateral to the lesion, while deficits to the body will be contralateral.

STROKES AND STROKE SYNDROMES

Locked-In Syndrome

Caused by a basilar artery stroke.

- Total paralysis resulting from damage to the corticospinal tract and most cranial nerves. Cortical functions are intact.

Medial Midbrain Stroke (CNs III and IV)

Presents with crossed findings of eye movements.

- Ptosis
- Mydriasis (dilated pupil)
- "Down and out" pupil (oculomotor nerve palsy)
- Weber syndrome
  - Ipsilateral oculomotor nerve palsy
  - Contralateral hemiplegia (due to damage to the corticospinal tract)

Lateral Pontine Syndrome (CNs V–VIII)

Caused by a lesion in the AICA.

- Loss of protopathic sensations contralaterally in the extremities
- Loss of protopathic sensations ipsilaterally in the face
- Ipsilateral Horner syndrome
- Ipsilateral cerebellar deficits
- May have loss of taste in the anterior two-thirds of the tongue (CN VII)

- May have a loss of facial sensation (CN VII)
- May have complete deafness if CN VIII is affected

Medial Pontine Syndrome (CNs V–VIII)

Associated with occlusions of branches off the basilar artery.

- Facial asymmetry
- Horizontal gaze palsy
- Internuclear ophthalmoplegia (secondary to medial longitudinal fasciculus involvement)

Lateral Medullary Syndrome (CNs IX–XII)

Associated with PICA strokes.

- Loss of contralateral protopathic sensations (pain, itch, tickle, and temperature) in the extremities
- Loss of ipsilateral protopathic sensations in the face
- Ipsilateral Horner syndrome
- Ataxia
- Vertigo
- Nystagmus
- Difficulty chewing, swallowing, and speaking

Medial Medullary Syndrome (CNs IX–XII)

Caused by a lesion in the medial medulla. Specifically, the anterior spinal artery is usually involved.

- Contralateral hemiparesis of the body but not the face
- Contralateral loss of epicritic sensation (light touch, light vibration, two-point discrimination, and astereognosis (the ability to recognize objects by touch that are being held)
- Ipsilateral tongue weakness

Table 15.4 Intervention Recommendations for Patients More Than 6 Months after Acute CVA

Gait training:

- Clinicians should use virtual reality training interventions coupled with walking practice for improving walking speed and distance in individuals more than 6 months following acute-onset central nervous system (CNS) injury as compared with alternative interventions.
- Clinicians should use moderate- to high-intensity walking training interventions to improve walking speed and distance in individuals more than 6 months following acute-onset CNS injury as compared with alternative interventions.
- Clinicians should not perform body weight-supported treadmill training for improving walking speed and distance in individuals more than 6 months following acute-onset CNS injury as compared with alternative interventions.
- Clinicians should not perform walking interventions with exoskeletal robotics on a treadmill or elliptical devices to improve walking speed and distance in individuals greater than 6 months following acute-onset CNS injury as compared with alternative interventions.
- Clinicians should not perform sitting or standing balance training directed toward improving postural stability and weight-bearing symmetry between limbs to improve walking speed and distance in individuals more than 6 months following acute-onset CNS injury as compared with alternative interventions.
- Clinicians should not use sitting or standing balance training with additional vibratory stimuli to improve walking speed and distance in individuals more than 6 months following acute-onset CNS injury as compared with alternative interventions.
- Clinicians may consider static and dynamic (non-walking) balance strategies when coupled with virtual reality or augmented visual feedback to improve walking speed and distance in individuals more than 6 months following acute-onset CNS injury as compared with alternative interventions.

STROKE TREATMENT SPECIFICS

Use of Ankle Foot Orthoses (AFO) and Functional Electrical Stimulation (FES)

According to Johnston et al.:[27]

- Both AFO and FES lead to improvements poststroke.
- In chronic stroke, FES can have a greater impact on quality of life (QOL) than an AFO. A period of 12–24 weeks of home use may be needed before seeing gains in QOL.
- Clinicians should provide AFO or FES for individuals with foot drop due to chronic poststroke hemiplegia who have goals to improve QOL.
- Clinicians should provide an AFO or FES for individuals with decreased lower extremity motor control due to poststroke hemiplegia who have goals to improve:

  - Gait speed (recommendation strength: strong—acute or chronic).
  - Other mobility (recommendation strength: strong—acute or chronic).
  - Dynamic balance (recommendation strength: strong—acute or chronic).
  - Walking endurance (recommendation strength: moderate for acute stroke, strong for chronic stroke).

- Clinicians should not provide an AFO or FES for individuals with decreased lower extremity motor control due to an acute or chronic poststroke hemiplegia who have primary goals to improve plantar flexor spasticity (recommendation strength: moderate).
- Clinicians may provide an AFO with decreased stiffness for individuals with decreased lower extremity motor control due to acute or chronic poststroke hemiplegia who have goals to allow activation of the anterior tibialis and gastrocnemius/soleus muscles while walking

with the AFO (recommendation strength: moderate).

- Clinicians should provide FES for individuals with decreased lower extremity motor control due to chronic poststroke hemiplegia who have goals to improve activation of the anterior tibialis muscle while walking without FES (recommendation strength: moderate).
- Clinicians may provide an AFO or FES for individuals with decreased lower extremity motor control due to acute or chronic poststroke hemiplegia who have goals to improve ankle dorsiflexion at initial contact and during loading response and swing (recommendation strength: weak).

Interventions to Improve Locomotion

Recommendations with strong evidence from the clinical practice guideline to improve locomotor function following chronic stroke (full recommendations are located on the ANPT website) are included in Table 15.4.[28]

REFERENCES

1. Parkinson's Foundation Contributors. *Statistics*. Parkinson's Foundation; 2024. https://www.parkinson.org/understanding-parkinsons/statistics
2. Ferreira-Sánchez MDR, Moreno-Verdú M, Cano-de-la-Cuerda R. Quantitative Measurement of Rigidity in Parkinson's Disease: A Systematic Review. Sensors (Basel). 2020 Feb 6;20(3):880. doi: 10.3390/s20030880. PMID: 32041374; PMCID: PMC7038663.
3. Willis AW, Roberts E, Beck JC, et al. Incidence of Parkinson disease in North America. *NPJ Parkinsons Dis*. Dec 15 2022;8(1):170.
4. Kassavetis P, Kaski D, Anderson T, Hallett M. Eye movement disorders in movement disorders. *Movement Disorders Clin Practice*. 2022;9(3):284–595. Doi:10.1002/mdc3.13413
5. Chua WY, Wang JDJ, Chan CKM, Chan LL, Tan EK. Risk of aspiration pneumonia and hospital mortality in Parkinson disease: a systematic review and meta-analysis. *Eur J Neurol*. Dec 2024;31(12):e16449.
6. Keus SH, Bloem B, Hendriks EJ, Bredero-Cohen AB, Munneke M. Evidence-based analysis of physical therapy with recommendations for practice and research. *Movement Disorders*. 2007;22(4):451–460.
7. Morris ME. Movement disorders in people with Parkinson disease: a model for physical therapy. *Physical Therapy*. 2000;80(6):578–597.
8. ParkinsonNet Contributors. *European Physiotherapy Guideline for Parkinson's Disease*. ParkinsonNet; 2024. https://www.parkinsonnet.com/guidelines/
9. Osborne JA, Botkin R, Colon-Semenza C, et al. Physical therapist management of parkinson disease: a clinical practice guideline from the American physical therapy association. *Phys Ther*. Apr 1 2022;102(4) pzab302. doi:10.1093/ptj/pzab302
10. Hu ZD, Zhu SG, Huang JF, et al. Carpets with visual cues can improve gait in Parkinson's disease patients: may be independent of executive function. *Eur J Med Res*. Nov 16 2023;28(1):530.
11. Burrai F, Apuzzo L, Zanotti R. Effectiveness of rhythmic auditory stimulation on gait in Parkinson disease: a systematic review and meta-analysis. *Holist Nurs Pract*. Mar–Apr 01 2024;38(2):109–119. doi:10.1097/hnp.0000000000000462
12. Contributors NIoNDaS. *Multiple Sclerosis*. National Institutes of Health; 2024. https://www.ninds.nih.gov/health-information/disorders/multiple-sclerosis
13. Heesen C, Böhm J, Reich C, Kasper J, Goebel M, Gold SM. Patient perception of bodily functions in multiple sclerosis: gait and visual function are the most valuable. *Mult Scler*. Aug 2008;14(7):988–991. doi:10.1177/1352458508088916
14. Kaddoura R, Faraji H, Othman M, et al. Exploring factors associated with falls in multiple sclerosis: insights from a scoping review. *Clin Interv Aging*. 2024;19:923–938.
15. Razazian N, Kazeminia M, Moayedi H, et al. The impact of physical exercise on the fatigue symptoms in patients with multiple sclerosis: a systematic review and meta-analysis. *BMC Neurol*. Mar 13 2020;20(1):93.

16. Heine M, van de Port I, Rietberg MB, van Wegen EE, Kwakkel G. Exercise therapy for fatigue in multiple sclerosis. *Cochrane Database Syst Rev*. Sep 11 2015;2015(9):CD009956.

17. Kim Y, Lai B, Mehta T, et al. Exercise training guidelines for multiple sclerosis, stroke, and Parkinson disease: rapid review and synthesis. *Am J Phys Med Rehabil*. Jul 2019;98(7):613–621.

18. Du L, Xi H, Zhang S, *et al*. Effects of exercise in people with multiple sclerosis: a systematic review and meta-analysis. *Front Public Health*. 2024;12:1387658.

19. Stevens CJ, Singh G, Peterson B, Vargas NT, Périard JD. The effect of cooling garments to improve physical function in people with multiple sclerosis: A systematic review and meta-analysis. *Mult Scler Relat Disord*. Oct 2023;78:104912. doi:10.1016/j.msard.2023.104912

20. American Association of Neurological Surgeons Contributors. *A Neurosurgeon's Guide to Stroke*. AANS.org; 2024. https://www.aans.org/patients/conditions-treatments/a-neurosurgeons-guide-to-stroke/

21. *Temporal Lobe*. The Cleveland Clinic. Accessed 10/08/2023, 2023. https://my.clevelandclinic.org/health/body/16799-temporal-lobe

22. Hui C, Tadi P, Khan Suheb MZ, Patti L. *Ischemic Stroke*. StatPearls Publishing; Updated 2024. https://www.ncbi.nlm.nih.gov/books/NBK499997/

23. Matos Casano HA, Tadi P, Ciofoaia GA. *Anterior Cerebral Artery Stroke*. StatPearls Publishing LLC; 2024.

24. Cereda C, Carrera E. Posterior cerebral artery territory infarctions. *Front Neurol Neurosci*. 2012;30:128–131. doi:10.1159/000333610

25. Brandt T, Steinke W, Thie A, Pessin MS, Caplan LR. Posterior cerebral artery territory infarcts: clinical features, infarct topography, causes and outcome. Multicenter results and a review of the literature. *Cerebrovasc Dis*. May–Jun 2000;10(3):170–182. doi:10.1159/000016053

26. Brainstem Stroke Mnemonics. *Memorable Neurology Lecture 15*. Memorable Neurology; 2021.

27. Johnston TE, Keller S, Denzer-Weiler C, Brown L. A clinical practice guideline for the use of ankle-foot orthoses and functional electrical stimulation post-stroke. *J Neurol Phys Ther*. Apr 1 2021;45(2):112–196. doi:10.1097/npt.0000000000000347

28. Hornby TG, Reisman DS, Ward IG, et al. Clinical Practice Guideline to Improve Locomotor Function Following Chronic Stroke, Incomplete Spinal Cord Injury, and Brain Injury. *J Neurol Phys Ther*. Jan 2020;44(1):49–100. doi:10.1097/npt.0000000000000303

Quick Reference

ASCENDING AND DESCENDING NEURAL TRACTS

See Table 16.1.

CRANIAL NERVES

See Tables 16.2 and 16.3.

OCULOMOTOR

See Tables 16.4 to 16.7.

VESTIBULAR

EWALD'S LAWS

1. A stimulation of the semicircular canal causes a movement of the eyes in the plane of the stimulated canal.
2. In the horizontal semicircular canals, an ampullopetal endolymph movement causes a greater stimulation than an ampullofugal one.
3. Ampullopetal endolymph flow (movement toward the ampulla) causes less vestibular excitement than endolymph flow away from it in the vertical canals (anterior and posterior semicircular canals).

ALEXANDER'S LAW

The spontaneous nystagmus of a patient with a vestibular lesion is more intense when the patient looks in the direction of the quick phase.

VESTIBULAR REFLEXES

- *VOR*: Vestibulo-ocular reflex (the vestibular system working with the eye motion)
- *VSR*: Vestibulospinal reflex (the vestibular system working with the spinal muscles)
- *VCR*: Vestibulocollic reflex (the vestibular system working with the neck muscles)

BEDSIDE VESTIBULAR FUNCTION TESTS

- *Head impulse*: Positive when corrective saccades are noted post-head impulse to find the target; the deficient side is in the direction of the head turn.
- *Head shake*: Positive when post-head shake nystagmus are observed. Nystagmus beat toward the stronger ear, and vertical nystagmus are a central sign.
- *Dynamic visual acuity*: Only recommended when instrumented. The software will alert you to a vestibular deficit. If done manually, at least a two-line difference in acuity from static acuity and dynamic acuity represents a likely vestibular deficit.

DOI: 10.1201/9781003524441-16

Table 16.1 Ascending/Descending Neural Tracts

Funiculus	Important Ascending Sensory Tracts
Anterior funiculus	• Anterior spinothalamic tract
Lateral funiculus	• Dorsal (posterior) spinocerebellar tract • Ventral (anterior) spinocerebellar tract • Spinotectal tract • Lateral spinothalamic tract
Posterior funiculus	• Fasciculus gracilis • Fasciculus cuneatus
Funiculus	Important Descending Motor Tracts
Anterior funiculus (Medial motor systems)	• Anterior corticospinal tract (pyramidal tract) • Tectospinal tract (extrapyramidal tract) • Vestibulospinal tract (extrapyramidal tract) • Reticulospinal tract (extrapyramidal tract)
Lateral funiculus (Lateral motor systems)	• Lateral corticospinal tract (pyramidal tract) • Rubrospinal tract (extrapyramidal tract)
Posterior funiculus	• None

Table 16.2 Cranial Nerve Origins/Exits

CN	Origin	Exits the Skull Via
I	Roof of nasal cavity (olfactory mucosa)	Olfactory foramina of the cribriform plate of the ethmoid bone to the olfactory bulb below the frontal lobe
II	The retina	Optic canal to the optic chiasm
III	Midbrain (at the level of the superior colliculus)	Superior orbital fissure (inside of annulus of Zinn)
IV	Midbrain (at the level of the inferior colliculus)	Superior orbital fissure (outside of annulus of Zinn)
V	Pons (primarily; also, midbrain, medulla, and spinal cord)	1. V1 branch: Superior orbital fissure (outside of annulus of Zinn) 2. V2 branch: Foramen rotundum 3. V3 branch: Foramen ovale
VI	Pons (inferior part) at pontomedullary junction	Superior orbital fissure (inside of annulus of Zinn)
VII	Pons (primarily)	1. Internal acoustic meatus (internal auditory canal) 2. Stylomastoid foramen
VIII	Pontomedullary junction (some nuclei are in the pons while others are in the medulla)	Internal acoustic meatus (internal auditory canal)
IX	Medulla (primarily)	Jugular foramen
X	Medulla	Jugular foramen
XI	Medulla (cranial part) (primarily) Cervical Spinal Cord (C1–C5) (spinal part)	1. Jugular foramen (the cranial component and some spinal component) 2. Foramen magnum (spinal component)
XII	Medulla (primarily)	Hypoglossal canal of the occipital condyles

Table 16.3 Cranial Nerves and Their Functions

CN	Nerve	Sensory or Motor	Function
I	Olfactory	Sensory	Relays information regarding smell
II	Optic	Sensory	Relays vision information
III	Oculomotor	Motor	• Responsible for motor innervation to four of the six extraocular eye muscles (superior and inferior recti, inferior oblique, and medial rectus) • Controls pupil size and accommodation for near vision
IV	Trochlear	Motor	Innervates the superior oblique muscle
V	Trigeminal	Sensory and motor	The largest CN has three divisions: 1. V1 branch: Ophthalmic (sensory information from the scalp, forehead, conjunctiva, and upper eyelids) 2. V2 branch :Maxillary (sensory information from the checks, upper lip, skin of the nose, nasal cavity) 3. V3 branch: Mandibular (sensory information from the ears, lower lip, and chin) Innervates muscles of the mastication and ears (tensor tympani, tensor veli palatini)
VI	Abducens	Motor	Innervates the lateral rectus muscle
VII	Facial	Sensory and motor	• Relays information regarding taste form most of the tongue (anterior two-thirds of tongue) • Relays information from the outer part of the ear (touch, pain, temperature) • Innervates muscles of facial expression, closing the eyelid, the stapedius (middle ear), and some of the jaw muscles (mastication) • Innervates glands for salivation, nasal glands, palatine glands, and tear production (lacrimal glands)
VIII	Vestibulocochlear	Sensory	• Cochlear portion: Relays information regarding sound • Vestibular portion: Relays information regarding balance, head motion and position
IX	Glossopharyngeal	Sensory and motor	• Relays information regarding taste from the back part of the tongue • Relays touch, pain, temperature, and taste from the posterior one-third of the tongue • Relays sensory information from the sinuses, tonsils, pharynx, soft palate, part of the ear, and part of the nasopharynx • Relays information from the baroreceptors and chemoreceptors of the carotid sinus • Innervates the stylopharyngeus muscle of the throat for voluntary pharynx elevation during swallowing and speaking • Innervates the parotid gland

(Continued)

Table 16.3 (Continued) Cranial Nerves and Their Functions

CN	Nerve	Sensory or Motor	Function
X	Vagus	Sensory and motor	• The main parasympathetic nerve (~90% of parasympathetic outflow) • Relays sensations from the ear canal and parts of the throat • Relays sensations from chest and trunk organs (e.g., heart, lungs, liver, spleen, stomach, gall bladder, pancreas, kidneys and intestines) • Relays information from the aortic arch including baroreceptors, and the partial pressures of O_2 and CO_2 • Relays taste information from the root of the tongue and epiglottis • Innervates throat muscles for swallowing, speech and coughing • Innervates muscles of organs in the chest and trunk, including digestive tract, and sweating
XI	Accessory	Motor	Innervates muscles of the neck (rotation, flexion, extension) and elevates and retracts the scapulae
XII	Hypoglossal	Motor	Innervates most of the tongue muscle: • Intrinsic muscles: Curls tongue • Extrinsic muscles: Elevated, depresses, protracts tongue

TESTS OF BENIGN PAROXYSMAL POSITIONAL VERTIGO (BPPV)

• Modified Dix–Hallpike (anterior/posterior canals)
• Side-lying test (anterior/posterior canals)
• Roll test (lateral canals)

TESTS OF SOMATOSENSATION

• Light touch
• Vibration
• Weber two-point discrimination
• Proprioception: Threshold to detect passive movement, joint position matching
• Romberg
• mCTSIB

NEURO EXAMINATION

• HINTS examination
• Cerebellar screens
• Muscle tone
• Deep tendon reflexes
• Corticospinal tract screens: Babinski, Clonus
• Memory

• Functional tools: TUG, grip strength, 5 Times Sit-to-Stand

MUSCLES OF THE EYE, NECK, TRUNK, AND LOWER EXTREMITY AFFECTING BALANCE

Here is a list of muscles that are used to balance or support other muscles that we use to balance, as well as those that move our head/neck and eyes.

Muscles of the Neck

See Tables 16.8 and 16.9.

Muscles of the Trunk

See Tables 16.10 and 16.11.

Muscles of the Pelvic Floor

See Table 16.12.

Muscles of the Lower Extremity

See Table 16.13.

Table 16.4 Extraocular Eye Muscles

Four Rectus Muscles	Abbreviation	CN	Action(s)	Origin	Insertion
Superior rectus[1]	SR	III	• Primary: Rolls eyes up (elevation) • Secondary: Adduction • Tertiary: Intorsion	The annulus of Zinn (common tendinous ring) in the posterior eye socket	The anterior, superior eye
Inferior rectus[2]	IR	III	• Primary: Rolls eyes down (depression) • Secondary: Adduction • Tertiary: Extorsion		The anterior, inferior eye
Medial rectus[3]	MR	III	Rolls eyes in (adduction)		The anterior, medial eye
Lateral rectus[4]	LR	VI	Rolls eyes out (abduction)		The anterior, lateral eye
Two Oblique Muscles					
Superior oblique[5]	SO	IV	Inferolateral eye motion (down and out) • Primary: Intorts • Secondary: Depresses • Tertiary: Abducts	The periosteal covering of the sphenoid above the annulus of Zinn Passes along the medial border of the roof of the orbit he tendon passes through the trochlea "pulley"	The posterior, inferolateral eye posterior to the superior rectus muscle
Inferior oblique[6]	IO	III	• Primary: Extorts • Secondary: Elevates • Tertiary: Abducts	The orbital floor, lateral to the nasolacrimal groove in the anterior eye socket	The posterior inferolateral surface of the eye posterior to the lateral rectus

Table 16.5 Eye Motions

Eye Motions	Goal
Saccades Smooth pursuit Vergence	Direct the eyes
Fixation Vestibulo-ocular reflex Optokinetics	Hold the images steady

Table 16.6 Visual Fields

Visual Field Area	Typical Degrees of Vision of Each Eye
Nasal	60 degrees medially
Superior	60 degrees upward
Inferior	70 to 75 degrees downward
Temporal	100 degrees laterally

Table 16.7 Visual Pathway Damage

Visual Field Cut Description	Visual Representation	Visual Pathway Damage Location and Causes
Total blindness of one eye called an anopsia		Complete lesion in the optic nerve anterior to the optic chiasm ipsilateral to vision loss Causes: • Papilledema secondary to increased cerebrospinal fluid pressure • Blockage of central artery of the retina • Optic neuritis secondary to multiple sclerosis
Ipsilateral nasal hemianopia		Monocular and ipsilateral vision loss secondary to a lesion of the nerves carrying nasal field information when it occurs anterior to the optic chiasm Causes: • Aneurysms of the internal carotid artery
Bitemporal heteronymous hemianopia		A lesion in the optic chiasm (seen with tumors to the pituitary) Causes: • Pituitary adenoma • Aneurysm at the junction of the anterior cerebral artery and anterior communicating artery
Contralateral homonymous hemianopia		Lesions to optic tracts Causes: • Occlusion of anterior choroidal artery • Occlusion of thalamogeniculate artery
Contralateral homonymous lower quadrantanopia		Lesions to the non-Meyer's loop of the optic radiation Causes: • Typically, by lesions as the pathway passes through the parietal lobe
Contralateral homonymous upper quadrantanopia		Lesions to the Meyer's loop of the optic radiation Causes: • Infarct to the inferior division of the inferior cerebral artery
Contralateral homonymous hemianopia with macular sparring		Lesions to the primary visual cortex Causes: • Lesions to the primary visual cortex

Table 16.8 Muscles of the Neck

Muscle	Action(s)	Innervation
Posterior Neck		
Splenius capitis	Supports head in erect position Unilateral contraction: • Lateral head and neck flexion • Head rotation ipsilaterally Bilateral contraction: • Extension of head and neck	Posterior rami of middle and lower cervical spinal nerves
Semispinalis capitis	Unilateral contraction: • Rotation of head and contralaterally Bilateral contraction: • Extension of the head and neck	Greater occipital nerve
Semispinalis cervicis	Unilateral contraction: • Lateral flexion of the neck • Contralateral rotation Bilateral contraction: Extension of cervical spine	Dorsal rami of cervical spinal nerves
Rectus capitis posterior major	Unilateral contraction: • Ipsilateral head rotation • Ipsilateral head side-flexion	Suboccipital nerve or dorsal ramus of cervical spinal nerve (C1)
Rectus capitis posterior minor	Extension of head	
Obliquus capitis superior	Unilateral contraction: Ipsilateral lateral head flexion Bilateral contraction: Head extension	
Obliquus capitis inferior	Ipsilateral rotation of atlantoaxial joint	
Lateral Neck		
Anterior scalene	Unilateral contraction: • Neck lateral flexion (ipsilateral) • Neck rotation (contralateral) • Elevates rib 1 Bilateral contraction: Neck flexion	Anterior rami of C4–6
Middle scalene	Neck lateral flexion Elevates rib 1	Anterior rami of C3–8
Posterior scalene	Neck lateral flexion Elevates rib 2	Anterior rami of C6–8
Anterior Neck		
Rectus capitis anterior	Stabilizes atlantooccipital joint Assists flexion of head on neck	C1, C2
Rectus capitis lateralis	Stabilizes head Weakly assists with lateral head flexion	Anterior rami of C1
Rectus capitis posterior minor	Extension of head	Suboccipital nerve Dorsal ramus of C1
Rectus capitis posterior major	Unilateral contraction: Ipsilateral side-flexion and rotation of the head Bilateral contraction: Head extension at C1–C2	

(Continued)

Table 16.8 (Continued) Muscles of the Neck

Muscle	Action(s)	Innervation
Longus capitis	Bilateral contraction: Head flexion Ipsilateral contraction: Ipsilateral head rotation	Anterior rami of C1–C3
Longus colli	Bilateral contraction: • Neck flexion • Ipsilateral neck lateral flexion Unilateral contraction: • Neck contralateral rotation	Anterior rami of C2–C6
Platysma	• Depresses mandible • Depresses angle of mouth • Tenses skin of lower face and anterior neck	Facial nerve (CN VII)
Sternocleidomastoid	Unilateral contraction: • Contralateral head rotation • Ipsilateral neck side-flexion Bilateral contraction (C1–C2 level): • Extension of head and neck Bilateral contraction (inferior cervical vertebrae): • Flexion of cervical spine • Elevates clavicle and manubrium	• Accessory nerve (CN XI) • Anterior rami of C1–C3
Digastric	Depresses mandible Elevates hyoid bone during swallowing Elevates hyoid bone during speaking	• Anterior belly: Alveolar nerve (CN V) • Posterior belly: Facial nerve (CN VII)
Mylohyoid	Forms floor of oral cavity Elevates hyoid bone and floor of mouth Depresses mandible	Alveolar nerve (CN V3)
Geniohyoid	Elevates hyoid bone Draws hyoid bone anteriorly	Anterior ramus of spinal nerve C1 (via hypoglossal nerve)
Stylohyoid	Elevates hyoid bone Draws hyoid bone posteriorly	Facial nerve (CN VII)
Sternohyoid	Depresses hyoid bone (from elevated position)	Ansa cervicalis (anterior rami of C1–C3)
Sternothyroid	Depresses larynx	
Omohyoid	Depresses hyoid bone Draws hyoid bone posteriorly	
Thyrohyoid	Depresses hyoid bone Elevates larynx	Hypoglossal nerve (anterior ramus of C1)

Table 16.9 Muscles of the Eye and Orbit

Orbital		
Orbicularis oculi	Orbital part: Closes eyelids tightly Palpebral part: Closes eyelids gently	Temporal and zygomatic branches of facial nerve (CN VII)
Corrugator supercilii	Depresses medial portion of eyebrow Moves skin between eyebrows (glabella)	Temporal branches of facial nerve (CN VII)
Depressor supercilii	Depresses medial portion of eyebrow Moves skin of glabella	
Procerus	Depresses medial end of eyebrow Wrinkles skin between eyebrows (glabella)	Temporal, lower zygomatic or buccal branches of facial nerve (CN VII)
Muscles of the Middle Ear		
Stapedius	Dampens vibrations from the tympanic membrane	Facial nerve (CN VII)
Tensor tympani	Tenses tympanic membrane Pulls handle of malleus medially	Mandibular nerve (CN V)
Extraocular		
Superior rectus	Rolls eye superiorly in the orbit Intorsion of the eye during adduction Adduction of the eye	Oculomotor nerve (CN III)
Inferior rectus	Rolls eye inferiorly in the orbit Extorsion of the eye during adduction Adduction of the eye	Oculomotor nerve (CN III)
Medial rectus	Rolls eye nasally in the orbit (adduction)	Oculomotor nerve (CN III)
Lateral rectus	Rolls eye temporally in the orbit (abduction)	Abducens nerve (CN VI)
Superior oblique	Primary: Inward torsion (intorsion) Secondary: Depresses eye Tertiary: Abducts eye	Trochlear nerve (CN IV)
Inferior oblique	Primary: Outward torsion (extorsion) Secondary: Elevates eye Tertiary: Abducts eye	Oculomotor nerve (CN III)

Table 16.10 Muscles of the Trunk

Suboccipital Muscles		
Muscle	Action(s)	Innervation
Rectus capitis posterior minor	Atlantooccipital joint: Head extension	Posterior ramus of C1
Rectus capitis posterior major	Bilateral contraction: Atlantooccipital joint head extension	
Obliquus capitis inferior	Unilateral contraction: Atlantoaxial joint head rotation (ipsilateral)	
Obliquus capitis superior	Unilateral contraction: • Atlantoaxial joint head rotation (contralateral) • Head lateral flexion (ipsilateral) Bilateral contraction: • Atlantooccipital joint head extension	
Superficial Trunk Muscles		
Trapezius muscle	Descending: • Scapulothoracic joint: Draws scapula superomedially/Atlantooccipital joint/upper cervical vertebrae: Extension of head and neck, lateral flexion of head and neck (ipsilateral) • Atlantoaxial joint: Rotation of head (contralateral) Transverse part: • Scapulothoracic joint: Draws scapula medially Ascending part: • Scapulothoracic joint: Draws scapula inferomedially	• Motor: Accessory nerve (CN XI) • Sensory: Anterior rami C3–C4 (via cervical plexus)
Latissimus dorsi muscle	Arm internal rotation Arm adduction Arm extension Assists in respiration	Thoracodorsal nerve (C6–C8)
Levator scapulae muscle	Scapulothoracic joint: • Draws scapula superomedially • Rotates glenoid cavity inferiorly Cervical joints: • Lateral flexion of neck (ipsilateral)	Anterior rami of spinal nerves C3–C4, dorsal scapular nerve (C5)
Rhomboid major muscle	Draws scapula superomedially Rotates glenoid cavity inferiorly Supports position of scapula	Dorsal scapular nerve (C5)
Rhomboid minor muscle		
Intermediate Trunk Muscles		
Serratus posterior superior	Elevates ribs	2nd–5th intercostal nerves

(Continued)

Table 16.10 (Continued) Muscles of the Trunk

Suboccipital Muscles		
Muscle	Action(s)	Innervation
Serratus posterior inferior	Depresses ribs Draws ribs inferoposteriorly	Anterior rami of T9–T12 (aka 9th–11th Intercostal nerves + subcostal nerve)
Deep Trunk Muscles		
Superficial		
Splenius capitis	Bilateral contraction: Extends head/neck Unilateral contraction: Lateral flexion and rotation of head (ipsilateral)	Lateral branches of posterior rami of C2–C3
Splenius cervices	Bilateral contraction: Extends neck Unilateral contraction: Lateral flexion and rotation of neck (ipsilateral)	Lateral branches of posterior rami of lower cervical spinal nerves
Intermediate		
Erector spinae: Iliocostalis	Bilateral contraction: Spinal extension Unilateral contraction: Lateral spinal flexion (ipsilateral)	Lateral branches of posterior rami of spinal nerves
Erector spinae: Longissimus	Bilateral contraction: Extension of spine Unilateral contraction: Lateral flexion of spine (ipsilateral) Longissimus capitis only: • Unilateral contraction: Lateral flexion and rotation of head (ipsilateral) • Bilateral contraction: Extension of head and neck	
Erector spinae: Spinalis	Unilateral contraction: Lateral flexion of cervical and thoracic spine (ipsilateral) Bilateral contraction: Extension of cervical and thoracic spine	
Transversospinal: Semispinalis capitis, cervicis, thoracis	Unilateral contraction: • Lateral flexion of head, cervical and thoracic spine (ipsilateral) • Rotation of head • Cervical and thoracic spine (contralateral) Bilateral contraction: • Extension of head, cervical and thoracic spine	Semispinalis capitis: • Descending branches of greater occipital nerve (C2) • Spinal nerve C3 Semispinalis cervicis/Thoracis: Medial branches of posterior rami of spinal nerves

(Continued)

Table 16.10 (Continued) Muscles of the Trunk

Suboccipital Muscles		
Muscle	**Action(s)**	**Innervation**
Transversospinal: Multifidus cervicis, thoracis, lumborum	Unilateral contraction: • Lateral flexion of spine (ipsilateral) • Rotation of spine (contralateral) Bilateral contraction: • Extension of spine	Medial branches of posterior rami of spinal nerves
Transversospinal: Rotatores breves and longi	Unilateral contraction: • Contralateral rotation of thoracic spine Bilateral contraction: • Extension of thoracic spine	
Deep		
Interspinales: Cervicis, thoracis, lumborum	Extension of cervical spine Extension of lumbar spine	Posterior rami of spinal nerves
Intertransversarii	Assists in lateral flexion of the spine Stabilizes spine	Anterior cervical intertransversarii: • Anterior and posterior rami of cervical spinal nerves Lumbar intertransversarii: • Anterior rami of lumbar spinal nerves
Levatores costarum	Elevation of ribs Rotation of thoracis spine	Posterior rami of T1–T12

Table 16.11 Muscles of the Anterior Thorax

Thoracic Cage		
Pectoralis major	Shoulder joint: • Arm adduction • Arm internal rotation • Arm flexion (clavicular head) • Arm extension (sternocostal head) Scapulothoracic joint: • Draws scapula anteroinferiorly	Lateral and medial pectoral nerves (C5–T1)
Pectoralis minor	Draws scapula anteroinferiorly Stabilizes scapula on thoracic wall	Medial pectoral nerve (C8–T1)
Serratus anterior	Draws scapula anterolaterally Suspends scapula on thoracic wall Rotates scapula (draws inferiorly angle laterally)	Long thoracic nerve (C5–C7)
Subclavius	Anchors clavicle Depresses clavicle	Nerve to subclavius (C5–C6)
External intercostals	Elevate ribs during forced inspiration Supports intercostal spaces Supports thoracic cage	Intercostal nerves
Internal intercostals	Depresses ribs during forced expiration Supports intercostal spaces Supports thoracic cage	
Innermost intercostals		
Subcostals		
Transversus thoracis	Depresses costal cartilages	
Diaphragm (respiratory)	Depresses costal cartilages Primary muscle of inspiratory breathing	• Phrenic nerves (C3–C5) • Sensory innervation of peripheries via 6th–11th intercostal nerves
Abdominal Wall		
External abdominal oblique	Unilateral contraction: • Trunk lateral flexion (ipsilateral) • Trunk rotation (contralateral) Bilateral contraction: • Trunk flexion • Compresses abdominal viscera • Expiration	• Intercostal nerves (T7–T11) • Subcostal nerve (T12) • Iliohypogastric nerve (L1)
Internal abdominal oblique	Unilateral contraction: • Trunk lateral flexion (ipsilateral) • Trunk rotation (ipsilateral) Bilateral contraction: • Trunk flexion • Compresses abdominal viscera • Expiration	• Intercostal nerves (T7–T11) • Subcostal nerve (T12) • Iliohypogastric nerve (L1) • Ilioinguinal nerve (L1)
Transversus abdominis	Unilateral contraction: • Trunk rotation (ipsilateral) Bilateral contraction: • Compresses abdominal viscera • Expiration	Intercostal nerves (T7–T11), subcostal nerve (T12), iliohypogastric nerve (L1), ilioinguinal nerve (L1)

(Continued)

Table 16.11 (Continued) Muscles of the Anterior Thorax

Thoracic Cage		
Rectus abdominis	Trunk flexion Compresses abdominal viscera Expiration	Intercostal nerves (T7–T11), subcostal nerve (T12)
Pyramidalis	Tenses linea alba	Subcostal nerve (T12)
Quadratus lumborum	Unilateral contraction: • Lateral flexion of trunk (ipsilateral) Bilateral contraction: • Fixes rib 12 during inspiration • Trunk extension	Subcostal nerve (T12), interior rami of spinal nerves L1–L4

Table 16.12 Muscles of the Pelvic Floor

	Muscles		Action(s)	Innervation
Superficial	Transverse perineal		Supports the pelvic floor Expulsion of semen in males Expulsion of the last drops of urine	Perineal nerve (pudendal nerve) (S2–S4)
	Bulbospongiosus		Males: • Facilitates urination • Facilitates erection • Facilitates ejaculation Females: • Facilitates erection of the clitoris Both: • Supports the perineal body	
	Ischiocavernosus		Maintains erection in males/females	
Deep	Levator ani	Iliococcygeus	Supports pelvic floor Opens/closes the levator hiatus	Nerve to levator ani (S4) Pudendal nerve (S2–S4)
		Pubococcygeus		
	Coccygeus		Supports pelvic viscera Flexes coccyx	Anterior rami of S4 and S5
	Puborectalis		Prevents pelvic organ prolapse Assists in maintaining continence Supports/guides the presenting fetus in childbirth	

Table 16.13 Muscles of the Lower Extremity

Gluteus maximus	Extension of thigh External rotation of thigh Abduction (superior part) of thigh Adduction (inferior part) of thigh	Inferior gluteal nerve (L5–S2)
Gluteus medius	Abduction of thigh	Superior gluteal nerve (L4–S1)
Gluteus minimus	Internal rotation (anterior part) of thigh Pelvis gluteus stabilization	
Tensor fasciae latae	Hip joint: • Thigh internal rotation of thigh • Weak thigh abduction Knee joint: • Leg external rotation • Weak leg flexion/extension • Stabilizes hip joint • Stabilizes knee joint	
Inner Hip		
Iliacus	Thigh external rotation	Femoral nerve (L2–L4)
Psoas major	Thigh abduction (from flexed hip)	Anterior rami of spinal nerves L1–L3
Psoas minor	Stabilizes head of femur in acetabulum	
Obturator externus	External rotation of thigh	Obturator nerve (L3, L4)
Obturator internus	Abduction of thigh (from flexed hip)	Nerve to obturator internus (L5, S1)
Superior gemellus	Stabilizes head of femur in acetabulum	
Inferior gemellus		Nerve to quadratus femoris (L4–S1)
Piriformis		Nerve to piriformis (S1–S2)
Quadratus femoris	Thigh external rotation Stabilizes head of femur in acetabulum	Nerve to quadratus femoris (L4–S1)
Anterior Thigh		
Sartorius	Hip joint: • Flexion of thigh • Abduction of thigh • External rotation of thigh Knee joint: • Flexion of leg • Internal rotation of thigh	Femoral nerve (L2–L4)
Rectus femoris	Hip joint: Flexion of thigh Knee joint: Leg extension	
Vastus intermedius	Leg extension	
Vastus lateralis		
Vastus medialis		
Posterior Thigh		
Semimembranosus	Hip joint: Thigh extension, thigh internal rotation	Tibial division of sciatic nerve (L5–S2)
Semitendinosus	Knee joint: Leg flexion, leg internal rotation Stabilizes semitendinosus pelvis	

(Continued)

Table 16.13 (Continued) Muscles of the Lower Extremity

Biceps femoris	Hip joint: • Extension of thigh • External rotation of thigh Knee joint: • Flexion of leg • External rotation of leg Stabilizes pelvis	Long head: Tibial division of sciatic nerve (L5–S2) Short head: Common fibular division of sciatic nerve (L5–S2)
Medial Thigh		
Pectineus		Femoral nerve (L2, L3) Obturator nerve (L2, L3)
Adductor magnus	Thigh: • Flexion • Adduction • External rotation (adductor part) • Extension • Internal rotation (ischiocondylar part) Pelvis stabilization	Adductor part: Obturator nerve (L2–L4) Ischiocondylar part: Tibial division of sciatic nerve (L4)
Adductor minimus	Adduction of thigh External rotation of thigh	Obturator nerve (L2–L4)
Adductor longus Adductor brevis	Thigh: • Flexion • Adduction • External rotation Pelvis stabilization	
Gracilis	Hip joint: • Flexion of thigh • Adduction of thigh Knee joint: • Flexion of leg • Internal rotation of leg	Obturator nerve (L2–L3)
Anterior Leg		
Tibialis anterior	Talocrural joint: • Dorsiflexion Subtalar joint: • Inversion • Supports medial longitudinal arch of foot	Deep fibular nerve (L4, L5)
Extensor hallucis longus	Metatarsophalangeal and interphalangeal joint: First toe extension Talocrural joint: Dorsiflexion	Deep fibular nerve (L5, S1)
Extensor digitorum longus	Toes 2–5 metatarsophalangeal and interphalangeal joints: Toe extension Talocrural joint: Dorsiflexion Subtalar joint: Foot eversion	
Fibularis tertius	Talocrural joint: Dorsiflexion Subtalar joint: Eversion	

(Continued)

Table 16.13 (Continued) Muscles of the Lower Extremity

Lateral Leg		
Fibularis longus	Talocrural joint: Flexion Subtalar joint: Eversion Supports longitudinal and transverse arches of foot	Superficial fibular nerve (L5, S1)
Fibularis brevis	Talocrural joint: Plantar flexion Subtalar joint: Foot eversion	
Posterior Leg		
Gastrocnemius	Talocrural joint: Plantar flexion Knee joint: Leg flexion	Tibial nerve (S1, S2)
Soleus	Talocrural joint: Foot plantar flexion	
Plantaris	Talocrural joint: Foot plantar flexion Knee joint: Knee flexion	
Popliteus	Unlocks knee joint; Knee joint stabilization	Tibial nerve (L5–S2)
Tibialis posterior	Talocrural joint: Plantar flexion Subtalar joint: Inversion Supports medial longitudinal arch of foot	Tibial nerve (L4, L5)
Flexor digitorum longus	Toes 2–5 metatarsophalangeal and interphalangeal: Toe flexion Talocrural joint: Plantar flexion Subtalar joint: Inversion	Tibial nerve (L5–S2)
Flexor hallucis longus	Metatarsophalangeal and interphalangeal joint: First toe flexion Talocrural joint: Foot plantar flexion Subtalar joint: Foot inversion	Tibial nerve (S2, S3)
Foot		
Abductor hallucis	Metatarsophalangeal joint: • First toe abduction • First Toe flexion Support of longitudinal arch	Medial plantar nerve (S1–S3)
Flexor hallucis brevis	Metatarsophalangeal joint: First toe flexion Support of longitudinal arch	Medial plantar nerve (S1, S2)
Adductor hallucis	Metatarsophalangeal joint: • First toe adduction • First toe flexion Support of longitudinal and transverse arches	Lateral plantar nerve (S2, S3)
Flexor digitorum brevis	Metatarsophalangeal joints 2–5: Toe flexion Supports longitudinal arch	Medial plantar nerve (S1–S3)
Quadratus plantae	Metatarsophalangeal joints 2–5: Toe flexion	Lateral plantar nerve (S1–S3)
Lumbricals (there are four)	Metatarsophalangeal joints 2–5: • Toe flexion • Toes adduction Interphalangeal joints 2–5: Toes extension	Lumbrical 1: Medial plantar nerve (S2, S3) Lumbricals 2–4: Lateral plantar nerve (S2, S3)

Table 16.13 (Continued) Muscles of the Lower Extremity

Plantar interossei (there are three)	Metatarsophalangeal joints 3–5: • Toe flexion • Toes adduction Interphalangeal joints 3–5: Toes extension	Lateral plantar nerve (S2, S3)
Dorsal interossei (there are four)	Metatarsophalangeal joints 2–4: • Toe flexion • Toe abduction Interphalangeal joints 2–4: Toe extension	
Lateral Plantar		
Abductor digiti minimi	Metatarsophalangeal joint: • 5th toe abduction • 5th toe flexion Supports longitudinal arch of foot	Lateral plantar nerve (S1–S3)
Flexor digiti minimi brevis	Metatarsophalangeal joint: 5th toe flexion	Lateral plantar nerve (S2–S3)
Opponens digiti minimi	Metatarsophalangeal joint 5: • Toe abduction • Toe flexion	
Dorsal Foot		
Extensor digitorum brevis	Distal interphalangeal joints: Toe 2–4 extension	Deep fibular/peroneal nerve (L5, S1)
Extensor hallucis brevis	Metatarsophalangeal joint: First toe extension	

REFERENCES

1. Caleb L, Shumway C, Motlagh M, Wade M. *Anatomy, Head and Neck, Eye Superior Rectus Muscle.* StatPearls Publishing; 2021. https://www.ncbi.nlm.nih.gov/books/NBK526067/
2. Caleb L, Shumway C, Motlagh M, Wade M. *Anatomy, Head and Neck, Eye Inferior Rectus Muscle.* StatPearls Publishing; 2021. 2023. https://www.ncbi.nlm.nih.gov/books/NBK518978/
3. Caleb L, Shumway C, Motlagh M, Wade M. *Anatomy, Head and Neck, Eye Medial Rectus Muscles.* StatPearls Publishing; 2021. https://www.ncbi.nlm.nih.gov/books/NBK519026/
4. Cabrera AF, Suarez-Quintanilla J. *Anatomy, Head and Neck, Eye Lateral Rectus Muscle.* StatPearls Publishing; 2021. https://www.ncbi.nlm.nih.gov/books/NBK539721/
5. Adbelhady A, Patel B, Aslam S, Aboud DA. *Anatomy, Head and Neck, Eye Superior Oblique Muscle.* StatPearls Publishing; 2021. https://www.ncbi.nlm.nih.gov/books/NBK537152/
6. Gupta N, Patel B. *Anatomy, Head and Neck, Eye Inferior Oblique Muscles.* StatPearls Publishing; 2021. https://www.ncbi.nlm.nih.gov/books/NBK545253/

Index

For Product Safety Concerns and Information please contact our EU
representative GPSR@taylorandfrancis.com
Taylor & Francis Verlag GmbH, Kaufingerstraße 24, 80331 München, Germany

9 781638 220817